MONUMENTAL MYTHS OF THE MODERN MEDICAL MAFIA AND MAINSTREAM MEDIA AND THE MULTITUDE OF LYING LIARS THAT MANUFACTURED THEM

"If you tell the truth, you don't have to remember anything."

~ Mark Twain

WHAT OTHERS ARE SAYING ABOUT THE BOOK:

"In <u>Monumental Myths</u>, Ty Bollinger welcomes you into a scenic tour of some of the most outrageous events in our modern history - and he is an excellent tour guide. You'll move at a good pace, knocking back topic after topic with gusto. You won't be bogged down with the kind of tedious excess that is the death of most PBS-endorsed political guidebooks, but neither will you lose essential and enlightening detail. And Ty's good-humored, common-sense but well-reasoned approach will keep you involved (and smiling) throughout, wanting to see what big lie gets skewered next. The events are covered, major and minor, from JFK to GMO, Boston to Waco, aspartame to Oklahoma City, fluoride to Monsanto-land, MLK, chemtrails and beyond. The book functions as a kind of 'greatest hits,' or sportsman's guide to a 'World Series of Conspiracy.' Ty brings that feeling to his work: the love of a good sports writer for a game. The game here is our history of national and international deception, played by the jackals who've manipulated their way into power. Most authors take on one issue to excess, burying us in useless and irrelevant data, without drawing our eye to the hundred similar (or identical) events on the horizon. But what we really want - and what Ty delivers - is a compendium, a means to compare and contrast the lies of history: how much better it is to have it all laid out in one, colorful, entertaining volume. And what's wrong with being entertaining? The bad guys don't know what to do when the truth-tellers crack wise and get funny - it throws them off their pitch. So much the better for the truth-seekers that we

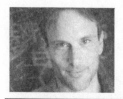

keep our sense of humor - and Ty certainly does. Even when the material goes into dark country, even when we're faced with acts of willful destruction so callous, brutal and monstrous you'd think we'd just lay down and give up, Ty marshals us on by shining a light on the things that make us human: our curiosity, wit and humor, compassion, integrity, critical thinking; and, thank goodness, the thing that governments and media ignore - our irreplaceable common sense."
~ Liam Scheff ~ Author of <u>Official Stories</u>, LiamScheff.com

"Why did <u>Monumental Myths</u> need to be written? To fill the monumental gaps in the real history not taught to most Americans! And Ty Bollinger is just the man for the job, covering a comprehensive array of events from perspectives unapproved by any government agency, but guaranteed to cure your historical deficiency diseases. The time is right and the people are finally hungry enough to see through the empty calories fed to us by the mainstream media. What Ty has done with this

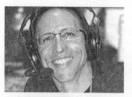

book is to satisfy the most voracious of appetites for those who are the hungriest to know what has gone wrong over the last 100+ years right up until today. With great breadth, depth and humor, prepare to have your historical and contemporary chakras aligned to see through some of the most monumental myths that, up until this point, have misled generations of freedom-loving people into 'misinformational' bondage. I can't thank Ty enough for putting all of this information into one book!"
~ Robert Scott Bell ~ Syndicated host of the "Robert Scott Bell Show"

*"If you do not know who Ty Bollinger is ... you should. If you live in a world where you wear blinders so you have a very narrow focal point, and you like it, do **not** read this book. If you think the grassy knoll is a place for a nice picnic in Dallas, do **not** touch this book. If you think you can get the best health care in the world by following the current system, 'Don't Worry. Be Happy,' and do **not** read this book. As the author of sixteen books on health, translated into eight languages, I could not put this put book down. I think Ty has been secretly taping conversations that I have over*

lunch every Thursday with two very smart friends … one a top lawyer and the other a top computer programmer. You may want to curl up with a cup of decaffeinated fair trade coffee (my preference would be moringa oleifera, but that is another matter) and read a book that is just like having a conversation with a good friend. 'Conspiracy theorist' or 'reality historian'? Only you can be the judge after reading his latest work but those that know Ty, as you will after reading this book, know the truth."

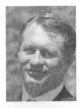

~ Dr. Howard W. Fisher ~ Anti-aging researcher and author of 16 books

"Ty Bollinger approaches health and wellness in a no nonsense fashion. He's a must read for anyone who wishes to live longer and healthier. His latest book, _Monumental Myths_, is a veritable buffet for so-called conspiracy theorists."

~ George Noory ~ Host of the Internationally-syndicated "Coast to Coast AM"

"In typical 'Ty' fashion, Ty Bollinger puts together another book that provides so much incredibly valuable information; it could have easily been the subject of a dozen volumes. However, this one is his best yet! The entertainment and intrigue this book provides is only surpassed by the crucial necessity of the information it empowers you with and the resulting awakening associated exclusively with the dawning of truth. This book optimizes the phrase, 'with knowledge, comes power.' But beware! Once you have experienced the 'light,' you can never go back into the 'darkness.' If even 10% of the population knew the truth behind these myths, which Ty exposes with surgical precision, our nation would not tolerate those responsible and the course of our great nation would once again be set on the right path! I can't recommend this book enough! Buy two copies and give one away!"

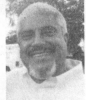

~ Dr. Rashid Buttar, DO ~ International best-selling author of The 9 Steps To Keep The Doctor Away; Ranked among the "top 50 doctors in the USA"

"Ty Bollinger has done it again! In his latest book, _Monumental Myths_, Ty has provided the reader with a complete volume of topics which have not been truthfully covered by the mainstream media. If you are already familiar with JFK, GMO, Oklahoma City, Monsanto and MLK (and more), then prepare to have your knowledge grow by leaps and bounds as well as be entertained with Bollinger's satirical sense of humor and witty writing skills. However, if you're like most people who are only familiar with the 'official stories,' then prepare to have your mind blown to 'smithereens.' Despite having known Ty Bollinger the entirety of my adult life, he never ceases to amaze me with his creativity, courage, ambition, integrity, and intellect. Reading this book is the next best thing to having a one-on-one conversation with Ty regarding some of the most interesting purported 'conspiracy theories' known. If you're willing to open your mind to 'uncomfortable truths' and accept the possibility that you've been spoon-fed 'comforting lies' for your entire life, then prepare to see conspiracy 'theory' become conspiracy 'reality' right in front of your eyes as you read this amazing book. Looking back at how we were trained in medical school, the profound influence of Big Pharma on our education, our minds, and ultimately our practice of medicine becomes crystal clear. If those of us in the USA who are most capable and intelligent are not willing to accept the obvious truth and act upon it, then who will save this country from the tyranny of corporate fascism? This book is your opportunity to open your mind and make a difference. Will you take the red pill or the blue pill?"

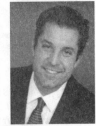

~ Dr. Irvin Sahni, MD ~ World-renowned orthopedic spine surgeon; LivingHerbsRx.com

"This is a dazzling and unexpectedly witty book. In his latest book, <u>Monumental Myths</u>, Ty Bollinger takes the reader on a stunning journey through a maze of the lead conspiracy topics of our times ...the huge 9/11 lie, deadly vaccines, the phony 'war on cancer,' the slaughter at Waco, Pat Tillman's murder, JFK, the Rockefellers, genocidal GMOs, sweet-death aspartame, the Boston bombings, Ruby Ridge, and the greatest catastrophe of them all ... Fukushima, just to name a few. In each case, Ty shreds the veil of often laughable lies we have been fed by the 'powers that be' and their vile, lap-dog liberal media. It won't take any reasonable reader long to realize most conspiracy 'theories' are actually conspiracy 'FACTS.' One monumental myth after another falls before Bollinger's swift sword of truth and you quickly realize that this author has done his research ... and then some. This book is not only packed with facts and dripping with great information but is also often hilarious to read thanks to Ty's sardonic sense of humor which illuminates nearly every page of this newest book offering. You'll be laughing as he dispatches myth after myth, despite the fact that the topics are deadly serious. This unique anthology is definitely a 'must have' book for

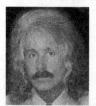 those of us who have a difficult time swallowing the lies continually spewed by the mainstream media. The book cover by David Dees is another stunning piece of artwork and makes a major statement all by itself. Order up a copy, put it on your coffee table, and you will have the ammo you need to provoke conversations with the people you care about and want to help wake up. Ty has done another great job in challenging us to actually think for ourselves ... the unmistakable sign of a truly extraordinary book." **~ Jeff Rense ~ Internationally-syndicated talk radio host and Editor-in-Chief of Rense.com**

"Ty Bollinger has done it again! He has been accused of telling truth in his new book and has been found guilty! Ty goes against the grain in <u>Monumental Myths</u> and presents the information in layman's terms. He will shock you with the **TRUTH!**" **~ "Doctor Drake" ~ Radio personality of the radio show called "Earth"**

"Americans are no longer being taught real history in school. And thanks to the controlled mainstream media, the only dish that is served on the nightly news is 'government approved' propaganda. Ty Bollinger remedies that in <u>Monumental Myths</u>, an extraordinary and entertaining book that provides a buffet of factual information on so-called 'conspiracy' topics such as false flags (like 9/11), Ruby Ridge, Waco, the Rockefellers, HIV-AIDS, the phony 'wars' (on terror,

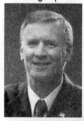 drugs, and cancer), and several strange 'suicides' like Vince Foster and Gary Webb, just to name a few. Throughout the book, Ty dispels the darkness and reveals the light of truth; and with truth comes freedom and liberty. As we read in John 8:32, 'and you shall know the truth, and the truth shall make you free.' In <u>Monumental Myths</u>, conspiracy 'theory' quickly becomes 'reality,' thanks to Ty's proficient writing skills, exhaustive research, and clever sense of humor. This is a 'must have' book and will provide the reader with indispensable information to engage in critical conversations with those people who are still 'asleep' on these matters. Great job, Ty!" **~ Dr. Chuck Baldwin ~ Pastor of Liberty Fellowship & co-author of <u>Romans 13: The True Meaning of Submission</u> and <u>To Keep or Not To Keep: Why Christians Should Not Give Up Their Guns</u>**

"Ty Bollinger's latest work, <u>Monumental Myths</u>, exposing the Medical Mafia and Big Pharma has traveled one step too far; a true hero to this country has the courage to go that dangerous one more step! Bollinger knows all the rules, but the rules do not know him." 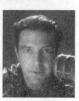 **~ Chad Holsclaw aka "Doctor Truth" ~ Co-host of "Earth" Radio**

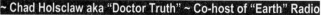

DEDICATION

This book is dedicated to my lovely, brilliant, wonderful, beautiful wife, Charlene – my "Princess" – and my precious, adorable children – Brianna, Bryce, Tabitha, and Charity. ♥♥ You are the reason that I get up every morning and do what I do. I love you all very much and thank God for each of you. ♥♥

Thank you Princess for reading through the entire book and helping me with the editing! ♥♥ Those of you that homeschool your children will be interested to know that Charlene used <u>Monumental Myths</u> as a *"what really happened"* history book and read it to the children as part of their homeschool lessons.

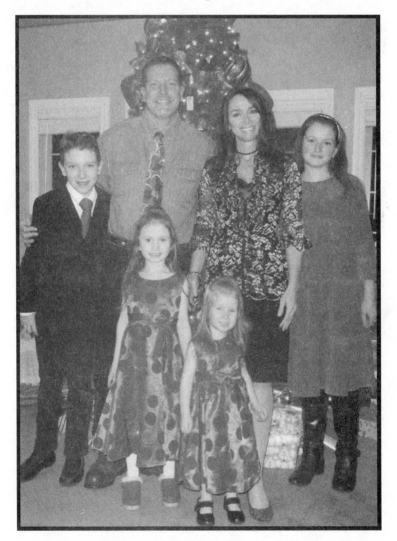

SPECIAL "KUDOS"

Special huge, enormous, whopper "thanks" and gigantic, colossal "kudos" go to my good buddy, Liam Scheff, and his tremendous trailblazing book, <u>Official Stories</u>. Liam's book was immensely impactful and inspiring; it motivated me to finish <u>Monumental Myths</u>, which I have been writing and muddling with for a couple of years.

I really appreciate all of the amazing information I gleaned from his chapters on JFK, 9/11, and HIV-AIDS. Liam is a brilliant writer, an exceptionally amusing and witty person, and quite frankly, a veritable virtuoso who speaks multiple languages and whose brain, if it actually had legs, could run circles around 99.9% of the population's brains, if those brains also had legs.

OK, OK, I know ... enough of the hypotheticals and hyperbole.

Anyway, I guess what I'm trying to say is that Liam is ne'er if e'er analogous to a run-of-the-mill American Neanderthal with a "teeny tiny" vocabulary and infinitesimal frontal lobe.

So, Liam, I want to say *"Thank you my friend"* ...
"Merci mon ami" ...
"Vielen Dank, dass sie mein freund" ...
"¿Tiene hambre?" ...

Wait, did I just ask you if you were hungry in Spanish? Sorry, I meant to say, *"Gracias mi amigo."*

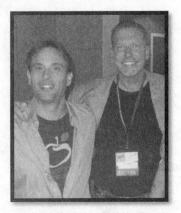

With Liam at the 2013 Health
Freedom Expo in Chicago

MONUMENTAL MYTHS OF THE MODERN MEDICAL MAFIA AND MAINSTREAM MEDIA AND THE MULTITUDE OF LYING LIARS THAT MANUFACTURED THEM

Ty M. Bollinger

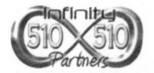

Published by: Infinity 510² Partners

Foreword by John B. Wells
Preface by Mike Adams
Esteemed Support from Robert Scott Bell

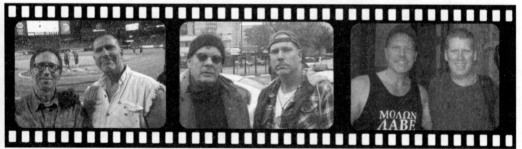

With Robert Scott Bell at a Braves game in Atlanta   With John B. Wells on Nov 22, 2013 in Dallas   With Mike Adams at the March vs. Monsanto in Austin

THANK YOU JOHN & MIKE & RSB!

You are an inspiration to me, and I really appreciate all three of you. In your own ways, you all are responsible for "waking up" literally millions of people to the truth and dispelling the monumental myths that abound in today's world. Keep the faith, fellas, and please remember that your diligent work is not going unnoticed.

"My people are destroyed for lack of knowledge."
~ Hosea 4:6

"And you shall know the truth,
and the truth shall set you free."
~ John 8:32

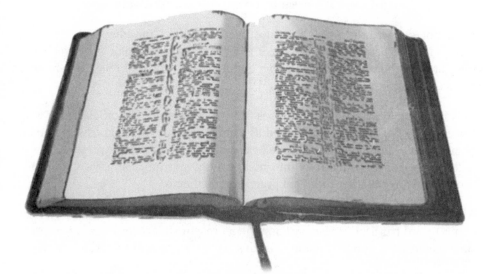

"Wherefore putting away lying, speak every man truth
with his neighbor: for we are members one of another."
~ Ephesians 4:25

"Have nothing to do with the fruitless deeds of
darkness, but rather expose them."
~ Ephesians 5:11

To order more copies of this book,
please visit the following website:

WWW.MYTHBUSTERSBOOK.COM

**Before you read this book, I must give you the
following FDA mandated warning and disclaimer:**

I am not a doctor; thus, I have not been formally "miseducated." I am not
certified in medicine; therefore, there is no certificate or diploma disgracing the
interior of my home or office and no monument to the biggest revenue generating
fraud ever perpetrated on human kind.

This book is for educational purposes only. It represents the official view of the
voices in my head. It is not intended as a substitute for the diagnosis, treatment,
or advice of a qualified, licensed medical professional. The facts presented in the
following pages are offered as information only, not medical advice, and in no
way should anyone infer that I am practicing medicine.

A conscious effort has been made to only present information that is both
accurate and truthful. However, I assume no responsibility for inaccuracies in my
source materials, nor do I assume responsibility for how this material is used.

The statements in this book have not been evaluated by the FDA (the "Federal
Death Administration"), the AMA ("American Murder Association"), "Big
Pharma," or the rest of the "Medical Mafia."

"There is no such thing, at this date of the world's history, in America, as an independent press. You know it and I know it. There is not one of you who dares to write your honest opinions, and if you did, you know beforehand that it would never appear in print. I am paid weekly for keeping my honest opinion out of the paper I am connected with. Others of you are paid similar salaries for similar things, and any of you who would be so foolish as to write honest opinions would be out on the streets looking for another job. If I allowed my honest opinions to appear in one issue of my paper, before twenty-four hours my occupation would be gone.

The business of the journalists is to destroy the truth, to lie outright, to pervert, to vilify, to fawn at the feet of mammon, and to sell his country and his race for his daily bread. You know it and I know it, and what folly is this toasting an independent press?

We are the tools and vassals of rich men behind the scenes. We are the jumping jacks, they pull the strings and we dance. Our talents, our possibilities and our lives are all the property of other men. We are intellectual prostitutes."

~ John Swinton
New York Times, 1880

TABLE OF CONTENTS

FOREWORD 15

PREFACE 18

INTRODUCTION 21

Section 1 - "Trust Us ... We're Lying" 33

Chapter 1 - The M.D. "Emperors" 35

Chapter 2 - The Rockefellers 45

Chapter 3 - Planned Parenthood 53

Chapter 4 - Hospitals & Iatrogenocide 59

Chapter 5 - Chemtrails 63

Section 2 - More Medical Mafia Myths 69

Chapter 6 - The Germ Theory 71

Chapter 7 - Cholesterol 77

Chapter 8 - Aspartame 83

Chapter 9 - Mercury in Your Mouth 93

Chapter 10 - Vaccines 99

Chapter 11 - Chemotherapy 119

Section 3 - Some Wars Aren't Meant To Be Won 127

Chapter 12 - The War on Cancer 129

Chapter 13 - The War on Terror 135

Chapter 14 - The War on Drugs 147

Section 4 - Initials, Acronyms & Assassinations — 159

Chapter 15 - JFK — 161

Chapter 16 - JFK, Jr. — 189

Chapter 17 - MLK — 199

Chapter 18 - The "FED" — 213

Chapter 19 - GMO — 225

Chapter 20 - HIV & AIDS — 233

Section 5 - False Flags, Massacres & Staged Events — 247

Chapter 21 - History of False Flags — 249

Chapter 22 - 9/11 — 255

Chapter 23 - Waco — 295

Chapter 24 - Oklahoma City — 311

Chapter 25 - Boston Marathon — 327

Chapter 26 - Ruby Ridge — 345

Chapter 27 - Sandy Hook — 355

Section 6 - Casualties of War — 371

Chapter 28 - Pat Tillman — 373

Chapter 29 - Gary Webb — 383

Chapter 30 - Vince Foster — 393

Section 7 - "F" Bombs — 409

Chapter 31 - Fluoride — 411

Chapter 32 - Fukushima — 421

Chapter 33 - Fast & Furious — 433

CONCLUSION — 441

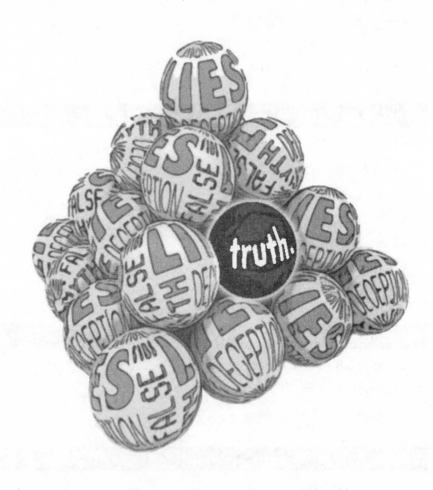

FOREWORD

John B. Wells

The Mayan Calendar, which ended on 21 December 2012 was anticipated by some to be the end of more than just the inscriptions on a primitive stone wheel. Many believed it was to be the end of everything regarding the world as we have known it. Apprehension was high among some. Expectation and anticipation in some, denial in others. Even those who believed nothing would happen or change could not deny that there was a global vigil. Would there be a cataclysmic event? A magnetic reversal of the poles? A collision with Nibiru? All over the world, people were preparing to experience the end of humanity itself, with a mixture of regret and relief.

It seemed as though we as citizens of Earth felt that all the systems we've become accustomed to were failing. Overreaching technology, financial machinations and conflicting social structures were and remain straining to endure. And we, whom these systems were to serve, find ourselves feeling strained to endure them.

The world did end. The sky did fall. Global civilization did collapse into anarchy and chaos. But not in the way we had imagined.

The world of those who have profited from fear and the reassurance that they had a ready solution to that fear; those who supplied the 'bullets and the bandages', their world ended.

The year was 2012 and it was spent in preparation for an awakening. We may have thought 2012 was the end of something or the beginning of something. But it was both. It was the beginning of the end of ignorance. Ignorance based in trust. Ever increasing clarity and understanding of how the most seemingly complex apparatus can be reduced to a few simple components to reveal the illness behind the symptoms. That the complexity of our world social order is a contrived illusion and deliberate deception.

The curtains are being pulled back, the screens dropped, the mirrors shattered and the smoke cleared away revealing that so many things we trusted, looked up to with admiration or even awe, things we believed were done in our best interest, on our behalf and to our benefit are misrepresentations, chicanery or bare faced lies. In the final analysis, the illness is the same as it ever was. **It is the love of money.**

Few would argue that health is the most important part of the human experience. Loss of money, property, even reputation are things which can be reversed. It is the loss of health that compromises survival, let alone success. Emotional distress from the loss of a loved one's health can damage or ruin our own. In Ty Bollinger's case it was the awakening to, and the inspiration for his work.

The family doctor's house call became the telephone delivered cliché, "Take two aspirin and call me in the morning" which really means "many causes, but only one remedy and if this doesn't work, you're probably going to get a lot sicker". Medical 'miracles' are performed every day by brilliant surgeons, researchers and doctors. Yet the health of the public at large is getting worse and worse. An octogenarian will usually tell you that diseases like cancer, diabetes, autism and immune disorders were not common in the time they lived. Diseases of their day were eventually eradicated by antibiotics. But as we have over-medicated our civilization, we are reaching the end of the effectiveness of antibiotics and new 'superbugs' attack our weakened immune systems.

I would submit to you that in the same way criminals are let out of prison, it being known that they will commit more crimes to pay more attorney fees and related costs, this is all the result of protecting an investment. There is a lot of money to be made in pharmaceuticals. Billions upon billions of dollars. Every year. Year after year.

With all of the 'advances in modern medicine' that we have been witness to, or have had witness borne by the media, what other possible reason could there be for these deadly illnesses to continue to visit us?

In his title, *"Monumental Myths of The Medical Mafia and Mainstream Media,"* Bollinger has not minced words. The rest of the title, *"and the Multitude of Lying Liars That Manufactured Them,"* completes his monumental thesis statement.

It isn't pleasant to find out you've been hoodwinked, fooled, and lied to, made a fool of, had advantage taken and separated from your money only to return for more abuse. The best medicine is the hardest to take, but you must take it if you want to regain your health. The best medicine, of course, is knowledge. And the greatest knowledge always comes at a very high price.

Rather than braving engagement with the public, I spent All Hallows Eve watching a documentary I chanced upon celebrating one of the greatest farces ever perpetrated on the public. The seventy-fifth anniversary of a legendary radio broadcast.

The public reaction to Orson Welles' broadcast of H.G. Wells' "War Of The Worlds" illustrates the point of this foreword perfectly. 'Martians' became 'Germans' in the panicked minds of the public. Though the word 'Germans' was never spoken in the broadcast. Germany as an adversary was something they knew. But as the broadcast continued and the rumors changed, were people then willing to accept a Martian invasion? Yes, even more so. Because a Martian invasion was an unknown horror that made the known horror less threatening.

Was it irresponsible to put this into their minds? That was the very dangerous question being asked by the newspapers and the higher-ups at CBS, and Welles' career hung in the balance. It didn't take long until the resolution was simply: if we are that gullible then we deserve to be deceived. The whole thing was genius. The perpetrator was a genius. Fame and fortune followed.

But the character of the country and the world is different now, isn't it?

~ John B. Wells
All Saints Day 2013

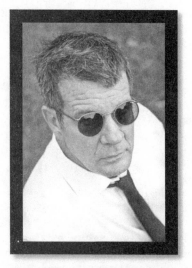

www.CaravantoMidnight.com
Weekend Host of the Nationally
Syndicated "Coast to Coast AM"

PREFACE
Mike Adams

Most of what you've been taught about health and medicine isn't factually true. It's based on a genuine mythology grounded in corporate interests: drug companies that want to sell you a dozen prescription medications, processed food companies that want to sell you their high-profit factory productions and medical institutions that want you to remain a long-term repeat customer for life.

To achieve these profit interests, food companies, drug companies and medical institutions have devised a seductive mythology that has been pounded into the consciousness of consumers everywhere. This mythology includes some real whoppers such as, *"fresh eggs are bad for you"* or *"cholesterol causes heart attacks."*

But it's even more insidious than that. One of the most dangerous medical myths is the false idea that you are born "deficient" in vaccines, psychiatric drugs and blood pressure medications, and that the only way you can be a normal, healthy human being is to subject your body to endless, high-profit interventions that just coincidentally happen to keep you sick and the drug companies wealthy.

This book, <u>Monumental Myths</u>, by Ty Bollinger takes you on a breath-taking tour of today's most prominent myths, shattering them one by one in the interests of helping humanity wake up to reality.

It's time for our world to transcend these myths and awaken to the higher truth that we have all been lied to. There is a better way to approach disease prevention and health care, and it doesn't involve making chemical companies rich while the people suffer. Instead, it's based on powerful nutritional therapies, healthy exposure to natural sunlight, regular exercise, restful sleep, stress reduction, mind-body practices, holistic treatment modalities and natural medicines derived from plants.

No one does a better job of exposing the false mythology of modern medicine (plus the chemical industry and processed food industry) than Ty Bollinger. In this book, you'll see dozens of medical myths blown wide open and readily dismissed as pure hokum. Remember, the industry of modern medicine falsely claims to be based on the "gold standard of evidence-based medicine" but is actually based on layer upon layer of contrived mythologies designed to extract money from the economy under the guise of "health care."

If we hope to move forward as a civilization, we must rid ourselves of the burden of "false thinking," and this book is a powerful tool in helping us achieve that goal. In place of false thinking, we must embrace higher truths such as:

- Your body wants to be healthy and is genetically programmed to do so.

- You are being systematically and intentionally poisoned through foods, medicines and propaganda. You must realize this in order to free yourself from it.

- Plants synthesize tens of thousands of powerful, medicinal compounds that can be harnessed to enhance human health. Any system of medicine which does not embrace the powerful healing potential of plants will never be able to deliver lasting health.

- Most humans today are wildly malnourished and lacking vitamins and plant-based nutrients, which is one reason why chronic disease is devastating our civilization (and our economy). Providing those nutrients often results in seemingly "miraculous" healing.

- There is more to a human being than the mere physical. Mind-body interactions are real. Intention affects physiology. Any system of medicine that does not account for the presence of the mind can never be a complete system of medicine because it is missing a huge piece of the puzzle for lifelong health.

- The simple avoidance of toxic chemicals in foods, medicines and even household products is, all by itself, a powerful strategy for radically improved health and longevity.

- Real science does not allow itself to get bogged down by the corporate-driven science of our modern era. Real science transcends the false "science" of Big Pharma and the toxic food industry to reveal powerful, higher truths about the amazing healing potential of the human body.

And the biggest truth of all, when it comes to medicine, is this:

The very **REASON** you are being systematically poisoned with mercury in vaccines, heavy metals in food and toxic chemicals in countless products is because the system wants you to remain truly lobotomized so that you cannot achieve real awareness. This has been called "dumbing down" but it's actually more like a "shutting off" of higher cognitive function so that you are disconnected from your true potential as a spiritually-aware human being. The purpose of this is to make sure people can never achieve the level of awareness required to question their reality (and the myths it is built upon) or challenge authority.

Modern food, medicine and chemical industries are both, in essence, systems of mind control. This book helps you reclaim control of your own mind so that you can experience true freedom and health at a level most never encounter.

This gets us to the real "miracle" that you can unleash with the help of this book: Once you cast off the systematic poisons while vastly increasing your body's natural defenses and detoxification pathways, you will experience a quantum leap expansion in your awareness, intelligence and quality of life. You will escape "the Matrix" of mind suppression that has been caused by toxic elements, synthetic chemicals, heavy metals and mind-altering drugs, and you will unleash renewed creativity, brilliance, vitality, optimism and personal power.

This book, in other words, is really a gateway to personal freedom. Read it, follow it and free your mind. From there, your possibilities are endless.

~ Mike Adams, the "Health Ranger"

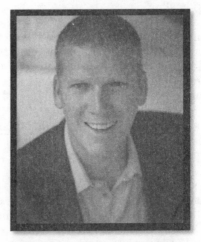

Editor of www.NaturalNews.com
Director of the Natural News Forensic Food Lab
(Labs.NaturalNews.com)

INTRODUCTION

Thank you for reading this book. No, I don't have it available on CD or DVD. You're going to have to actually read ... you **can** read, can't you? Anyway, I hope that it makes you think and stimulates discussion with others. That's why I wrote it. If you are still "sleeping" (metaphorically speaking), then I hope this book "wakes you up."

In this book, we're going to be examining numerous topics, including chemotherapy, fluoride, aspartame, vaccines, the "war on drugs," the siege on Waco, the Boston marathon bombings, 9/11, iatrogenocide, HIV, GMO, the AMA, JFK, JFK Jr., MLK, the FED, and the TSA. Hey, what's with all the acronyms? I guess they just sounded good together.

Check out the table of contents. You'll see that this book is chock full of a whole mess of diverse subjects and events. What do they all have in common? I'm glad you asked...

We have been lied to about all of them.

I initially woke up to the "Medical Mafia" while I was researching and writing my first book, <u>Cancer–Step Outside the Box</u>, which I published in 2006. You see, from 1996 to 2004, I lost several close family members to cancer, including my mother and father. Rather than just complain about the loss of my loved ones, I decided to **do** something. I decided to research and investigate – two tasks that I performed repeatedly while I was doing graduate work at Baylor University.

So, over the next several years, I researched and investigated one topic – **cancer** – for literally thousands of hours. What I discovered not only shocked me, but it outraged me as well: Non-toxic, effective, natural treatments for cancer are being systematically suppressed and cancer patients are dying due to lack of this vital knowledge. **Why?** Because the Medical Mafia and their "leg breakers" (like the FDA and FTC) control the flow of information and regulate the "approved" treatments.

After I published the book, I was contacted by a brilliant doctor in California with whom I had consulted numerous times while writing the book. He told me that he had a DVD to send me. I asked him what the topic of the DVD was, and he told me that it was about 9/11.

"What about 9/11?" I asked.
"It was an inside job," he replied.
"You're crazy!" I retorted, quite indignantly.
To which he graciously replied, *"You thought I was sane enough to quote me numerous times in your book, so the least you can do is watch the DVD with an open mind. Then, if you still think I'm crazy, then so be it."*

Fair enough. He had a good point. Many people had also called me "crazy" after I published my cancer book, so I decided to watch the DVD. But down deep in my soul, as I watched with my wife, Charlene, I wanted to prove, once and for all, that this doctor was a "nutter," a "tin foil hat" wearing lunatic.

Guess what? After 90 minutes of watching, we both were standing by the TV with our jaws about to hit the floor. He was right. We just stared at each other, each of us with a sick feeling in the pit of our stomachs. We felt betrayed. We felt deceived. We felt cheated. We felt misled. We were alarmed. And we were sickened by the fact that, for the first time in our lives, we realized that the USA wasn't what we always thought it was. We recognized that we were being constantly lied to by the very people that we trusted. We realized that the "official story" about 9/11 is about as believable as the Easter Bunny, Keebler Elf, Santa Claus, and fairies with wings of pixie dust. It's a monumental myth ... a ruse ... a fable ... a "tall tale" concocted to deceive the masses. And it worked like a charm on me and my wife – we swallowed it *"hook, line, and sinker"* – at least for a while. But sooner or later, we all must wake up from the dream.

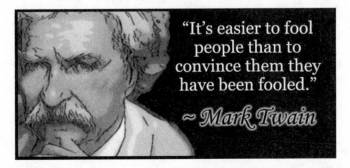

"It's easier to fool people than to convince them they have been fooled."

~ Mark Twain

As is common with folks when they first "wake up," we went out and told everybody about it, foolishly believing that they, too, would want to know the truth. Little did we know that many people **love** being deceived and living in the matrix. We swiftly learned that there are folks who do **not** want to "wake up," because the truth is too painful. Our own friends and family literally laughed at us, got angry at us, ignored us, gossiped about us, and even ostracized us. We were called every name in the book – "insane" ... "conspiracy kooks" ... "lunatics" ... "truthers." While we're on the subject, I consider it a badge of honor when someone calls me a "truther." Why? Because the antithesis of a truther is a ... **LIAR**. So, yes, please do call me a truther. I **am** a truther. I **love** the truth.

We were told that we "hate America" because we dared to question the official story. I can't count the number of people that called me a "traitor" for daring to dissent and asking tough questions. I was even told by a relative that I was insane and needed to go see a psychiatrist! OK, so let me get this straight. Since I asked questions about the official 9/11 fairytale, I was mentally unstable? Huh? I would assert that someone who actually **believes** the 9/11 fairytale is the mentally unstable person. Nevertheless, the facts and the truth didn't stop the cruelty or the name-calling. It was painful, and it actually still is painful, but we press on spreading the truth, knowing that there are still millions of Americans who are living in a fantasy world and they need to be shaken and forcibly waked up.

That's my goal. To help folks wake up from their slumber and unplug from the matrix. To help them realize that almost every "official story" over the past century is nothing more than a "monumental myth" fabricated by those who want to control us and keep us asleep, deceived, and obedient. I want people to start thinking for themselves and draw their own conclusions about current events, rather than mindlessly believing (and then regurgitating) the talking points spewed forth by the "press-titute" teleprompter-reading bobble-head mutant "reporters" in the controlled mainstream media.

You think I'm exaggerating? **Nay nay!** Take for instance the KTVU-FOX news report on the crash of the Asiana Airlines crash in July of 2013. In the report, the anchor incorrectly (and ridiculously) identified the airline pilots as *"Sum Ting Wong"*..."*We Tu Lo*"..."*Ho Lee Fuk*"...and *"Bang Ding Ow."* No, I'm not kidding. This really happened. This incident not only confirms my theory that many local news anchors are chosen using a low-IQ lottery from a list of head injury patients, but it also confirms my claim that the mainstream media is nothing more than a bunch of teleprompter reading idiots. I'll bet the producer's name was *"Sum Dum Guy."*

Now, before I go any further, I want to make it crystal clear that throughout the book, when I refer to the mainstream media as *"bobble-head bleached blondes"* and *"press-titutes"* and *"teleprompter readers"* (amongst other slangs and pejoratives) that I am **not** talking about everyone in the media. There are some excellent investigative reporters doing great work, and there are some media anchors and talk-show hosts that are "on our team." Ben Swann, Amber Lyon, Carol Alt, and Judge Andrew Napolitano immediately come to mind, just to name a few. Those who have "sold out" know who they are, and those who are legitimate, sincere, and honest also know who they are.

Anyway, after we "woke up" to 9/11, we began to question other "official stories" that we reckoned might be nothing more than "monumental myths." And that's when the floodgates were opened wide and we learned about Waco, Oklahoma City, Ruby Ridge, the Rockefellers, the phony "wars" on cancer and terror and drugs, as well as the assassinations of John F. Kennedy, Martin Luther King, and the list goes on and on and on. I think you get the point, though. It was a turning point in our lives, as we realized that almost everything we had ever believed to be true was actually a lie. And, of course, those lies are spread by liars.

Many of the liars have been photographed with their "hand in the cookie jar" (figuratively, of course). They've been "busted." Oddly enough, many of the lying liars continue in their path of deception – like President Obama, for example. He's a pathological liar and lies all the time. Well, not necessarily all the time ... just when he opens his mouth. Actually, he's not a pathological liar. This would indicate that he is incapable of telling the truth, and I don't believe for a second that our "duplicitous despotic dictator" has told thousands of lies since 2008 because he is incapable of telling the truth. No, I believe the more accurate term for Barry Soetoro (aka Barak Hussein Obama) is "sociopath." What makes a sociopathic liar different from a pathological liar is that he employs lying for the specific purpose of manipulating others. This explanation fits Obama like a glove, as he must certainly be the most manipulative and insincere President in history. And some of the lies he's told are ... for lack of a better term ... "monumental."

Take, for instance, the literally dozens of times he told 300+ million Americans, "... *if you like your current healthcare plan, you will be able to keep your healthcare plan ... **period**.*" As you all know by now, it turns out that was a prevarication ... a lie ... an untruth ... whatever you want to call it; caught on videotape, by the way. But rather than admit that he lied to the American people, on November 4, 2013, Obama "doubled down" and told another "whopper" lie to cover up the initial "whopper" lie, telling about 200 of his most ardent and enthusiastic supporters that he **never** promised what video recordings show him promising at least 29 times. He told the crowd, "*What we said was you could keep it **IF** it hasn't changed since the law was passed.*" Really? Needless to say, that claim is not supported by any of the 29 videotaped statements, which don't include any mention of his newly invented "*if it hasn't changed*" exception. "*Would you like some fries with your whoppers, Mr. President?*"

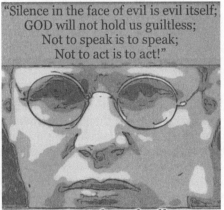

"Silence in the face of evil is evil itself;
GOD will not hold us guiltless;
Not to speak is to speak;
Not to act is to act!"

~ *Dietrich Bonhoeffer*

In 2008, Obama was able to manipulate the majority of trusting (i.e. naïve) Americans by engaging in an around-the-clock campaign of breathtaking lies. And, even today, after bringing the USA to the brink of total collapse and being repeatedly caught with his hand in the cookie jar, he still has nearly half of the American voters bamboozled. And please don't write me and say, *"You're a racist."* Give me a break. Put that "race card" back in your pocket, will you? There's not a racist bone in my body. The fact of the matter is that if you know that someone is lying and cheating and you choose not to expose them, then it's a sin, regardless of the color of their skin. I'm no racist, but I **am** a truth-teller, even when the truth is not "politically correct."

And it's not just Obama. Bush was a liar, too. So was Clinton. So was Bush's "daddy." Most of our "beloved leaders" are sociopathic liars. In reality, lying is a common trait of sociopaths, dictators, politicians, authoritarian leaders, and the mainstream media. Remember that the so-called "nightly news" (i.e. propaganda) is primarily lies, and it really helps if the "respected expert" (i.e. lying anchor) actually believes them. That way they can sleep at night ... in their coffins.

So why do we continue to believe the lying liars? It reminds me of ancient Rome. *"Falsus in uno, falsus in omnibus,"* translated *"false in one thing, false in everything,"* is a Roman legal principle indicating that a witness who willfully falsifies one matter is not credible on any matter. Remember this principle as you read this book. Also remember the Latin phrase, *"cui bono?"* which simply means *"who benefits?"* This is the very first question to be asked in any investigation. If you can figure out the answer to this question, you will be "hot on the tracks" of discovering who might have "allowed" an event to occur and/or who might have actually "made" it happen. Most of the time, the lies are so preposterous that even a small child, who has not been brainwashed, can figure out the truth.

Lying is the pillar of the state and lying is the cornerstone of the Medical Mafia. Some lies (i.e., *fluoride is good for your teeth*) are more clever than others, some lies (i.e., *mercury fillings are safe*) are easier to swallow, and some lies (i.e., *fires from airplane collisions brought down the Twin Towers on 9/11*) are downright ridiculous. But in the end, the "sheeple" love to believe the lies, they embrace them; they **need** them so they can return to their trance and fantasize about "America's Next Top Model" and "The Kardashians" and "Real Housewives." I mean, who wants to hear unpleasant truths when there are so many comforting lies?

More Latin? More Rome? **YES!** *"Panem et circenses"* ... translated means *"bread and circuses."* The phrase came from the satirist Juvenal of ancient Rome, who was disgusted and repulsed by the Romans' lust for entertainment. You see, in the first two centuries A.D., Rome faced a cavernous gulf between rich and poor. Its economy was stagnant. Slaves acquired by conquest built most of its bridges, roads, and aqueducts. As this cheaper labor replaced Roman citizens, hoards of unemployed, idle, hungry people filled the city.

The Caesars created make-work and part-time jobs, subsidized housing and doled out grain. Faced with incredible pessimism and ennui, typical Romans spent most of their time attending gladiator games, chariot races, and public executions. In the Roman Empire, it was bread and chariot races and gladiatorial games that filled the belly and distracted the mind of the Romans, allowing emperors to rule as they saw fit, brutalizing them vis-à-vis imperial expansion and domestic policing.

Sound familiar? There's much truth to the view that people can be kept submissive as long as you fill their bellies and give them violent spectacles to fill their free time. Heck, in light of the recent NSA "spying" scandal, we can see that Americans are sheepishly silent even when the government invades their privacy and illegally spies upon them. Few would disagree that "bread and circuses" typify the USA. Give your typical American "male" plenty of jejune entertainment, beer, pizza, American Idol, Victoria Secrets' models, MMA, NASCAR, NCAA football, and the NFL, and you could probably molest his children without him even caring.

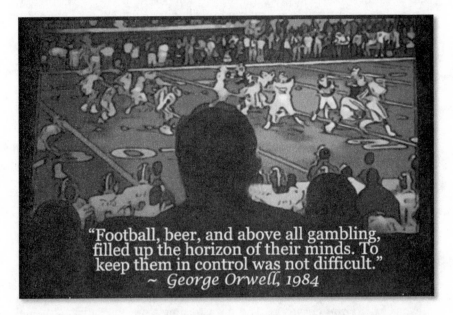

"Football, beer, and above all gambling, filled up the horizon of their minds. To keep them in control was not difficult."
~ *George Orwell, 1984*

I believe that America also suffers from a lack of empathy. The "Golden Rule" in the Bible is to treat others the way you want to be treated. But when Ron Paul brought this up at a 2012 debate (in the "Bible belt" of South Carolina) and applied it to the USA's multitude of unconstitutional wars of aggression overseas, he was "**booed**" loudly. Truth is that we are simply not encouraged to put ourselves in the place of others. You know, walk a mile in their shoes.

For example, how many Americans fancy the idea of a foreign power operating drones in our sovereign skies, launching missiles at gun-toting Americans suspected by this foreign power of being "terrorists" or "militants"? Yet we operate drones in places like Afghanistan, Pakistan, and Yemen, killing suspected "militants" with total impunity. Even when innocent women and children are killed, which happens quite regularly, our "emperors" and the mainstream media don't encourage us to have compassion for them. We are basically told to think of them as "collateral damage." **Regrettable?** Perhaps, but otherwise inconsequential. As I write this book, the Obama administration is increasingly couching vicious military intervention in "humanitarian" terms. Invading sovereign nations, deploying troops, murdering innocent civilians, and tipping wars in our favor is done in the name of "defeating tyranny" and "spreading democracy." Take, for instance, Khadafy in Libya. Is Assad of Syria next?

As you read the book, please be aware of the Hegelian Dialectic, which is *"thesis, antithesis, synthesis"* also known as *"problem, reaction, solution."* In other words, a problem is manufactured usually with a ready-in-the-wings antithesis (reaction) at an extreme so that the resulting synthesis (solution) can take society further toward a knee-jerk direction that it doesn't really want to go. It works like this: You want to introduce something you know the people won't like. This may be more power to the police, a further erosion of basic freedoms, or even a war. You know that if you offer these policies openly the people will react against them. So you first create a **PROBLEM**, such as a "terrorist" plot, an economic collapse, a nuclear bomb threat, or the threat of an impending war. You make sure someone else is blamed for this problem rather than the real people behind it all. So you create a "patsy" (like Lee Harvey Oswald, Timothy McVeigh, James Earl Ray, Osama Bin Laden, the Tsarnaev brothers, or Sirhan Sirhan) and you use the controlled mainstream media to tell people what they should think about your manufactured event and who they should blame for it.

This brings us to stage two, the **REACTION** from the people. After 9/11, the typical response was, *"I'm so mad about those Muslims! What is the government going to do about this?"* This allows them to then openly offer the **SOLUTION** to the problems they have just created, such as new legislation which advances the agenda of centralization of global power or the erosion of more basic freedoms.

I've been doing research on some of these topics for almost 20 years, while some of the newer material I have only researched for a couple of years. I read and research all the time, from multiple and diverse sources. Why? Because it's important to see both sides of an argument before you jump to conclusions. Do the proponents present "clear and convincing" evidence to support their position? OK, then maybe it's feasible. Or do they merely attack the character of those on the "other side" and call them names like "lunatic" or "conspiracy theorist"?

Please understand that it is currently standard practice in the USA to simply dismiss any piece of information that punches a hole in any widely accepted explanation of a disturbing event by tagging the new explanation as a "conspiracy theory." It's time to put an end to this name-calling nonsense once and for all. It is absolutely accurate to say that conspiracies exist all around us every day of our lives and in all walks of life. As a matter of fact, conspiracies are a very common part of life. Children conspire to play jokes on their friends, football teams conspire (in the huddle) to outmaneuver their opponents; the rich conspire with one another to get richer; governments conspire about virtually everything.

As a matter of fact every single person who has ever been convicted of a crime by a jury is the subject of a conspiracy theory; only in these cases a jury has accepted the theory as truth after seeing the evidence. The fact is that any time two or more people are involved in setting private plans to do anything, you have a conspiracy. Conspiracies happen every day. It's a fact. In light of this information, there are basically three types of people who repudiate and deny the existence of "high level" conspiracies: 1) the ignorant, 2) fools, and 3) the actual conspirators.

Don't believe everything in this book because I said it. Go study the topic for yourself, then come to your own conclusion. But on the flip side of the coin, please don't believe everything the Kool-Aid drinking blonde bimbo bobble-head media anchor tells you either. That's why God gave you a brain. Use it. Please. And please don't be offended if I step on your toes once or twice (or a dozen times) in this book. If I don't step on your toes, you probably don't have any feet.

Some (most) of the information in this book is going to go against everything you've been told to believe. Many of the subjects are "known" to be nothing more than "conspiracy theories." The liars (I mean "experts") on TV will tell you that if you even think about questioning the "official story," then you are a wild-eyed, paranoid, tinfoil-hat-wearing, dog-abusing, baby-hating, nut job. If you love the USA and/or freedom, butterflies, rainbows, unicorns, puppy dogs, rock and roll, Santa Claus, the Easter Bunny, baseball, hotdogs, apple pie, and your grandma, then you will never ever express doubts about any part of the "official story" ... to anyone ... **ever**.

Quite to the contrary, history is replete with instances of heroes who dared to question the "official story" and/or the "status quo" and were ostracized, persecuted, banished, and even killed for their courage to "buck the system."

For example ...

Remember Ignaz Semmelweis? You know? The Hungarian physician who was persecuted for urging doctors to wash their hands prior to delivering babies? For this he was expelled from both the hospital and the medical society. His life ended in an insane asylum. No doubt he felt like he was living in the "matrix."

Remember DDT? In the 1940s and 1950s, the synthetic pesticide dichlorodiphenyltrichloroethane (better known as DDT) was used to kill bugs that spread malaria and typhus in several parts of the world. Advertisements for the DDT ran in magazines and on the radio with the ironic slogan *"DDT is good for Me-e-e!"* Apparently it wasn't that good for you ... since it was banned by the US government in 1972.

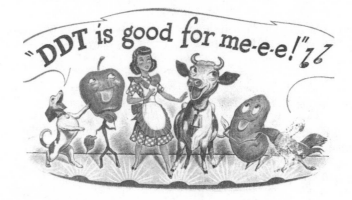

Remember thalidomide? Thalidomide was used in the late 1950s and early 1960s to combat morning sickness, but led to children being born without limbs. But don't worry about it. No big deal. The German inventor issued an apology. I guess that makes everything OK.

I could continue, but I think you get the point: Most of the "government sanctioned facts" we are expected to accept as true are nothing more than monumental myths told by double-dealing liars. Winston Churchill may have referred to the Russians as *"riddles wrapped in a mystery inside an enigma,"* but I fancy using alliteration in reference to the "untruths" and outright "shams" of the malevolent Medical Mafia and mendacious mainstream media. Most of their official stories are nothing more than a *"furtive foothill of foul-smelling feces wrapped in a fairytale inside a fable of fabrications and falsehoods."* Try that on for size!

At the end of the day, rather than *"in God we trust,"* perhaps the new national motto of the USA should be: *"Stuff yourself with food, root for your favorite professional sports team; dismiss anyone who questions the government as 'unpatriotic' and cheer on the imperial war machine.*" Modern day America is like "ancient Rome meets <u>1984</u> meets *The Hunger Games.*" It's the perfect storm. That's why it's imperative for us to wake up as many people as possible, while there is still time. Remember, as history demonstrates, most truths actually get ridiculed before they are accepted. That's a fact. The purpose of this book is to expose the lies and reveal the truth. There are no footnotes and only a few dozen URLs, but you can find major research sources and recommendations in the "Resources" section at the end of each chapter. Check 'em out.

The tone will be informal, sarcastic at times, on many occasions solemn, and occasionally amusing. I think it's an enjoyable and stimulating read, but hey, I'm the author, so I'm prejudiced. So please turn off the "boob tube" and snuggle up on the sofa (or toilet), and prepare to be enlightened (or at least entertained) by the topics in this book.

Be sure to put on your "truth digging gloves" because we are going to be turning over stones and searching for truth. As they say, *"Search for the truth amongst the lies and you will find it."*

You know what else they say? *"You can't win for losing"* ... *"it is what it is"* ... *"awesome"* ... *"spoiler alert"* ... *"kick the can down the road"* ...

Sorry, I got off on a tangent there. What was I saying? Oh yes ... you know what they say ...

"The truth shall set you free!"

The book will bust some myths, destroy some idols, and create some heroes. **Black** will become white and white will become **black**. At times, the truth will almost appear to be an optical illusion, but that's only because we've been conditioned to not recognize it.

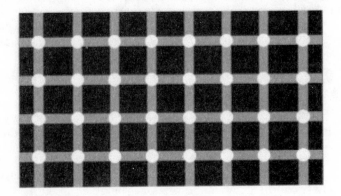

Grab a nice cold glass of water (you might actually need a shot of whisky) before I give you the **red** pill. And please swallow it. Then buckle your seatbelt and prepare to unplug from the "matrix," go further down the "rabbit hole" than you've ever gone before and permanently leave Kansas!

WARNING: In the words of Morpheus in The Matrix, *"This is your last chance. After this, there is no turning back. You take the* **blue** *pill – the story ends, you wake up in your bed and believe whatever you want to believe. You take the* **red** *pill – you stay in Wonderland and I show you how deep the rabbit-hole goes."*

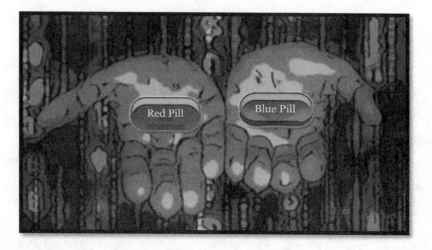

You think I didn't see it? I saw it. Yes, indeed. I definitely saw you take the **red** pill.

OK, what are you waiting for? Get to reading …

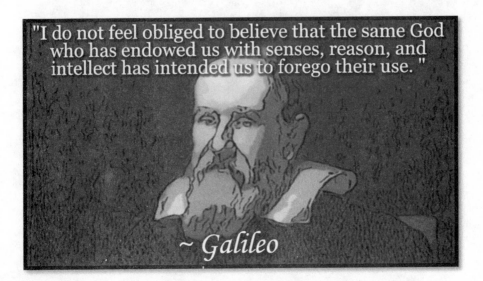

"I do not feel obliged to believe that the same God who has endowed us with senses, reason, and intellect has intended us to forego their use. "

~ Galileo

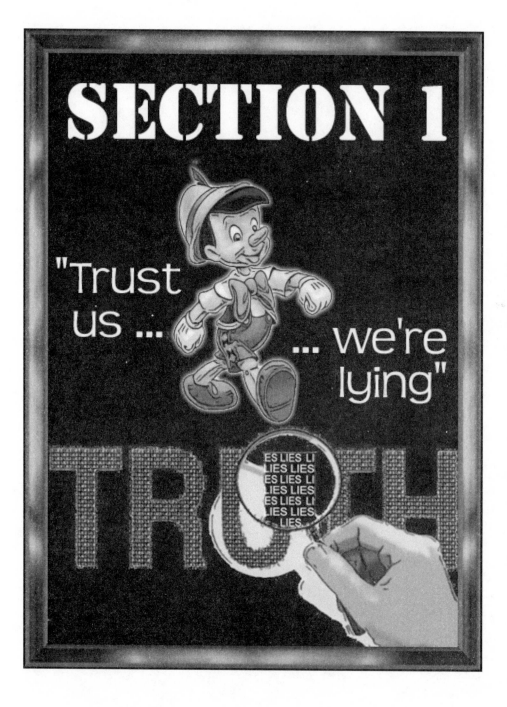

Chapter 1

~ THE M.D. "EMPERORS" ~

MONUMENTAL MYTH

Medical doctors ("M.D.s") are intellectually superior to homeopaths, herbalists, naturopaths, chiropractors, etc. The therapeutics of modern (conventional) M.D. directed medicine is the most popular because they are the most effective for treating sickness and disease. When you are sick and go to the doctor, you are going to the person who knows what to do to help you get better. When the doctor diagnoses what your problem is, and then pulls out his or her prescription pad and writes you a prescription for a drug that will take care of the problem, you should be relieved.

CAN YOU HANDLE THE TRUTH?

In the words of my good buddy, Robert Scott Bell, the medical industry is nothing short of a *"Church of Biological Mysticism"* with medical doctors the equivalent of *"high priests."* I like that phrase and comparison, and will be elaborating and expanding upon it throughout the book. Despite the fact that M.D.s repeatedly practice "voodoo" medicine and quack science, modern medicine often calls itself "conventional medicine" while pejoratively referring to other systems of medicine as "alternative."

But modern medicine has only been around a little over 100 years, while traditional medical systems (such as Chinese and Ayurvedic medicine) have been around over 3,000 years. Homeopathy has been around 200 years, chiropractic and naturopathic medicine have been around over 100 years, and of course, people have been using herbs and dietary remedies since the beginning of recorded history.

The reality is that the M.D. "emperors" are buck naked. I know, I know, right now they may be marching down the street with an entourage of "sheeple" following them who are delusional and pretending that they are actually wearing purple silk robes and golden-threaded paraphernalia. But the day is coming when the entire world will be asking the question: *"Why are the M.D. 'emperors' naked?"*

I'll tell you why. The "emperors" of modern medicine (aka the M.D.s) have driven the "bus" of medicine over a hazardous cliff, down the mountain, into a perilous swamp, right in the middle of the alligators that haven't eaten in a long, long time. **Why do I say this?** In order to understand the current state of affairs of medical practice in the USA, it's vital to understand exactly how we got here. So, let's put on our history caps, jump into the time capsule, and go all the way back over 100 years to the turn of the 20th century.

When Dr. George H. Simmons began in 1899 what became a twenty-five year reign as head of the American Medical Association (AMA), it was a weak organization with little money and little respect from the general public. The advertising revenue from its medical journal, the *Journal of the American Medical Association* (*JAMA*), was a paltry $34,000 per year. The AMA realized that competition was causing physicians' incomes to dwindle, as the number of medical schools had increased from around 90 (in 1880) to over 150 (in 1903).

Chiropractic had just been introduced into the mainstream, homeopathy was thriving, herbalists were flourishing, all the while regular doctors were unable to profit from their medical practices. With the state governments reluctant to create laws restricting the various healing arts, Simmons hired Joseph McCormack (the secretary of the Kentucky State Board of health) to "rouse the profession to lobby." With McCormack leading the charge, the AMA began to bolster their ranks, preaching ethics (like not competing with other physicians or publishing your prices) and decrying "quackery" (anything that competed with regular medicine).

Simmons was shrewd enough to have the AMA establish a *Council on Medical Education* in 1904. This council's stated mission was to "upgrade medical education" – a noble goal. However, the *Council on Medical Education* had actually devised a plan to rank medical schools throughout the country, but their guidelines were dubious, to say the least. For instance, just having the word "homeopathic" in the name of a medical school reduced their ranking because the AMA asserted that such schools taught "an exclusive dogma."

However, by 1910, the AMA was out of money and didn't have the funds to complete the project. The Rockefellers had joined forces with the Carnegie foundation to create an education fund, and they were approached by N. P. Colwell (secretary of the *Council on Medical Education*) to finish the job they had started, but could no longer fund. Rockefeller and Carnegie agreed. Simon Flexner, who was on the Board of Directors for the Rockefeller Institute, proposed that his brother, Abraham, who knew nothing about medicine, be hired for the project. On a side note, although their names are not very well known, the Flexner brothers have probably influenced the lives of more people and in a more profound way than any other brothers in the last century, with the possible exception of Wilbur and Orville Wright. After going bankrupt attempting to run a boarding school, Abraham Flexner was hired by the Carnegie Foundation for the Advancement of Teaching. The Rockefellers and Carnegies had traditionally worked together in the furtherance of their mutual goals, and this certainly was no exception. The Flexner brothers represented the lens that brought both the Rockefeller and the Carnegie fortunes into sharp focus on the medical profession.

Their plan was to "restructure" the AMA and "certify" medical schools based solely upon Flexner's recommendations. The AMA's head of the *Council on Medical Education* traveled with Flexner as they evaluated medical schools. Eventually, Flexner submitted a report to The Carnegie Foundation entitled "Medical Education in the United States and Canada," which is also known as the "Flexner report." Not surprisingly, the gist of the report was that it was far too easy to start a medical school and that most medical schools were not teaching "sound medicine."

The medical sociologist Paul Starr wrote in his Pulitzer Prize-winning book (The Social Transformation of American Medicine): "*The AMA Council became a national accrediting agency for medical schools, as an increasing number of states adopted its judgments of unacceptable institutions.*" Further, he noted: "*Even though no legislative body ever set up ... the AMA Council on Medical Education, their decisions came to have the force of law.*" With the AMA grading the various medical colleges, it became predictable that the homeopathic colleges, even the large and respected ones, would eventually be forced to stop teaching homeopathy or die. And that's exactly what happened.

Published in 1910, the Flexner report (quite correctly) pointed out the inadequacies of medical education at the time. No one could take exception with that. It also proposed a wide range of sweeping changes, most of which were entirely sound. No one could take exception with those, either. However, Flexner's recommendations emphatically included the strengthening of courses in pharmacology and the addition of research departments at all "qualified" medical schools.

It is what followed in the wake of the Flexner report that reveals its true purpose in the total plan. With public backing secured by the publication of the Flexner report, Carnegie and Rockefeller commenced a major upgrade in medical education by financing only those medical schools that taught what they wanted taught. In other words, they began to immediately shower hundreds of millions of dollars on those medical schools that were teaching "drug intensive" medicine.

Predictably, those schools that had the financing churned out the better doctors. In return for the financing, the schools were required to continue teaching course material that was exclusively drug oriented, with no emphasis put on natural medicine. The end result of the Flexner report was that all accredited medical schools became heavily oriented toward drugs and drug research. In 1913, Simmons and the AMA went on the offensive even more strongly by their establishment of the "Propaganda Department," which was dedicated to attacking any and all unconventional medical treatments and anyone (M.D. or not) who practiced them.

The purpose was to dominate the oil and chemical (which eventually became the "pharmaceutical") markets, and the Flexner report gave both of these tycoons the "ammunition" they needed to achieve that goal. In the end, the Rockefeller/Carnegie plan was a smashing success. Those medical schools that did not conform were denied the funds and the prestige that came with those funds, and were forced out of business.

By 1925, over 10,000 herbalists were out of business. By 1940, over 1500 chiropractors would be prosecuted for practicing "quackery." The 22 homeopathic medical schools that flourished in 1900 dwindled to just 2 in 1923. By 1950, all schools teaching homeopathy were closed. In the end, if a physician did not graduate from a Flexner approved medical school and receive an M.D. degree; he or she couldn't find a job.

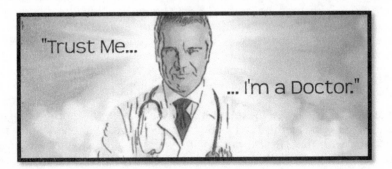

The Flexner report was the commencement of a conspiracy to limit and eventually eliminate competition from natural, non-pharmaceutical, non-patentable treatments for disease. This is why today M.D.s are so heavily biased toward synthetic drug therapy and know little about nutrition. They don't even study health; they study disease. Modern doctors are taught virtually nothing about nutrition, wellness or disease prevention.

Expecting a medical doctor to guide you on health issues is sort of like expecting your CPA to pilot a jet airliner. It's simply **not** an area in which they have been trained. That's not to say M.D.s aren't intelligent people. Most of them have high IQs. But even a genius can't teach you something they know nothing about. And, yes, doctors can be fooled, "snookered" and "bamboozled" too, just like the rest of us.

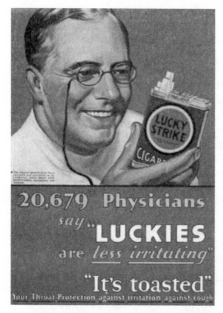

Case in point: Back in the 1920s, the public was becoming increasingly worried about the deleterious health consequences of cigarette smoking. Cigarettes were called "coffin nails" and people started talking about "smoker's hack." Executives for "Big Tobacco" were worried, so they began to use doctors (actors of course) in their advertisements to reassure folks that cigarettes were nothing to be concerned about.

During the 1920s, Lucky Strike was the dominant cigarette brand. This brand, made by American Tobacco Company, was the first to use the image of a physician in its advertisements. "*20,679 physicians say 'Luckies are less irritating,*" the deceiving ads proclaimed.

The advertising firm that promoted Lucky Strikes had sent physicians free cartons of the cigarettes and asked them whether Lucky Strikes were less irritating to "sensitive and tender" throats. The slogan at the bottom of the ads read, "*Your throat protection against irritation and cough.*" The ad to the left appeared in *The Magazine of Wall Street* for July 26, 1930. In the small print on the left it says "*The figures quoted have been checked and certified to by Lybrand, Ross Bros. & Montgomery, Accountants & Auditors.*"

By the mid-1930s, Lucky Strike had some competition. A new advertising campaign for Philip Morris referred to research conducted by physicians. One ad (on the previous page) actually claimed that after prescribing Philip Morris brand cigarettes to patients with irritated throats, "*every case of irritation cleared completely or definitely improved.*" There was an interesting paradox in the cigarette ads. For instance, in one ad a company would make the claim that cigarettes aren't harmful and then in another ad they would say something like "*our cigarettes are less harmful than the other brands.*"

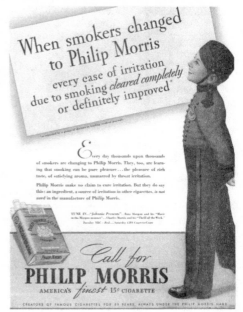

But, hey, the ads were working. People were smoking like chimneys and Big Tobacco was blissful. Business was booming! Something that made them even happier was when the *JAMA* published its first cigarette advertisement in 1933, stating that it had done so only "*after careful consideration of the extent to which cigarettes were used by physicians in practice.*" Remember the paradox that I just mentioned? It wasn't confined to cigarette companies. The *JAMA* also participated in the strange brew of "double think" because at the same time it was running cigarette ads, it also published the first major study to causally link smoking to lung cancer. What to believe? Who knows? Doctors promoted cigarettes in *JAMA* ads, while *JAMA* research indicated a lung cancer link. Are you confused yet? I suppose in the land of unicorns and pixie dust, this actually might make sense, but not in the land of reality. Anyway, as I previously mentioned, although the doctors in these advertisements were always actors and not real doctors, the image of the doctor continued to permeate cigarette ads for several decades.

Along comes RJ Reynolds Tobacco Company! In medical journals and in the mainstream media, one of the most infamous cigarette advertising slogans was associated with RJR's Camel cigarettes: "*More doctors smoke Camels than any other cigarette.*" These ads pictured doctors in labs, sitting back at their desk or speaking with patients. The campaign began in 1946 and ran for almost a decade in magazines and on the radio.

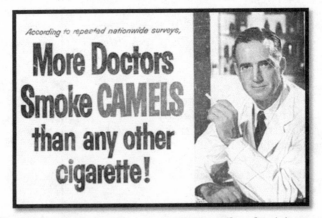

The Camel ads included this message: "*Family physicians, surgeons, diagnosticians, nose and throat specialists, doctors in every branch of medicine... a total of 113,597 doctors... were asked the question: 'What cigarette do you smoke?' And more of them named Camel as their smoke than any other cigarette! Three independent research groups found this to be a fact. You see, doctors too smoke for pleasure. That full Camel flavor is just as appealing to a doctor's taste as to yours... that marvelous Camel mildness means just as much to his throat as to yours.*"

The first research to make a statistical correlation between cancer and smoking was published in 1930 in Cologne, Germany. In 1938, Dr. Raymond Pearl of Johns Hopkins University reported that smokers do not live as long as non-smokers. The tobacco industry dismissed these early findings as "anecdotal" while at the same time recruiting doctors to endorse cigarettes.

Did doctors **really** believe that smoking was good for you? You betcha. They were mesmerized and brainwashed just like everybody else. It was almost like they were on a bad "acid trip" or had smoked too much crack! There were big cigarette ad campaigns in medical journals. For example, there is an ad showing a physician writing on a prescription pad which states, *"For your patients with sore throats and cough, Phillip Morris cigarettes."*

But remember...**every myth eventually gets busted!** On Jan. 11, 1964, Surgeon General Luther Terry announced the findings of the Surgeon General's Advisory Committee on Smoking and Health. The report, *Smoking and Health: Report of the Advisory Committee to the Surgeon General of the United States*, concluded that there was a link between lung cancer and chronic bronchitis and cigarette smoking. In a press conference, Terry said, *"It is the judgment of the committee that cigarette smoking contributes substantially to mortality from certain specific diseases and to the overall death rate."* By the end of 1965, the tobacco industry was required to put warning labels on its products and advertisements to warn the public of the health risks associated with smoking.

After a couple hundred years of tobacco use, tobacco companies would lose several more major battles throughout the next few decades, including the ban on television ads in 1970 when President Nixon signed the Public Health Cigarette Smoking Act. Despite all this, over 50 million Americans still smoke and almost half a million die prematurely as a result of tobacco products.

In his book, The Cigarette Century: The Rise, Fall and Deadly Persistence of the Product that Defined America, Allan M. Brandt (Harvard medical historian) documented the role that medical "research" played in the cigarette debate. After studying research, court transcripts, and formerly restricted Big Tobacco memoranda, he summed up the misleading nature of "expert" medical testimony in tobacco litigation: *"I was appalled by what the tobacco expert witnesses had written. By asking narrow questions and responding to them with narrow research, they provided precisely the cover the industry sought."*

It is important to understand this little history lesson in order to understand better how the field of medicine has come to be what it is now, and to debunk the myth that M.D.s are demi-gods and they should be worshipped as omniscient in their field. In essence, due in large part to the Flexner report, we have a clandestine medical dictatorship.

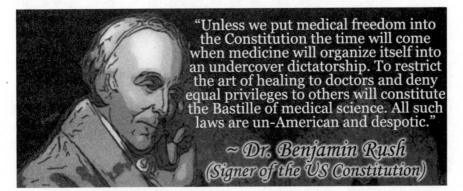

"Unless we put medical freedom into the Constitution the time will come when medicine will organize itself into an undercover dictatorship. To restrict the art of healing to doctors and deny equal privileges to others will constitute the Bastille of medical science. All such laws are un-American and despotic."

~ Dr. Benjamin Rush
(Signer of the US Constitution)

In this medical dictatorship, what we constantly find is a series of myths, cons, and frauds perpetrated against "we the people," masterminded by profit-seeking medical groups conspiring with multinational corporations (like Big Pharma, Big Agra, and Big Tobacco) to maximize profits at the expense of public health. Although the myths have changed (i.e. the AMA isn't pushing cigarettes anymore), thanks to the Flexner report, the Medical Mafia is still pushing deadly drugs that will one day be regarded to be just as absurd as smoking.

Let's get real here, folks. Drug intensive therapy is miserably outdated, ineffective, and downright dangerous. Nobody with half a brain actually believes that drugs help people heal. Drugs harm. Drugs kill. Drugs cause addiction. I predict that in the near future (or maybe, like "Star Wars," in a distant galaxy far, far away), scientists will look back on medicine today with astonishment at how an industry with such malicious and greedy intentions could have gained so much influence. In the words of Dr. Richard Shulze, ND, *"We're going to look back at this century and we're going to laugh eventually, but we'll cry first. This is one of the most barbaric periods. It's going to be called the 'Dark Ages' of Medicine."*

In summary, the Flexner report coupled with the enigmatic veil of secrecy and mystery which is associated with a "medical degree" and the bizarre propensity for most folks to defer to anyone in an apparent position of authority (regardless of whether or not it is merited) has resulted in a recipe for disaster. The bottom line is that M.D.s are in the "driver's seat of modern medicine's Maserati" only because of financial coalitions that were organized at the turn of the 20th century. Or, an easier way to say it: M.D.s owe their pre-eminent medical and social status to **drug money**.

According to my friend, Dr. Robert J. Rowen, M.D., in his *Second Opinion Newsletter*, *"In my humble opinion, the best way to improve the health of the nation is to cease visiting conventional doctors for ANYTHING at all except emergency conditions. Statins are a scam. Treating for blood pressure when systolic is less than 160 has no significant benefit. Most vaccines are a total sham and highly toxic. You can replace most pain pills with natural substances avoiding burning a hole in your gut with NSAID chemicals. And adult diabetes is totally curable with diet and exercise. Back surgery has a 50% 'make-you-worse' rate, most knee arthroscopy is worthless in the long run, and cancer-screening treatment is a total catastrophe. ... It's vital we show everyone that this emperor (conventional medicine) has no clothes."*

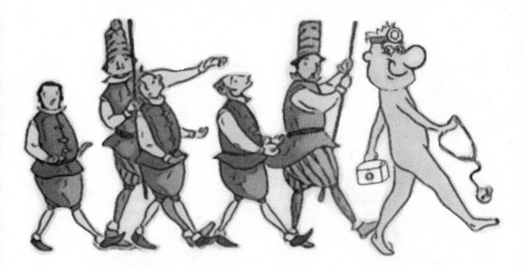

RESOURCES

Video
"Flexner Report" – http://vimeo.com/27003739

Books
The Social Transformation of American Medicine (Paul Starr)
The Cigarette Century: The Rise, Fall, and Deadly Persistence of the Product that Defined America (Allan M. Brandt)
Murder by Injection (Eustace Mullins)
The MD Emperor Has No Clothes (Dr. Peter Glidden, ND)
If Naturopaths are 'Quacks' ... Then I Guess I'm a Duck (Dr. Shauna Young)

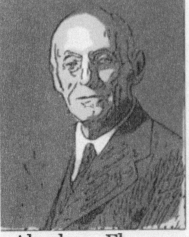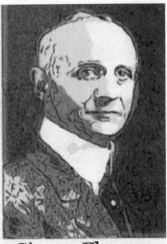

Abraham Flexner   Simon Flexner

Chapter 2

~ THE ROCKEFELLERS ~

MONUMENTAL MYTH

John D. Rockefeller created the structure of modern philanthropy. He believed in educating the poor and desired to give everyone the equal opportunity to learn. Over the past century, he and his family, including his children, grandchildren, and great-grandchildren worked diligently for the benefit all of mankind and should be considered champions for humanity. The Rockefellers are the epitome of philanthropists.

CAN YOU HANDLE THE TRUTH?

I've already mentioned John D. Rockefeller in the previous chapter. In addition to his impact on the AMA via the Flexner report, Rockefeller founded the American Cancer Society ("ACS") in 1913 at the New York Harvard Club. However, during this chapter, I want to really focus on the Rockefeller involvement with eugenics, which is the applied "pseudo-science" of social Darwinism.

Much of Charles Darwin's thinking was derived from the economic theories of British-born Thomas Malthus who, in his *"Essay on the Principle of Population"* asserted that human population tends to grow exponentially while the capabilities of agricultural resources tend to grow arithmetically. In other words, there are too many people and not enough food, so eventually there will be a massive "survival of the fittest" food crisis where the poor and weak die off and only the "well-to-do" survive. This "Malthusian catastrophe" is actually a bunch of hogwash; nevertheless it is one of the bases of the modern eugenics movement.

What is eugenics? It is the destructive pseudo-science and philosophy declaring man should intervene to alter human traits in an attempt to better the human race by preventing the reproduction of the "unfit" and "inferior races" and "useless eaters." Popular eugenics techniques include "selective breeding," marriage restriction, forced racial segregation, forced abortion, forced sterilization, human experimentation, killing of institutionalized populations (mentally defective and handicapped), infanticide, and genocide. Sir Francis Galton, the (half) cousin of Charles Darwin, is considered to be the *"father of eugenics."* He actually coined the term *"eugenics"* which comes from the Greek words *"eu"* (which means "good") and *"genēs"* (which means "generation" or "origin").

In 1863, Galton theorized that if talented people only married other talented people, the result would be measurably better offspring. But Galton didn't just theorize this; he wanted to put it into practice, so he carried out an "experiment" where the Galton, Darwin, Huxley, and Wedgwood families only bred with each other, in an attempt to create a "superhuman" breed. Sounds great, right? Well, it may have sounded great, but the reality is that within two generations, over 90% of their offspring either died at birth or were physically or mentally disabled. Their family tree actually got smaller, rather than expanding like a family tree normally does. On the subject of the Huxley family, Julian Huxley (the brother of Aldous who authored Brave New World) first used the term *"trans-humanism."* He was a member of the British Eugenics Society, eugenics being the foundation of trans-humanism.

Despite Galton's failed "4 family experiment," the eugenics movement continued to grow, especially in the USA, thanks to the funding provided by John D. Rockefeller, who, after creating the Rockefeller Foundation in 1913, quickly took charge of the Bureau of Social Hygiene and gave it the task of conducting "research and education on birth control, maternal health, and sex education." Via the National Research Council, which was the Rockefeller Foundation's "medical division," Rockefeller funded the horrible sex research of Alfred Kinsey, who, along with his fellow pedophiles sexually abused 2,000 infants and children. A year or two before he died, Kinsey circumcised himself with a pocketknife. Among his intimates was Dr. Ewen Cameron, the infamous CIA-funded mind control doctor who ran the MKULTRA program. Another of Kinsey's apparent influences was the occultist Aleister Crowley ("the Great Beast") known in the press as *"the wickedest man alive."*

In 1913, Cettie Rockefeller (Junior's mother and John D's wife) gave $25,000 to the Bureau of Social Hygiene to "promote instruction in social hygiene for female students around the country." The Bureau of Social Hygiene then funded Margaret Sanger's proposal for birth control clinical studies by the American Birth Control League (ABCL), which eventually became Planned Parenthood. She advocated limiting "dysgenic stocks" such as Negros, Hispanics, American Indians and Catholics, as well as "slum dwellers" such as Jewish immigrants. We will take a closer look at the pure, unadulterated evil and depravity of Margaret Sanger in the next chapter.

By 1927, eugenics was mainstream in the USA, with forced sterilization laws in 25 states. Believe it or not, in 1928, some of the first computers were put to use in the eugenics field, as Thomas Watson (founder of IBM) supplied punch card computers to Hitler and the Nazis for use in the death camps, with the inmates being tattooed with human ID numbers.

During that same period of time, the Rockefeller Foundation created the pseudoscientific medical specialty known as "psychiatric genetics," and using the foundation's funds, Rockefeller funded both of the Kaiser Wilhelm Institutes in Germany – the "Kaiser Wilhelm Institute for Psychiatry" and the "Kaiser Wilhelm Institute for Anthropology, Eugenics and Human Heredity." The Rockefellers' chief executive of these institutions was the fascist Swiss psychiatrist, Ernst Rudin, assisted by his protégés, Otmar Verschuer and Franz J. Kallmann.

Verschuer, a hero in American eugenics circles, functioned as a head of the Kaiser Wilhelm Institute for Anthropology, Eugenics and Human Heredity. Verschuer had a long-time assistant ... his name was Josef Mengele. Perhaps you've heard of him? Or maybe you're only familiar with his nickname – the *"Butcher of Auschwitz."* Mengele became medical commandant and experimented on concentration camp inmates at Auschwitz. His gruesome medical experiments included needles used to change eye color, the removal of limbs without anesthetics, sex changes, sterilization, and other unspeakable crimes. Tens of thousands were murdered and their organs, heads, limbs, and eyeballs were sent to the Rockefellers at the Kaiser Wilhelm Institute.

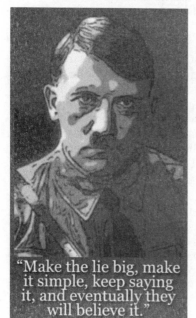

"Make the lie big, make it simple, keep saying it, and eventually they will believe it."

Rudin and his staff, as part of the "Task Force of Heredity Experts," chaired by Hitler's private army (the "SS") chief, Heinrich Himmler, crafted Germany's sterilization law. Described as an *"American model law,"* it was implemented in July 1933 and proudly printed in the USA in the September 1933 *Eugenical News* with Hitler's signature. In 1938, Kallmann wrote a book which was used as a rationalization to murder of over 250,000 mental patients and various "defective" people, most of them children. Dr. Alexis Carrel of the Rockefeller Institute (and a Nobel Prize winner) publically applauded Hitler for advocating the mass murder of mental patients and prisoners. Carrel also advocated the use of poison gas to get rid of "useless eaters."

Hitler actually studied American eugenics laws, and he tried to legitimize his anti-Semitism by "medicalizing" it and wrapping it in the more palatable pseudo-scientific facade of eugenics. Hitler was able to recruit more followers among reasonable Germans by claiming that science was on his side. But his eugenics ideas were actually "made in the USA" as is evidenced in <u>Mein Kampf</u>, published in 1924, where Hitler quoted American eugenic ideology and revealed a detailed knowledge of American eugenics.

Hitler proudly expressed to his comrades just how meticulously he followed the progress of the American eugenics movement, as he told a fellow Nazi, *"I have studied with great interest the laws of several American states concerning prevention of reproduction by people whose progeny would, in all probability, be of no value or be injurious to the racial stock."*

Rockefeller funded and sent leading US eugenicists (C.M. Goethe, Charles Davenport, and Harry Laughlin) to Germany to help "fine tune" Hitler's eugenics program. And "fine tune" it they did, with millions of innocent people being slaughtered in the camps. Yes, Rockefeller and his bankster cronies were up to their eyeballs in eugenics and mass extermination. But that's not even the tip of the iceberg. In addition to funding eugenics across the globe, Rockefeller's goal was to dominate the oil, chemical, and pharmaceutical markets, so in 1941, his company (*Standard Oil of New Jersey*) purchased a controlling interest in a huge German drug/chemical company called I.G. Farben, which was the single largest donor to the election campaign of Adolph Hitler. One year before Hitler seized power, I.G. Farben donated 400,000 marks to Hitler, his Nazi party, and the "SS." Accordingly, after Hitler's seizure of power, I.G. Farben was the single largest profiteer of the German conquest of the world during WW II. While millions of people were being imprisoned and murdered, I.G. Farben was profiting.

I.G. Auschwitz, a wholly-owned subsidiary of I.G. Farben, was the largest industrial complex of the world for manufacturing synthetic gasoline and rubber for the conquest of Europe. Auschwitz used the concentration camp prisoners as "slave labor" in their factory. But there was no "retirement plan" for the prisoners of Auschwitz. Those who were too frail or too ill to work were selected at the main gate of the Auschwitz factory and sent to the gas chambers. Even the chemical gas Zyklon-B used for the annihilation of millions of innocent people resulted from I.G. Farben's drawing boards and factories.

In 1941, Otto Armbrust (the I.G. Farben board member responsible for the Auschwitz project), stated to his colleagues, *"Our new friendship with the SS is a blessing. We have determined all measures integrating the concentration camps to benefit our company."* The I.G. Farben cartel used the victims of the concentration camps as human guinea pigs. Tens of thousands of them died during human experiments such as the testing of new and unknown vaccinations.

It should be noted that J.D. Rockefeller and Averell Harriman were business partners of Prescott Bush (yes, that's George W's grandfather) in Brown Brothers Harriman. In addition to funding and promoting eugenics, they supported and funded the Nazi rise to power. After World War II, the Rockefeller eugenics movement experienced a "facelift" to distance itself from the discredited Nazis, many of whom were brought to the USA in "Operation Paperclip."

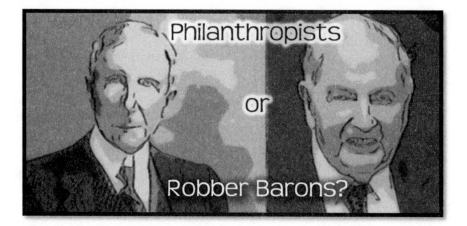

In the 1940s, Rockefeller also funded the Tavistock Institute for Human Relations, which hired Dr. Sigmund Freud to start the ball rolling, with their ultimate objective being to determine the most effective ways to manipulate and control the mass consciousness. Tavistock has, since then, trained individuals who have infiltrated and assumed the leadership roles in virtually every think tank, religion, corporation, governmental department, major university, and mainstream media outlet on earth.

In the 1950s, the Rockefellers reorganized the US eugenics movement and added population-control and abortion groups. Shockingly, during the 1950s, the American Eugenics Society forcibly sterilized over 64,000 "defective and undesirable persons!" Later, due to the backlash from being associated with crimes against humanity, the American Eugenics Society changed its name to the Society for the Study of Social Biology, which still remains today.

In its 1968 annual report, the Rockefeller Foundation acknowledged funding the development of so-called "anti-fertility vaccines" and their implementation on a mass-scale. Other measures to reduce US fertility were encouraged, such as encouraging increased homosexuality, utilizing "fertility control agents" in the water supply, encouraging women to work (to break up the family), abortion and sterilization on demand, and making contraception truly available and accessible to all.

In 1969, Dr. Lawrence Dunegan, M.D. attended a meeting of pediatric physicians in Pittsburgh where the speaker was Dr. Richard Day, national medical director of Planned Parenthood, which was funded by the Rockefeller Foundation. Dr. Day said that in the future there will be hard-to-cure diseases created, and that cures for nearly all cancers had been developed but were being hidden at the Rockefeller Institute so that populations would not increase.

In the 1990s, vaccines were created that contained stealth cancer viruses or other deadly pathogens that will either kill or sterilize. For instance, research was conducted by the National Institute of Immunology on the use of "carriers" such as tetanus toxoid and diphtheria to bypass the immune system and deliver the female hormone, hCG. **Why?** Because injection of hCG bound to tetanus causes sterilization or miscarriage, if given during pregnancy. In 1993, there was an enormous increase in miscarriages in Nicaragua; the same in Mexico during 1994, and then the Philippines during 1996. No investigations were performed in Nicaragua and Mexico, but the Philippines Medical Association discovered that hCG had been added to tetanus vaccine.

There was an article in *Vaccine Weekly* which detailed the fact that this hCG-laced tetanus vaccine was causing spontaneous abortion and miscarriage. There was also a *BBC* special on the same topic. Guess who funded the research by the National Institute of Immunology. You got it! The Rockefeller Foundation and the Population Council (which was funded by Rockefeller).

Are you getting the picture? The Rockefeller "game plan" is to control the population, energy, food, medicine, and finances of the entire globe in an effort to escort the US into a one-world government and global fascism.

RESOURCES

Websites
http://hnn.us/article/1796
http://www.naturalnews.com/eugenics.html
http://www.hartford-hwp.com/archives/27a/247.html

Books
War Against the Weak: Eugenics and America's
Campaign to Create a Master Race (Edwin Black)
Nazi Nexus: America's Corporate Connections
to Hitler's Holocaust (Edwin Black)

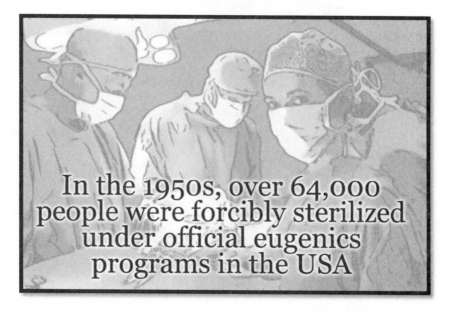

In the 1950s, over 64,000 people were forcibly sterilized under official eugenics programs in the USA

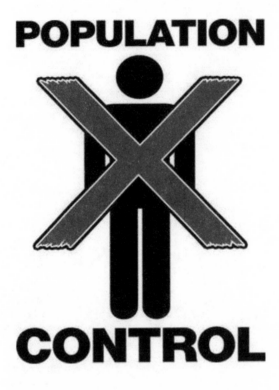

Chapter 3

~ PLANNED PARENTHOOD ~

MONUMENTAL MYTH

Planned Parenthood exists to empower individuals (women) to make independent, informed decisions about their sexual and reproductive lives. They provide information and health care and promote public policies that make those services available to all women. Planned Parenthood believes in strong, caring families and communities, where every child is cared for and loved, regardless of race or religion. Planned Parenthood and its workers are the "good guys" and they protect us from the dangers of "unwanted" children and unprotected sex.

CAN YOU HANDLE THE TRUTH?

Planned Parenthood is the nation's largest abortion chain, with a goal to enslave our young people into sexual addiction which drives the profit making service of abortion. Do you know the ultimate goal of Planned Parenthood is **population control**?

Although Planned Parenthood passes itself off as promoting women's health care, they push birth control pills identified by the World Health Organization as a Class 1 carcinogen. Cancer is the second highest cause of death in American women. Does this sound like Planned Parenthood cares about women's health?

One of the most powerful investigations completed to date showed Planned Parenthood's willingness to cover up the sex-trafficking of young girls. Planned Parenthood was caught coaching a man and woman, posing as a pimp and a prostitute, to obtain abortions, STD testing and birth control for their underage female sex slaves. Staffers instructed the "sex traffickers" to tell the girls to lie about their ages and the ages of their "boyfriends." They even coached the undercover operatives on how to receive discounts on birth control and abortions, and advised which facilities had less stringent standards. Once again, Planned Parenthood was caught on tape covering up abuse—showing they were more than willing to break state and federal laws in order to continue profiting from abortion, even if it meant driving young women back into the arms of their abusers.

Planned Parenthood facilities across the nation were phoned by an undercover investigator seeking to donate specifically to "lower the number of blacks in America" through abortions earmarked for African-American babies. Not one staffer at the 15 Planned Parenthood centers contacted declined the money, nor expressed shock at the request. Some actually agreed with the caller's racist agenda and one Director of Development went so far as to state she was "excited" over the request.

This is not really surprising though, especially in light of the fact that Planned Parenthood, which was previously known as the American Birth Control League, was founded by none other than Margaret Sanger. Ever heard of her? Sanger was a racist, eugenicist, and Satanist. In the last chapter about the Rockefellers, I defined eugenics. But just in case you forgot, eugenics is destructive pseudo-science and social movement that advocates "selective breeding" to better the human race by preventing the reproduction of the "unfit" and "inferior races." Sanger was specifically concerned with reducing the Negro population.

At a March 1925 international birth control gathering in New York City, a speaker warned of the menace posed by the "black" and "yellow" peril. The man was not a Nazi or Klansman; he was Dr. S. Adolphus Knopf, a member of the ABCL. Sanger's other colleagues included self-confessed and erudite racists. For example, Lothrop Stoddard (Harvard graduate and the author of *The Rising Tide of Color against White Supremacy*) described the eugenic practices of the Third Reich as "scientific" and "humanitarian." Dr. Harry Laughlin, another Sanger associate, spoke of purifying America's human "breeding stock" and purging America's "bad strains," which included the *"shiftless, ignorant, and worthless class of antisocial whites of the South."*

Not to be bested by her associates, Margaret Sanger supported the forced sterilization of those she designated as "unfit," a plan she said would be the *"salvation of American civilization."* That many Americans of African origin constituted people whom Sanger considered to be "unfit" cannot be easily refuted. As her organization grew, Sanger set up more clinics in the communities of other "dysgenic races" (such as Blacks and Hispanics).

Sanger turned her attention to "Negroes" in 1929 and opened another clinic in Harlem in 1930. At a 1932 Senate hearing, Margaret Sanger spoke of her goals: *"The main objectives of the [proposed] Population Congress is to … apply a stern and rigid policy of sterilization and segregation to that grade of population whose progeny is already tainted, or whose inheritance is such that objectionable traits may be transmitted to offspring."* http://www.blackgenocide.org

In 1939, Margaret Sanger wrote in a letter to Clarence Gamble, Founder of Pathfinder (one of the most militant, well-funded organizations promoting population control throughout the world) that her "Negro Project" (an effort to deliver birth control to poor African Americans) needed a black physician and black minister to "gain the trust" of the black community. Oh yes, Sanger had some interesting names for black folks, including "human weeds" and "reckless breeders." Nice lady. A real **class act**. Yes, you smell sarcasm.

Allow me to provide the full quote in context. *"We should hire three or four colored ministers, preferably with social-service backgrounds, and with engaging personalities. The most successful educational approach to the Negro is through a religious appeal. The minister's work is also important and also he should be trained, perhaps by the Federation [of eugenicists] as to our ideals and the goal that we hope to reach. We don't want the word to go out that we want to exterminate the Negro population and the minister is the man who can straighten out that idea if it ever occurs to any of their more rebellious members."*

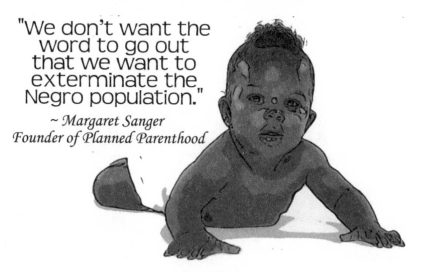

"We don't want the word to go out that we want to exterminate the Negro population."
~ *Margaret Sanger*
Founder of Planned Parenthood

In his book, <u>Killer Angel</u>, George Grant says: *"[Sanger] was thoroughly convinced that the 'inferior races' were in fact 'human weeds' and a 'menace to civilization.' ... [S]he was a true believer, not simply someone who assimilated the jargon of the times as Planned Parenthood officials would have us believe."* Not surprisingly, Sanger and many of the Planned Parenthood board members were also members of the American Eugenics Society.

According to the very latest research released by Protecting black Life (an outreach of Life Issues Institute), Planned Parenthood has 79% of its surgical abortion facilities located within walking distance of black American and/or Hispanic/Latino communities. They are the largest abortion provider in the USA, performing about 1/3 of all abortions in the country, performing more than 329,000 abortions a year (that's over 27,000 abortions a month, over 6,000 abortions a week, and over 900 abortions a day). That equates to one dead baby every 95 seconds! Those 330,000 murders (I mean "abortions") earned them an estimated $154 million dollars!

And guess what ... **you** are paying for these abortions. Yep. Planned Parenthood is financially backed by the US government, receiving 46% of its annual budget (almost $500 million per year) from taxpayer dollars.

That's right. Planned Parenthood uses almost half a billion taxpayer dollars to target black neighborhoods, perform late term abortions, and advise sex traffickers and pimps on how to secure taxpayer funded abortions for underage girls?

But Sanger didn't just hate black folks. She hated anyone who was "inferior" (whatever that means). She hated large families. She hated children. In light of the fact that she was an alcoholic and addicted to Demerol, she should have looked in the mirror before advocating the forced sterilization of the "insane and feebleminded."

Planned Parenthood's history is ugly and sordid, yet they openly embrace their past and carry forward that same agenda today.

"The most merciful thing that the large family does to one of its infant members is to kill it."

~ *Margaret Sanger*
Founder of Planned Parenthood

RESOURCES

Websites
http://www.blackgenocide.org/sanger.html
http://www.cwfa.org/articledisplay.asp?id=1466

Books
Killer Angel (George Grant)
Grand Illusions: The Legacy of Planned Parenthood (George Grant)

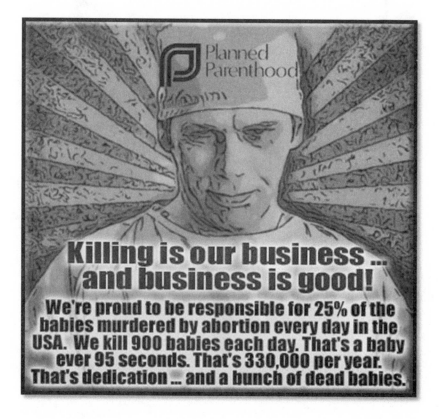

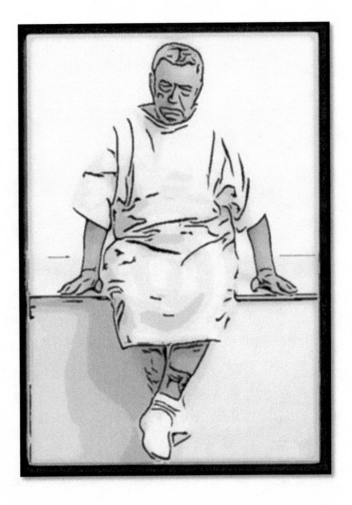

Chapter 4

~ HOSPITALS & IATROGENOCIDE ~

MONUMENTAL MYTH

Hospitals are generally clean, sanitized places where harmful pathogens would have a difficult time surviving. It is very unlikely to die from an unnecessary medical procedure, a resulting infection, or medical error. Doctors save far more lives than they harm and doctor-induced injuries and deaths are very rare.

CAN YOU HANDLE THE TRUTH?

If you want to stay healthy or get healthy, a hospital is the very last place you want to find yourself. Most hospitals are filthy places that are infested with antibiotic-resistant superbugs, serve disease-promoting foods, and lack vital sunlight. And multiple studies now show that potentially deadly mistakes with drugs or surgical procedures appear to be frighteningly common in US hospitals. No, I'm not talking about emergency rooms. If I had a severed hand, I would get to the emergency room as fast as possible and hopefully the doctor would be able to reattach the hand. Emergency room physicians do amazing jobs and oftentimes are paid only a fraction of what the "specialists" are paid, so I'm not knocking them at all. What I'm talking about is treatment for chronic, degenerative disease.

The term "iatrogenic" means "*caused by medical treatment.*" The first part of the word, "*iatro,*" comes from the Greek word "*iatros*" for medical or medicinal, while "*genic*" comes from "*genēs*" which means origin. Iatrogenic death occurs when people die due to errors or negligence by doctors. The reported yearly death rate from medical error is over 120,000. This compares to around 44,000 deaths from motor vehicles and only a few hundred from commercial aviation. You should be far more worried about dying in a hospital than from an airplane crash.

A host of new studies indicate that approximately 80% of medications, tests, and procedures are likely unnecessary. In other words, if doctors were baseball players, they would have a .200 batting average. Or if they were basketball players, they'd be shooting 20%. Have you ever heard of any professional basketball players who miss the mark that often? Other than Shaquille O'Neal when he's shooting free throws? Dr. Harvey Fineberg, M.D., president of the *Institute of Medicine* and former dean of the Harvard School of Public Health, has said that between 30% and 40% of our entire healthcare expenditure is paying for fraud and unnecessary treatment. According to Dr. Barbara Starfield of the Johns Hopkins School of Hygiene and Public Health, **250,000 deaths** per year are caused by medical errors. A study by Harvard University professor Lucian Leape found that one million patients are injured by errors during hospital treatment annually, with some **120,000 deaths**. One out of every 200 patients in hospitals in New York State had an iatrogenic death. Less than 10% of the medical mistakes are reported to hospital authorities. http://www.progress.org/fold107.htm

The Nutrition Institute of America funded an independent review of "government-approved" medicine that was published in 2006. Professors Gary Null and Dorothy Smith, along with doctors Carolyn Dean, Martin Feldman and Debora Rasio titled the report "Death by Medicine." In this report, the researchers found that America's leading cause of death isn't heart disease or cancer: **its conventional medicine.** They found that the iatrogenic death rate in the USA (death caused by doctors and/or medical treatments) is **783,936** a year! In comparison, there are only 31,940 deaths by firearms each year, 19,766 of which are suicides.

Deaths Per Year	Cause
106,000	Non-error, negative effects of drugs
88,000	Hospital infections
98,000	Medical error
115,000	Bedsores
37,136	Unnecessary procedures
108,800	Malnutrition
199,000	Outpatients
32,000	Surgery-Related
783,936	**Total deaths per year from iatrogenic causes**

So what's behind these death rates from adverse events?

Profit and politics – plain and simple.

In the words of Robert Scott Bell, modern medicine has become nothing more than the *Church of Biological Mysticism.*" I couldn't agree more. And the deadly nature of this pseudoscientific "church" is made crystal clear whenever there is a doctor's strike. In 1976 in Bogota, Columbia, there was a 52 day period in which doctors disappeared altogether except for emergency care. The death rate went down 35%. There was another doctor's strike during 1976 in Los Angeles. The death rate dropped 18%. During 1973, there was a doctor's strike in Israel. The death rate dropped 50%.

A 2008 review published in the prestigious journal, *Social Science & Medicine,* analyzed five separate incidents in which doctor strikes led to decreased mortality. Awkwardly, they also attempted to blame the lack of elective surgeries, but in the end, they were forced to admit that "*the literature suggests that reductions in mortality may result from these strikes.*" Are you getting the picture? Doctors are dangerous! It looks like the best way to reduce deaths may be to fire the doctors.

Statistics show that the average doctor is approximately **24 times** more deadly than the average gun owner, and that an average doctor has a 17% chance of killing at least one patient, every single year. Remember George Washington? Throughout his life, he only used what is now known as "alternative" medicine, until the last day of his life. He was apparently in so much pain that he finally allowed the high priests of the "*Church of Biological Mysticism*" to try a new "scientific" procedure on him called "bloodletting." It took them less than 24 hours to finish him off with their quackery.

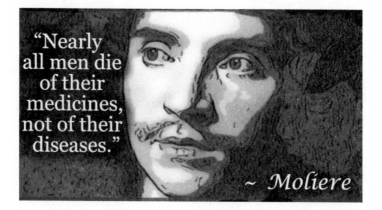

"Nearly all men die of their medicines, not of their diseases."

~ Moliere

Just because something is considered to be "common medical practice" doesn't mean that it's been proven effective. The Office of Technology Assessment (OTA) was created by Congress to analyze scientific and technical issues in America. From 1972 to 1995, the OTA conducted studies on health care and related topics, but they crossed the line when they produced an "unfavorable" report on the US healthcare system. As a result, the OTA was promptly disbanded. Why? You don't expect the government to fund an organization that is honest, do you? C'mon, especially when that honesty damages the multi-billion dollar healthcare industry. Wake up to the tyranny. *"Velcome to Amerika!"*

In 1978, the OTA issued a major research report that concluded *"only 10 to 20 percent of all procedures currently used in medical practices have been shown to be efficacious by controlled trial."* Want me to translate that for you? This means that between 80% and 90% of what doctors do to you is scientifically **unproven guesswork**. By the government's own definition, according to this OTA report, the majority of conventional medicine is "quackery."

While the popular belief is that the US healthcare system is the best in the world, it's actually more like the "wild west." Did you know that in most states, it is illegal for a doctor to recommend any vitamin, nutrient or food for the prevention or treatment of any disease? Doing so can cause a doctor to have his medical license permanently revoked. How irrational and archaic is that?

Care (not treatment) is the answer. Drugs, surgery and hospitals become increasingly dangerous for chronic disease cases. Facilitating our God-given healing capacity by improving our diet, exercise, and lifestyle is the key.

Bottom line: Unless you really need immediate critical care, try to avoid doctors and hospitals.

RESOURCES

Websites
http://www.progress.org/fold107.htm
http://www.webdc.com/pdfs/deathbymedicine.pdf

Books
Licensed to Kill: The Growing Epidemics of Iatrogenic
Disease and Bureaucratic Madness (Andrew Robbins)
Confessions of a Medical Heretic (Dr. Robert S. Mendelsohn, M.D.)

Chapter 5

~ CHEMTRAILS ~

MONUMENTAL MYTH

Those crisscrossing streaks of white clouds trailing behind jet aircraft, stretching from horizon to horizon, eventually turning the sky into a murky 'haze, are nothing more than normal contrails ("condensation trails"). They are merely water vapor.

CAN YOU HANDLE THE TRUTH?

Contrails are water vapor (H_2O) from jet engines that quickly freezes and becomes visible when there is sufficient relative humidity to slow dissipation. These ice crystals can appear to follow/trail/tail behind the plane before being absorbed into the atmosphere in 30 seconds or less. Such normal occurrences have been observed since the advent of jet and other high climbing airplanes in the 1940s. **Con**trails occur during specific atmospheric conditions or only in certain altitudes where it's cold enough (-40°F) to turn the water vapor to ice.

What are *"**chem**trails"* (chemical trails)? I'll bet that if you watch the sky for a few weeks, you will see them. Chemtrails are visible white aerosol like emissions from aircraft that are totally unrelated to the jet engine combustion process. They are often laid in a grid-like pattern by multiple planes where they disperse slowly taking on the appearance of odd, at first narrow, but widening, smoky clouds until merging together to form, if sufficiently numerous, an aerosol bank that obscures the blue sky and gives the appearance of a dirty white overcast.

Unlike normal contrails which quickly dissipate, **chem**trails (*"fake clouds"* as my children call them) sometimes take hours to dissipate and eventually fan out to a *"spider web"* type of haze that covers the entire sky. As these are formed from minute reflective metallic particulates they eventually reach the earth. It is understood that they are usually composed of aluminum, barium, lithium and strontium metals, as well as other pathogens, sometimes including biological ones.

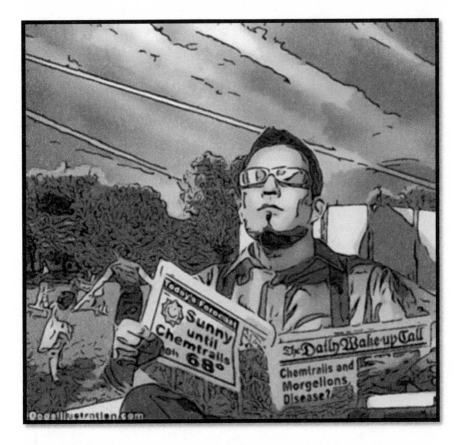

Until about 15 years ago, jets had never spewn emissions that hung over the skies for hours (unless they were low-flying small planes spraying crops). But today, our skies are checkered with white streaks that span from horizon to horizon and eventually turn a blue sky into a grey haze. Our innate intelligence tells us these are not mere vapor trails from jet engines. Even to my children, it's obvious that chemtrails are a spray of "material" or chemicals and not normal water vapor.

Scientific analysis of chemtrail particulates has indicated the presence of aluminum, barium, and strontium, amongst other heavy metals, at **thousands** of times the "safe" level. Even more alarming is the fact that most of these particles are less than 10 microns, which means that these particles bypass our lung's filters and enter the blood stream, causing radical changes in the endocrine and nervous systems, potentially causing heart attacks and strokes.

The degree of silence and cover-up of this toxic spraying is "Orwellian." Perhaps the most stunning aspect of this strange spraying in the sky is the lack of media coverage of such an obvious and intrusive phenomenon. Couple this massive chemical spraying with the campaign for "clean air" (and the absurd CO_2 emissions crack down) and you have "cognitive dissonance" at its best.

The two ideas are so contradictory the average citizen gives up trying to reconcile the two and goes into a state of rationalization. It's a known scientific method of cultural and social manipulation.

- Promise transparency ... *while hiding everything.*
- Declare war ... *and receive the peace prize.*
- Teach global warming ... *while the planet is cooling.*
- Protect our freedom ... *by giving up our liberty.*
- Save nations ... *by destroying them.*

Sadly, most people have become so "Pavlovian" that they can't even acknowledge anything that hasn't been formally introduced into the group consciousness. Having found "nirvana" here on earth, they have no need for critical thinking as long as the media tells them what they see and hear, and to accept the repetitions of its bobble-heads as their own and only thoughts. In true Hindu fashion of the three monkeys, they neither see, hear, nor speak of the evil that abounds.

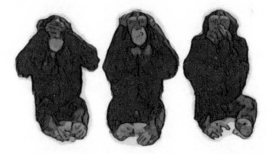

I would like anyone, believer or non-believer, to check out HR 2977 "The Space & Preservation Act of 2001." In this document the US government **openly admits** the existence of chemtrails and weather control weapons; also, to boot, mass mind control weapons and techtronic laser weapons. You also might want to read a *USA Today* article from Feb 25th, 2011 entitled "*Can Geoengineering Put the Freeze on Global Warming?*" The article admits that chemtrails and geoengineering do exist, but they're done to protect us from "global warming." Yeah right.

But the practice of geoengineering is nothing new. As early as the late 1940s, American mathematician John von Neumann was researching weather modification and its potential uses in climatic warfare for the US

Department of Defense. In the 1950s early cloud bursting experiments were performed by Wilhelm Reich and in 1956 Dr. Walter Russell was writing of the potential for complete weather control. In the 1960s, Dr. Bernard Vonnegut (brother of the famous writer) vastly improved the techniques then in use by employing silver iodide crystals in the cloud seeding mixture.

Still not convinced?

Here are a few US patents relating to chemtrails and geoengineering:

- Patent#1619183
- Patent# 2045865
- Patent# 2591988
- Patent# 3437502
- Patent# 3531310

The toxic effects of aluminum are a major culprit in many diseases (including Alzheimer's, Parkinson's disease, various dementias, Osteoporosis, and Schizophrenia). In children, behavioral problems such as ADD and ADHD have been associated with aluminum. Our nursing homes are loaded with people affected by Alzheimer's disease (the amyloid plaques associated with Alzheimer's have been found to contain aluminum at their core). As a matter of fact, over 60% of patients in nursing homes have some sort of dementia.

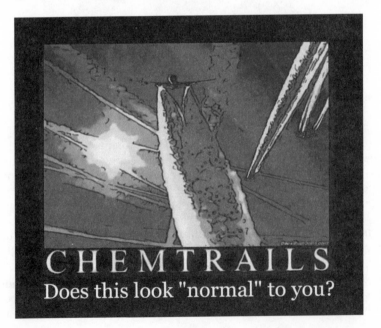

Oh, I can hear it now! *"The Government Wouldn't Do That!"*

Really? Tell that to the residents of St. Louis, who were subjected to military testing and radiological weapons testing back in the 1950s and 1960s. While the controlled mainstream media and government agencies try to whip you into a frenzy over CO_2 (plant food), a small amount of escaping Freon, hairspray, and flatulent cattle, millions of dollars are spent to fund the chemtrails project, which pollutes the planet and poisons its people.

At the 2013 Atlanta Music Liberty Fest, US Air Force veteran, Kristen Meghan, gave a groundbreaking presentation of what she discovered about chemtrails while serving in the Air Force. She learned that there was an operation at Warner Robbins AFB that "was exposing thousands of civilians to carcinogens" including strontium chromate. When she began to question her superiors, she was told to "shut up." She eventually left the military because they were silencing her.

I'll bet that the "powers that be" laugh themselves to sleep at night (in their coffins) thinking about the naiveté and willingness of the "sheeple" to accept and pay for their own destruction, being so enthralled by electronic trinkets, TV, sports, and celebrities that they have lost all aesthetic sense and cannot even be bothered to occasionally look up in the sky, being ever so happy with their enslavement.

Personally, I have found that **young** pilots are the most oblivious to chemtrails, being completely willing to believe whatever lame explanation is offered by the "disinfo" agents to explain why airplane "exhaust" lingers for hours and then covers the sky with a blanket of milky haze, when this phenomenon has never happened before in the history of airplanes. The older pilots seem to "get it" but the young "whippersnappers" oftentimes seem to be missing the ability to actually think logically and draw common-sense conclusions. Perhaps they have been so indoctrinated and brainwashed that they are incapable of rational thought processes? Maybe they are suffering from the effects of chemtrail fallout? Or perhaps they suffer from rampant arrogance and pride, thinking of themselves as one of the people who are "in the know." It reminds me of a line from an old Statler Brothers song: *"There was a time when I thought I could never be, wiser than I was, when I was twenty-three."*

Speaking of famous country music singers, in his song "What I Hate," Merle Haggard sings: *"What I hate is looking up seeing chemtrails in a clear blue sky today...[and] most folks don't seem to care at all. ... What I love is someone bright enough to see. ...Maybe we can change our neighborhood."* Although officials insist that the chemtrail programs are only in the discussion phase, evidence is abundant that they have been underway since about 1990, and the effect has been **devastating** to crops, wildlife, and human health. We are being sprayed with toxic substances without our consent and (adding insult to injury) they are **lying** to us about it.

So while we "humans" are routinely blamed for trashing the planet with consumerism and are going to be paying through the nose with individual carbon taxes, the "esteemed" scientists are advocating spraying the entire sky of the planet with toxic chemical and biological materials, ummmm, to save the planet (yeah, that's the ticket). A classic example of extreme Orwellian double-think, to say the least.

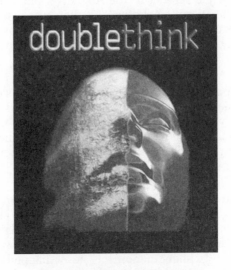

RESOURCES

Websites
http://www.freepatentsonline.com/1619183.pdf
http://www.freepatentsonline.com/2045865.pdf
http://www.freepatentsonline.com/2591988.pdf
http://www.freepatentsonline.com/3437502.pdf
http://www.freepatentsonline.com/3531310.pdf

Movies
"What in the World Are They Spraying?"
http://www.youtube.com/watch?v=jfokhstYDLA

"Why in the World Are They Spraying?"
http://www.youtube.com/watch?v=jofBcHoiuXo

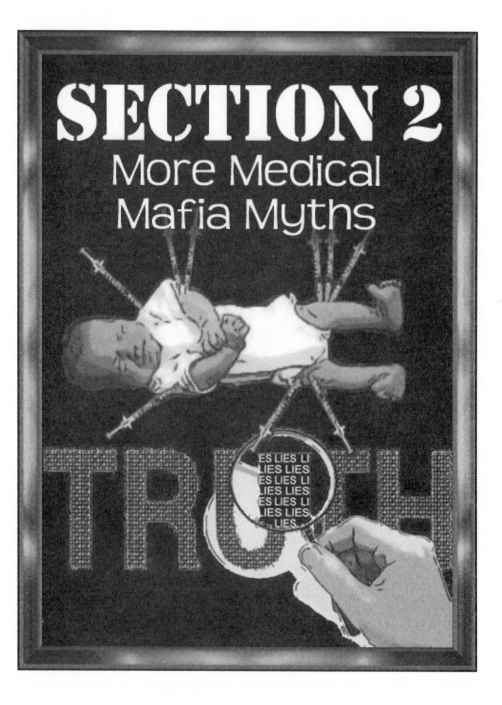

Chapter 6

~ THE GERM THEORY ~

MONUMENTAL MYTH

The germ theory of disease states that some diseases are caused by microorganisms ("germs"). These small organisms, too small to see without magnification, invade humans, animals, and other living hosts. Their growth and reproduction within their hosts can cause a disease. Microorganisms that cause disease are called pathogens, and the diseases they cause are called infectious diseases.

CAN YOU HANDLE THE TRUTH?

In 1860, French chemist Louis Pasteur fathered the "germ theory" (also called the "pathogenic theory") of disease causation, which makes the assumption that people get sick because of microscopic germs. These germs enter our body from the air or bodily fluids of another sick person and cause disease. According to the germ theory, a specific germ is responsible for each disease, thus it is the job of science to find the right drug or vaccine to kill off the offending bug without killing the patient.

The reality is germs **can** cause disease; however, they do not always. If the body has a compromised internal terrain (immune system) due to high stress, poor diet, lack of water, sleep, or exercise, or other illnesses, it is more likely to get "sick" from these germs. On the other hand if your body is strong and healthy the body will not get sick from these germs, because the body's immune system will kill them before they get a chance to cause disease. As the old saying goes, *"a half-truth is a whole lie."*

Based on the half-truth germ theory of disease, the medical industry began their relentless search for the perfect drug to combat each disease-causing germ, of which there are now over 10,000 distinct diseases recognized by the American Medical Association. And we have a new class of researcher – the "germ hunters."

With the germ theory of disease, no longer did we have to take personal responsibility for sickness caused by our own transgressions of the laws of health. Instead, we blamed germs that invaded the body. The germ theory effectively shifted our personal responsibility for health and well-being onto the shoulders of the medical profession who supposedly knew how to kill off the offending germs.

Louis Pasteur is credited with inventing the anthrax and rabies vaccines (among others), despite the fact that, when you crunch the numbers, it appears that the vaccines actually **spread** the diseases rather than **cured** them. This is nothing that couldn't be fixed with some "statistical voodoo" though. You see, Louis had the exact same modus operandi ("method of operation") as the Medical Mafia does today. As he was working on the vaccines and doing the necessary testing, he would get rid of the animals that came down with the diseases he was attempting to prevent.

As a matter of fact, Pasteur developed an exceedingly effective way of getting out of pickles, statistically speaking, when the numbers just weren't crunching correctly. According to her 1926 book, These Cults, Annie Riley Hale stated, "*Pasteur carefully screened his statistics, after some untoward deaths occurred during and immediately after treatment, by ruling that all deaths which occurred either during treatment or within 15 days of the last injection – should be excluded from the statistical returns. Because of this extraordinary ruling, the death rates in all Pasteur Institutes were kept at a low figure.*"

Did you catch that? Any animals that died within 15 days of injection were **removed** from the statistical sample! Ten cows injected with rabies vaccine. Eight die within 2 weeks. Two remain. You and I would say that the vaccine was 20% effective. **Nay nay!** According to Pasteur, the vaccine was 100% effective, since the 8 cows that died within 15 days don't count! What a crock of ... well ... you know ... bovine excrement.

Sounds like the "5 second rule" doesn't it? You know...the children's made-up rule that when food is dropped on the floor, if you pick it up within 5 seconds, there are no germs and it's OK to eat. Totally concocted and fabricated. Needless to say, because of his "15 day rule," Pasteur **always** got the results he wanted since he omitted the deaths due to vaccine injection. Does that sound scientific? Does that sound honest?

Fast forward one hundred fifty years. Nothing has changed. Scientists and doctors regularly discard test subjects (humans, animals) that contradict their intended results. Of course, they give it a fancy scientific name today – "confirmatory bias" – which is the tendency of people to search for and favor information that supports their predetermined beliefs, while excluding or discarding information to the contrary. Let's just say that if you have a "BS meter," it should be beeping loudly when you read the details of most "scientific" studies performed today, because they still employ methodologies similar to Pasteur's "15 day rule," although they'll never admit it.

Father of the "Germ Theory"

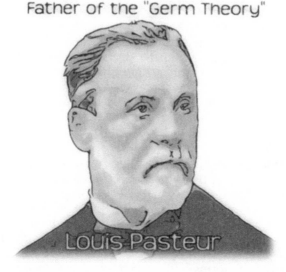

Louis Pasteur

Back to Pasteur. Had he lived today, he would likely have been thrown in jail for cruelty to animals. In his book <u>Official Stories</u>, my friend Liam Scheff describes the plethora of horrific acts committed by Pasteur during his research. *"Louis Pasteur's work centered on animals: dogs, rabbits, and sheep. He opened the skulls of dogs, cut out a piece of brain and put in a forkful of rabid dog's brain, to see what would happen. He developed a 'system' of grotesque, Frankenstein-like procedures: intracranial injections, opening animals' bodies and inserting foreign blood, tissue, saliva and pus in what can only be described as the surgical torture of animals. This wasn't an exceptional practice in his laboratory, it was his primary method."*

By the 1870s, the medical profession fully adopted his germ theory, and it was the universal acceptance of this theory and widespread fear of germs ("*bacteriophobia*") which resulted in frenzied efforts to avoid all germs. An entire new era of medicine was inaugurated, including pasteurization, the vile practice of vaccination, and the irrational fear of eating raw food. The germ theory was the beginning of bacteriophobia, which still exists today, and the medical community has swallowed it, hook line and sinker.

We **assume** the germ theory is true - right? I mean, it's been proven, right? Actually, the germ theory has more holes than a piece of Swiss cheese, and Pasteur knew it. A little research shows us that Pasteur loved hanging out with the "very important people" and he was a far better salesman than scientist. He rarely let his research keep him away from an opportunity to address royalty or medical society in the most "prestigious" university settings.

Historical records indicate, however, that Pasteur "borrowed" the research for some of his most famous discoveries (including the germ theory) and then capitalized on the celebrity of being there first. For instance, the first "Germ Theory of Infectious Disease" was published in 1762 (almost 100 years prior to Pasteur's theory) by a Viennese physician, Dr. M. A. Plenciz. We also now know that in the race for an anthrax vaccine, it was established that Pasteur actually stole the formula from a colleague named Toussaint.

One major "fly in the ointment" was Pasteur's contemporary, Antoine Beauchamp, who was at the time researching the diseases of silkworms and teaching at Lille University. His research showed that Pasteur was wrong on almost every count. Beauchamp promoted what is referred to as the "cellular terrain theory" of disease, in which he hypothesized that disease arises from microbes within the cells of the body. He believed that microbes can go through diverse stages of growth and they can mutate into various forms within their life cycle. In other words, he believed that the microbes were "pleomorphic" ("*pleo*" = many, "*morphic*" = forms).

His theory was that when the host organism (*i.e.*, person) became unbalanced and unable to maintain homeostasis, then these microbes would mutate and become pathogenic. In other words, it is the condition of the host organism that is the primary cause of disease. Beauchamp called these organisms "microzymas," meaning "small ferments." Beauchamp believed that the bacteria, microbes, viruses, and fungi that were being blamed as the cause of disease, were actually part of God's "clean-up crew," breaking down sick tissue and ultimately decomposing a no-longer-occupied body. He believed that the best way to avoid becoming overrun by harmful "germs" was to eat well, sleep well, and have access to clean water.

Claude Bernard, another French scientist, entered into the debate with the theory that it was actually the environment that is the determining factor in disease. He agreed with Beauchamp in his belief that microbes do mutate, but Bernard asserted that these mutations are all a result of the environment to which they are exposed. Therefore, Bernard's theory was that disease in the body is dependent upon the state of the internal biological terrain.

Modern science has proven that Bernard and Beauchamp were right. We now know that most of the time we have within us the bacteria and viruses that cause Staph, Strep, E. coli, the flu, etc. However, it is the simple presence of the "good bacteria" and the activity of our immune system that keeps these organisms in check. Truth be told, most bacteria and viruses tend to be "environment-specific." That's why some people get colds and others don't. That's why some survived the Bubonic Plague and others didn't. That's also why some doctors and nurses seem to be immune to disease even though they're surrounded by it every day.

What the medical industry so conveniently manages to avoid seeing, is that a germ infested body, is comparable to a fly infested trash can. Can they not see the folly of continuously reinventing the fly spray needed to kill the super fly that mutates? Would it surely not be so much easier to clean the trash can? To teach the owner of the trash can how to clean it and explain how to prevent it from getting dirty again? I guess that makes too much sense.

Why did Pasteur's never-proven "germ theory" prevail over Beauchamp's "cellular theory"? One reason was that Pasteur was a tireless promoter of himself and his theories, while Beauchamp preferred teaching and doing actual research. The other reason was **profit**. You see, Beauchamp's theory only required giving the people enough food, rest, and sanitation to keep their internal terrain in good condition. This was neither profitable nor popular among the captains of industry, then or now.

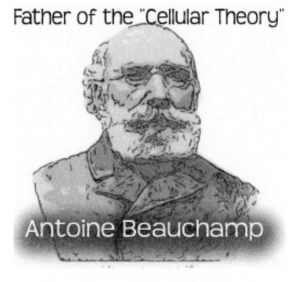

Father of the "Cellular Theory"

Antoine Beauchamp

But Pasteur's germ theory asserted that a perpetual war raged between our bodies and foreign invaders. And, as all CEOs know, if war means huge profits, perpetual war means perpetually huge profits. Pasteur's germ theory would be extremely lucrative for the kings, emperors, and the new class of "clerics" – the scientists. As a result, Beauchamp's findings were actively suppressed and Pasteur's were promoted.

In fact, Pasteur personally went to great lengths to disprove Beauchamp and Bernard's theory. Due largely to his wealth and political connections, he was able to convince the scientific community that his theory was correct, despite the fact that he had never been educated in science! Before he died, Pasteur instructed his family not to release some 10,000 pages of lab notes after his death. Not until 1975, after the death of his grandson, were these "secret" notes finally made public. Professor Gerald L. Geison, a historian from Princeton, made a thorough study of the lab notes. He presented his findings in an address to *The American Association for the Advancement of Science* in Boston in 1993. Dr. Geison's conclusions: Pasteur published much fraudulent data and was guilty of many counts of "scientific misconduct," violating rules of medicine, science, and ethics.

Interestingly, while on his deathbed, Pasteur admitted that his germ theory had flaws and that Bernard was correct. He said, *"Bernard was correct ...The terrain is everything."* I think his pride prohibited him from admitting that Beauchamp was also correct, as he had been Pasteur's nemesis for so long.

However, it was too little, too late. The mainstream scientists had already embraced his "half-truth" germ theory.

And on we go ...

RESOURCES

Websites
http://www.whale.to/a/b/pearson.html
www.dabas-berni.net/veseliba/PASTEUR_EXPOSED.doc

Books
Official Stories (Liam Scheff)
The Dream and Lie of Louis Pasteur (R. B. Pearson)

Chapter 7

~ CHOLESTEROL ~

MONUMENTAL MYTH

Cholesterol is *"public enemy number one."* When there is too much cholesterol in your blood, it builds up in the walls of your arteries, causing a process called atherosclerosis. High cholesterol is one of the major risk factors leading to heart disease, heart attack and stroke. Lowering your "bad cholesterol" will lengthen your life. All scientists and doctors support the idea that high cholesterol causes heart disease. Statin drugs are essential in controlling cholesterol levels and preventing heart disease.

CAN YOU HANDLE THE TRUTH?

Perhaps one of the biggest health myths propagated in western culture and certainly in the USA, is the misuse of an invented term "bad cholesterol" by the mainstream media and Medical Mafia. Moreover, a scientifically-naive public has been conned into a fraudulent correlation between elevated "bad" cholesterol (LDL) and cardiovascular disease.

You see, the cholesterol itself, whether being transported by low-density lipoproteins (LDL) or high-density lipoproteins (HDL), is **exactly** the same. Cholesterol is simply a necessary ingredient that is required to be regularly delivered around the body for the efficient healthy development, maintenance, and functioning of our cells. The difference is in the "transporters" (HDL and LDL). The fact is that both HDL and LDL are essential for the human body's delivery logistics to work effectively. Problems can occur, however, when the LDL particles are both tiny and their carrying capacity outweighs the transportation potential of available HDL, which can result in more cholesterol being transported around the body with diminished resources for returning excess capacity to the liver.

OK, OK, I know. I'm getting overly scientific here. Sorry.

Ask any American what causes heart disease, and 99% of the time the answer will be *"high cholesterol."* You see, the fact is that cholesterol has been vilified and is now regarded as a "terrifying" substance that must be lowered at all costs. However, if you speak with gerontologists that specialize in elderly medicine, you will quickly find that almost all of the most elderly patients have "high" cholesterol levels (according to the supposedly "normal" standards). But these patients are still alive and many of them are in very good health and are very active for their age.

Believing all of the cholesterol myths above, Americans decreased their intake of good fats and oils (like coconut oil, fish oil, olive oil) and started consuming more vegetable oils and margarine (a "transfat"). This diet has caused thousands of deaths from heart disease, as have the statin drugs which supposedly prevent heart disease, but in reality have numerous deleterious effects. Statins are considered to be "HMG-CoA reductase inhibitors", that is, they act by blocking the enzyme (HMG-CoA reductase) in your liver that is responsible for making cholesterol. There are over 900 studies proving the adverse effects of statin drugs, including anemia, cancer, chronic fatigue, acidosis, liver dysfunction, thyroid disruption, Parkinson's, Alzheimer's, and even diabetes!

Statins have been shown to increase your risk of diabetes through a few different mechanisms. The most important one is that they increase insulin resistance, which contributes to chronic inflammation (the common element of most diseases) and actually results in heart disease, which, ironically, is the primary reason for taking a cholesterol-reducing drug in the first place! Perhaps most importantly, cholesterol is not the cause of heart disease. Your body needs cholesterol.

What is cholesterol? It's a waxy, fat-like substance that's found in all the cells of our body. It has a hormone-like structure that behaves like a fat in that it is insoluble in water and in blood. Cholesterol travels through your bloodstream in small packages called "lipoproteins" which are made of lipids (fats) on the inside and proteins on the outside.

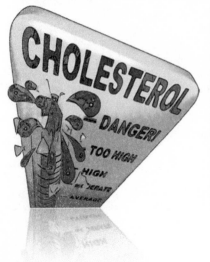

What you are almost never told is that cholesterol supports many extremely important functions in the maintenance of good health. Below is a small list of cholesterol's functions. Perhaps one of the most important functions of cholesterol is acting as an essential precursor to all of our steroid hormones, which play a crucial role in our health and without which we cannot live. Even low levels of these hormones can cause serious health problems.

The fact is that when cholesterol levels fall below 160 mg/dL, cholesterol deficiency symptoms may begin to be severe enough to be noticed. One of the first problems often noticed is adrenal insufficiency, which may cause allergic reactions (that have never occurred before) to foods or plants. Sex hormones may also become detrimentally affected, thus causing the person to become hypo-gonadal or to have severe imbalances (ratios of testosterone to estradiol) and have very low DHEA levels. All of these may lead to more serious diseases, some of which may be life threatening.

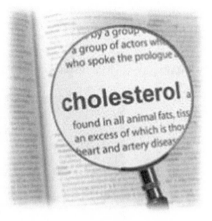

Optimal serum cholesterol levels actually help to prevent some types of cerebrovascular diseases and suboptimal cholesterol levels have been associated with an increased risk of cerebrovascular diseases. Cholesterol is also an essential component of cell membranes and, helps maintain the integrity of cell membrane fluidity (which is constantly changing do to fluctuations of dietary fat consumption). Cholesterol also plays a particularly important function as a major constituent of the myelin sheath, which acts as insulation of neurons. It should be noted that cholesterol is so important to bodily functions that the cell membranes actually manufacturer it in direct response to the body's demands.

Cholesterol plays a large role in the function of the immune system; low cholesterol levels may increase the risk of several types of cancer. Cholesterol is actually secreted by glands in the skin which help protect the skin from infections from detrimental bacteria and fungi. Cholesterol also acts as an antioxidant and possesses powerful antioxidant properties.

Cholesterol is also required to deal with stress, so you can see its importance in our Western society. Cholesterol accomplishes this task by being an essential constituent of all adrenal gland hormones. These hormones include adrenaline, cortisone, and cortisol which are released by the body in response to stress in order to counteract its effects.

It should also be noted that excessive stress causes production of high quantities of endogenous cholesterol. Remember that cholesterol is the precursor in the formation of all steroid hormones.

Perhaps most importantly, cholesterol is an essential component in the machinery that triggers the release of neurotransmitters in the brain. *"If you want Alzheimer's,"* says my good buddy, *"take lots of flu shots and take lots of cholesterol lowing medications, and you will guarantee a future that you won't remember anything."*

Well put, RSB. I agree completely.

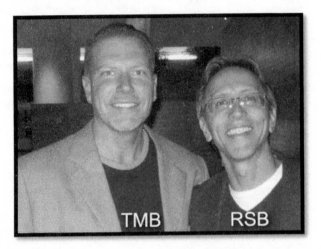

Mother's milk is especially rich in cholesterol and contains a special enzyme that helps the baby utilize it. Babies and children need cholesterol-rich foods throughout their growing years to ensure proper development of the brain and nervous system. Cholesterol is very concentrated in the brain, where it contributes to the functioning of "synapses" (tiny gaps between cells which allow nerves to communicate with each other). Cholesterol may also help to prevent depression, since low cholesterol (under 160 mg/dl) is associated with an increased risk of depression. Remember that cholesterol is the precursor of testosterone and testosterone has been shown to be one of the most effective antidepressants for both men and women.

According to recent research at Harvard, the primary causes of atherosclerosis (*hardening of the arteries which leads to heart disease*) are lesions and plaque in the arteries caused by **sugar** which causes insulin to be released. Insulin causes lesions in the endothelium of the arteries that become clogged with cholesterol. So, cholesterol gets the blame, but the real culprit is sugar. So, if you avoid sugar and simple carbs, cholesterol is not an issue.

In summary, cholesterol is vital to our survival, and trying to artificially lower it can have detrimental effects, particularly as we age. But the *"noddy science"* offered by marketing men, the Medical Mafia, and mainstream media to a generally scientifically-naïve public has led many people to believe that we should replace certain food choices with specially developed products that can help "lower cholesterol." But elevated cholesterol is **not** a risk factor for heart disease. Most of the people who suffer heart attacks have normal blood-cholesterol levels, while many with high cholesterol never have a heart attack.

In the end, Big Pharma continues to rake in enormous profits from selling expensive and dangerous cholesterol-lowering drugs to treat conditions (like atherosclerosis and heart disease) that are **not** caused by cholesterol.

So, the next time you see a cholesterol commercial on the propaganda box, please realize that you are being fed a big, fat, hairy, monumental myth aimed at convincing you to begin taking toxic prescription drugs, which will ruin your health and transform you into a lifelong customer of the "drug pushers" we call M.D.'s and their "mafia dons" in Big Pharma.

RESOURCES

Websites
http://cholesterol.mercola.com/
http://www.naturalnews.com/022960_medical_myths_cholesterol.html

Video
Robert Scott Bell – "Finally! The Truth About Cholesterol"
http://www.youtube.com/watch?v=V4xkXmakaUU

Books
Fat and Cholesterol are Good for You (Dr. Uffe Ravnskov, M.D.)
The Great Cholesterol Con (Malcolm Kendrick)
The Great Cholesterol Myth (Johnny Bowden & Stephen Sinatra, M.D.)

In Shakespeare's day, it was Hemlock.

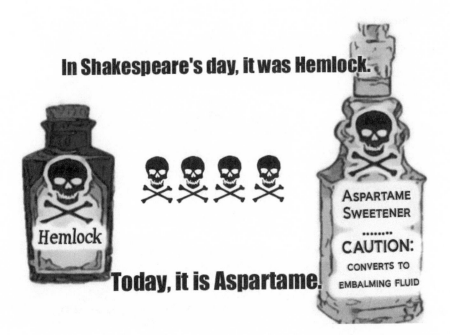

Today, it is Aspartame.

Chapter 8

~ ASPARTAME ~

MONUMENTAL MYTH

Aspartame is a harmless diet sweetener that helps you lose weight. Big Pharma giant, G.D. Searle Company (now Pfizer), patented aspartame in 1965, but was accused of fraud in one of its safety studies and sales were suspended, but no wrongdoing was discovered. After a review, the FDA finally approved aspartame for consumption in 1981 and for beverages in 1983. Folks who question the safety of aspartame are lunatics that belong in an asylum. After all ... it's "FDA approved."

CAN YOU HANDLE THE TRUTH?

Is aspartame dangerous? Does a bear have hair? Do trees have leaves? Does a phone have a tone? Does a ... OK, OK, I know. That's enough of the rhyming rhetorical questions. This artificial chemical sweetener has found its way into thousands of products including soft drinks, desserts, yogurt, chewing gum, gelatins, puddings, tabletop sweeteners, and even some brands of children's vitamins and sugar-free cough drops. Currently aspartame is consumed by over 200 million people around the world.

If you scoot on over to some of the "conventional" websites on aspartame, you'll find that it's typically peddled to be as harmless as a fluffy, white sheep having a sweet dream about a tiny leprechaun riding a lucky unicorn and finding a pot of gold at the end of an enchanted rainbow. You'll read that all the "aspartame alarmists" are nothing short of lunatics. You'll find testimonials by all sorts of "experts" and important people endorsing aspartame. But if you take a look at the history books, you'll soon realize that the "fluffy dreamy" tales about aspartame are actually a massive illusion of falsehood manufactured by the Medical Mafia's quack scientists and snake oil salesmen who were apparently having a wild "acid trip" when they began to sell the monumental myth that aspartame is safe for human consumption. Truth be told, aspartame (frequently marketed as NutraSweet®, Equal®, and AminoSweet®) is the most controversial food additive **ever** approved.

To understand why I say this, let's hop in the Delorean (or Pinto or riding lawnmower, for you "Duck Dynasty" fans) and travel back in time to 1965, where aspartame was accidentally discovered by James Schlatter, a chemist at G.D. Searle Company (Searle), who licked particles of a new ulcer drug from his fingers and discovered the sweet taste of aspartame. **Eureka**! But selling this chemical as a food additive to hundreds of millions of healthy people every day would mean many more dollars than limited sales to the much smaller group of ulcer sufferers. So, in 1967, Searle began the safety tests on aspartame which were necessary for applying for FDA approval of food additives. Early tests of the substance showed it produced microscopic holes and tumors in the brains of experimental mice, epileptic seizures in monkeys, and was converted by animals into dangerous substances, including formaldehyde.

In 1969, Searle hired Dr. Harold Waisman, a biochemist at the University of Wisconsin, to conduct aspartame safety tests on seven infant monkeys, who were fed aspartame mixed with milk. After 300 days, five of the monkeys had grand mal seizures and one died. (Remember the sprinter, Flo Jo, who drank Diet Coke and died of a grand mal seizure?) Dr. Waisman died before all of his studies were completed. In the spring of 1971, Dr. John Olney (a neuroscientist) informed Searle that his studies showed that aspartame caused holes in the brains of infant mice. Later that year, one of Searle's own researchers confirmed Dr. Olney's findings in a similar study. But Searle didn't care...they were after their cash cow!

In 1973, Searle applied for FDA approval and submitted over 100 studies they claimed supported the safety of aspartame. One of the first FDA scientists to review the aspartame safety data stated that *"the information provided (by Searle) is inadequate to permit an evaluation of the potential toxicity of aspartame."* According to the late Dr. Adrian Gross, Searle *"...took great pains to camouflage these shortcomings of the study. As I say filter and just present to the FDA what they wished the FDA to know, and they did other terrible things. For instance, animals would develop tumors while they were under study. Well, they would remove these tumors from the animals."* Nevertheless, on July 26, 1974, the FDA approved aspartame for limited use in dry foods, making available to the public for the first time the data supporting their decision. This data was subsequently reviewed by renowned brain researcher John Olney from Washington University in St. Louis, who filed the first objection against aspartame's approval.

Two years later in 1976, triggered by Olney's objection, the FDA began an investigation of Searle's laboratory practices. The investigation found their testing procedures shoddy, full of inaccuracies and *"manipulated"* test data. The investigators reported that they *"had never seen anything as bad as Searle's testing."* Then in 1977, a governmental task force uncovered that Searle had falsified data by submitting inaccurate blood tests. In another study, a closer look revealed that uterine tumors had developed in many of the test animals, and Searle admitted that these tumors were related to the ingestion of aspartame. The FDA formally requested that the US Attorney's office begin grand jury proceedings to investigate whether indictments should be filed against Searle for knowingly misrepresenting findings and *"concealing material facts and making false statements"* in aspartame safety tests.

While the grand jury probe was underway, Sidley & Austin, the law firm representing Searle, began job negotiations with the US Attorney in charge of the investigation, Samuel Skinner. In July 1977, Skinner resigned and took a job with Searle's law firm. The resignation of Skinner stalled the grand jury investigation for so long that the statute of limitations lapsed. Eventually, the grand jury investigation was dropped.

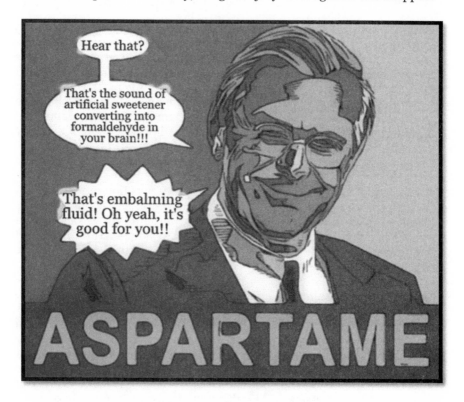

In 1979, the FDA established a Public Board of Inquiry (PBOI) to rule on safety issues surrounding aspartame. A year later, the PBOI concluded that aspartame should not be approved pending further investigations of brain tumors in animals, and based on its limited review, the PBOI blocked aspartame marketing until the tumor studies could be explained. Unless the FDA commissioner overruled the board, the matter was closed. But in 1980, Ronald Reagan was elected President of the United

States, and his transition team included Donald Rumsfeld, CEO of G. D. Searle.

According to a former G.D. Searle salesperson, Patty Wood-Allott, Rumsfeld told his sales force that, if necessary, *"he would call in all his markers and that no matter what, he would see to it that aspartame would be approved that year."* (Gordon 1987, page 499 of US Senate, 1987) Not surprisingly, the transition team picked Dr. Arthur Hull Hayes Jr. to be the new FDA Commissioner. Hayes was widely profiled as a man who believed that approval for new drugs and additives was too slow because *"the FDA demanded too much information."* He was definitely the right man for the job of getting aspartame approved for human consumption.

Within a couple of months, Hayes appointed a five-person "Scientific Commission" to review the claims on aspartame. In a 3–2 decision, the panel upheld the original ban, stating that the artificial sweetener was unsafe. But despite the panel's decision, Hayes later installed a sixth member on the commission who voted in favor of the making aspartame legal. The vote was now deadlocked. So what happened? Drum roll please .... Hayes personally broke the tie in aspartame's favor, overruling the conclusions of the PBOI and officially approving aspartame for all dry products. In 1982, Searle filed a petition that aspartame be approved as a sweetener in carbonated beverages and other liquids.

Almost immediately, the National Soft Drink Association urged the FDA to delay approval of aspartame for carbonated beverages pending further testing because aspartame is very unstable in liquid form. Despite the public outcry, in 1983, the FDA approved aspartame for soft drinks and the first carbonated beverages containing aspartame were sold for public consumption.

Shortly after aspartame was approved for beverages, complaints began to arrive at the FDA. Reactions such as dizziness, blurred vision, memory loss, slurred speech, headaches, and seizures were common with consumption of drinks containing aspartame. The complaints were more serious than the agency had ever received on any food additive. In just the first several years after aspartame was approved for beverages, the FDA received over 10,000 complaints about aspartame. In February of 1994, the US Department of Health and Human Services released the listing of adverse reactions reported to the FDA. Amazingly, aspartame accounted for more than 75% of all adverse reactions reported to the FDA's Adverse Reaction Monitoring System. By the FDA's own admission, fewer than 1% of consumers who have adverse reactions to products ever report it to the FDA. This balloons the 10,000 complaints to around a million!

In 1985, Dr. Adrian Gross told Congress that because aspartame was capable of producing brain tumors and brain cancer, the FDA should not have been able to set an "allowable" daily intake of the substance at any level. His last words to Congress were, *"And if the FDA violates its own law, who is left to protect the public?"* (August 1, 1985, *Congressional Record*, SID835:131) From 1985 to 1995, researchers did about 400 aspartame studies. Dr. Ralph G. Walton reviewed all the studies on aspartame and found 166 with relevance for human safety. Of those 166 studies, 74 were funded by Searle, 85 were independent, and 7 were funded by the FDA. The results will amaze you, but probably won't surprise you. Of the 74 studies funded by Searle, all of them gave aspartame a clean bill of health. However, of the 85 studies that were not funded by Big Pharma or the FDA, 84 of them found aspartame to be dangerous to one's health.

In the most comprehensive, longest-ever running study on aspartame as a human carcinogen (over two million person-years), researchers analyzed data from the Nurses' Health Study and the Health Professionals Follow-Up Study for a 22-year period. This landmark study was published in late 2012. Over 77,000 women and over 47,000 men were included in the analysis, for a total of almost 2.3 million person-years of data. Apart from sheer size, what makes this study superior to other past studies is the thoroughness with which aspartame intake was assessed. Every two years, participants were given a detailed dietary questionnaire, and their diets were reassessed every four years. Previous studies which found no link to cancer only assessed participants' aspartame intake at one point in time, as opposed to every two years (for two decades) in this study.

The findings were alarming, so say the least. **One diet soda** a day increases leukemia risk by 42% (in men and women), multiple myeloma risk by 102% (men only), and non-Hodgkin lymphoma risk by 31% (men only).

A 2012 University of Miami study, which was published in the *Journal of General Internal Medicine*, admitted that drinking **one diet soda** a day increases the risk of heart attack and strokes by a whopping 44%. This was no small study. The research involved over 2,500 participants over a period of ten years. Of course, this has been known for decades and is discussed in Dr. H. J. Roberts, M.D.'s medical textbook, Aspartame Disease: An Ignored Epidemic. Are you still craving that diet soda now? How about a stick in the eye? Or better yet, how about eating a bag of feces? Why do I mention poop? Because the patent for aspartame is available online and it confirms that the sweetener is made from the waste (i.e. "poop") produced by genetically modified E. coli bacteria! Yuck!

As if being "fecal matter" weren't enough to turn your stomach, aspartame is also considered to be an "excitotoxin." Since humans lack a blood-brain barrier in the hypothalamus, excitotoxins are able to enter the brain and cause damage by reacting with specialized receptors (neurons) in such a way as to lead to the destruction of certain types of brain cells. In other words, they excite your brain cells to death! Aspartame accounts for over 75% of the adverse reactions to food additives reported to the FDA. Many of these reactions are very serious, including seizures and death.

Using MEDLINE, Dr. Ralph G. Walton, MD, performed an analysis which indicated that 92% of non-industry sponsored studies reported one or more problems with aspartame in terms of its effects on health. These studies reported a range of side effects including fibromyalgia, brain tumors, memory loss, lymphoma, leukemia, and peripheral nerve cancer.

The truth of the matter is that the FDA has always known aspartame is a carcinogen. The late Dr. Adrian Gross (FDA toxicologist) told Congress that without a shadow of a doubt aspartame triggers brain tumors and brain cancers and violates the Delaney Amendment which forbids putting anything in food you know will cause cancer. As Dr. James Bowen told the FDA, the manufacturers of aspartame have damaged a generation of children and should be criminally prosecuted for genocide for the mass poisoning of the USA and hundreds of other countries of the world.

So what's in aspartame? Aspartame is made of three components, 50% phenylalanine, 40% aspartic acid, and 10% methanol (*wood alcohol*).

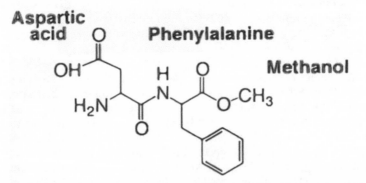

Phenylalanine is an amino acid typically found in the brain. Persons with the hereditary disorder phenylketonuria (PKU) are unable to metabolize phenylalanine. This results in dangerously high levels of phenylalanine in the brain, which is sometimes fatal. It has been shown that ingesting aspartame (especially along with carbohydrates) can lead to excess levels of phenylalanine in the brain even in persons who do not have PKU. In his testimony before the US Congress, Dr. Louis J. Elsas showed that high blood phenylalanine can be concentrated in parts of the brain and is especially dangerous for infants and fetuses. He also indicated that since it is metabolized much more efficiently by rodents than humans, testing and research on rats alone is not sufficient enough to denounce the dangers of aspartame for human consumption. Phenylalanine also depletes serotonin; thus, it triggers all kinds of psychiatric and behavioral problems, including depression. I have heard it said that many mental institutions are full of patients who are nothing but aspartame victims. Remember the character Marty McFly in "Back to the Future"? Were it not for the phenylalanine in aspartame, which interferes with the brain's uptake of L-Dopa, Michael J. Fox, a former Diet Pepsi spokesman, would likely never have been diagnosed with Parkinson's disease at age 30. It's very possible that he would be healthy today and still making movies (*"Back to the Future Part 17"*) were it not for his consumption of Diet Pepsi.

Aspartic acid is also a component of aspartame. My friend, Dr. Russell L. Blaylock, MD, a professor of neurosurgery at the Medical University of Mississippi, recently published a book thoroughly detailing the damage that is caused by the ingestion of excessive aspartic acid from aspartame. Dr. Blaylock makes use of almost 500 scientific references to show how excess free excitatory amino acids such as aspartic acid and glutamic acid (about 99% of MSG is glutamic acid) in our food supply are causing serious chronic neurological disorders and a myriad of other acute symptoms. Much like nitrates and MSG, aspartic acid can cause amino acid imbalances in the body and result in the interruption of normal neurotransmitter metabolism of the brain.

Methanol (wood alcohol) is a toxic poison. Some people may remember methanol as the poison that has caused some "skid row" alcoholics to end up blind or dead. Methanol is gradually released in the small intestine when the methyl group of aspartame encounters the enzyme chymotrypsin. Methanol breaks down into formic acid and formaldehyde ("embalming fluid") in the body. According to the EPA, methanol *"is considered a cumulative poison due to the low rate of excretion once it is absorbed. In the body, methanol is oxidized to formaldehyde and formic acid; both of these metabolites are toxic."*

The EPA's recommended limit of consumption of methanol is 7.8 milligrams per day, but a one liter bottle of a beverage containing aspartame contains over 50 mg of methanol. How many folks do you know that drink a liter of soda pop each day? Heck, I know folks who drink 2 or 3 liters per day! According to a 1990 report by Kathleen Nauss and Robert Kavet entitled, *"The Toxicity of Inhaled Methanol Vapors"* (published in *Critical Reviews in Toxicology*), chronic, low-level exposure to methanol has been seen to cause headaches, dizziness, nausea, memory lapses, blurred vision, ear buzzing, gastrointestinal issues, weakness, vertigo, chills, numbness, behavioral disturbances, insomnia, neuritis, tunnel vision, depression, heart problems, and pancreatic inflammation.

But don't many fruits and vegetables contain some methanol? Yes, they do, but they also contain a large amount of ethanol, which acts as a buffer and neutralizes methanol, thus preventing the conversion of methanol to formaldehyde. In aspartame, there is no such buffer.

Diketopiperazine (DKP) is a byproduct of aspartame metabolism and has been implicated in the occurrence of brain tumors. G.D. Searle conducted animal experiments on the safety of DKP. The FDA found numerous experimental errors occurred, including *"clerical errors, mixed-up animals, animals not getting drugs they were supposed to get, pathological specimens lost because of improper handling,"* and many other errors. These sloppy laboratory procedures may explain why both the test and control animals had 16 times more brain tumors than would be expected in experiments of this length.

Despite all the evidence and research which indicates that the ingredients of aspartame are toxic poisons, I know that there are still folks who will say: *"But I need aspartame to help me lose weight."* **Honk! Wrong!** Think again! Research actually indicates that aspartame increases your hunger and can actually impede your weight loss. Phenylalanine and aspartic acid can cause spikes in insulin levels and force your body to remove the glucose from your blood stream and store it as fat. Aspartame also inhibits the production of serotonin and prevents your brain from signaling to your body that you are full. This can lead to food cravings and make it more difficult for you to lose weight.

Truth be told, aspartame triggers every kind of birth defect from autism to cleft palate, and it is also an "abortifacient," which is defined as a drug that induces abortion. It's normal for young girls to look forward to marriage and children. However, many young girls sip on diet soda not realizing that aspartame is an endocrine disrupting agent which changes the menstrual flow and causes infertility. So, when the FDA tells us that aspartame has been proven to be safe, rest assured that it is basing its findings on the fraudulent Searle studies (*i.e.,* they are "lying through their teeth"). Then, when the *JAMA*, examining the FDA findings (which are based on the fraudulent Searle studies), announces that *"the consumption of aspartame poses no health risk for most people,"* don't believe it! **Aspartame kills.**

Believe it or not, aspartame was once on a Pentagon list of biowarfare chemicals submitted to Congress! Yummy! I don't know about you, but that fact alone is enough to make me avoid this "contaminated chemical concoction" like the Plague! As a matter of fact, the toxic effects of aspartame are documented by the FDA's own data. In 1995, the FDA was forced (under the Freedom of Information Act) to release a list of 92 aspartame symptoms reported by tens of thousands of victims. It appears this is only the tip of the iceberg.

Oh yes, I almost forgot the "icing on the corruption cake." In 1985, G.D. Searle was absorbed by Monsanto. Donald Rumsfeld reportedly received a $12 million bonus.

And the wretched tale of "fake food" and "malicious experimentation" on the human race continues onward …

RESOURCES

Websites
http://www.naturalnews.com/aspartame.html
http://aspartame.mercola.com/
http://www.ncbi.nlm.nih.gov/pubmed/23097267
http://www.ncbi.nlm.nih.gov/pubmed/16507461
http://www.ncbi.nlm.nih.gov/pubmed/17805418

Videos
"The Truth About Aspartame" – Dr. Russell Blaylock, M.D.
http://www.youtube.com/watch?v=lqIFDoOwSFM

"Sweet Misery: A Poisoned World"
http://www.youtube.com/watch?v=ZI7_8FDzuJE

Books
Excitotoxins: The Taste That Kills (Dr. Russell Blaylock, M.D.)
Sweet Poison (Dr. Janet Starr Hull)
Aspartame Disease: An Ignored Epidemic (Dr. H. J. Roberts, M.D.)

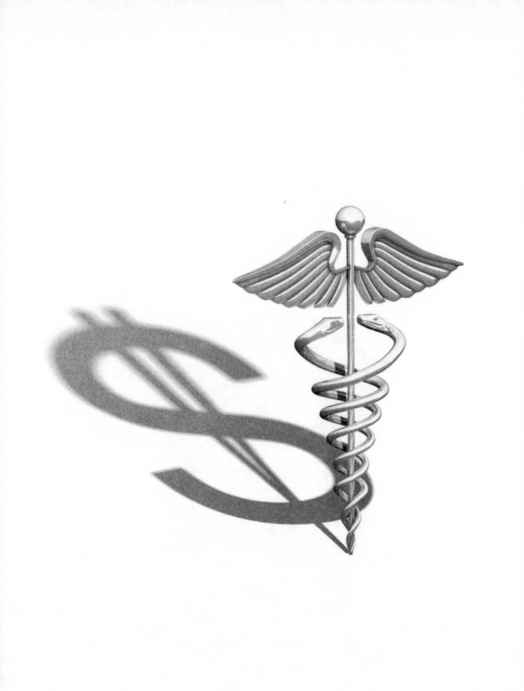

Chapter 9

~ MERCURY IN YOUR MOUTH ~

MONUMENTAL MYTH

Evidence shows that dental amalgam fillings create no major health problems. Newly developed techniques have demonstrated that minute levels of mercury **are** released from amalgam fillings, but no health consequences from exposure to such low levels of mercury have ever been demonstrated. Mercury toxicity is nothing to be concerned about. As a matter of fact, mercury is good for you and helps cognitive function.

CAN YOU HANDLE THE TRUTH?

Dental amalgam is a medieval, pre-Civil War product that is 50% mercury and is still frequently used in dental fillings. Half of all North American dentists still use amalgam for its quick and easy profits, then pass the bill for damages (health and environmental) on to the rest of us. Mercury is nothing short of a "Pandora's Box" of toxic poison peddled by industry lobbyists, the Medical Mafia, and supported by dubious pseudoscientific studies.

As a result, regrettably, dentists are still taught in dental school that the mercury in amalgams is "bound" with the other metals and doesn't leak, which is why half of them still believe it's safe. Yet, you can actually measure the mercury vapor coming off the tip of the root of an amalgam-filled tooth. The fact that mercury vapor can be measured at the tip of a tooth's root is absolute proof that these amalgam fillings **do** leak.

Every time you chew, mercury (in the form of nonreactive mercury vapor) is released from the amalgam-filled teeth and travels from your mouth to your lungs, then to your brain via your bloodstream. A common enzyme in your body called "catalase" converts (oxidizes) mercury vapor into a **very toxic** form of mercury and traps it inside your cells, where it becomes a "biochemical train wreck" in your body, causing your cell membranes to leak, and inhibiting key enzymes your body needs for energy production and removal of toxins.

So how much mercury is in your mouth? There is approximately ½ gram of mercury in each dental filling. You may think that since you only have a couple of mercury fillings it's not a big deal. **Think again**. To put this in perspective, the amount of mercury contained in one average size filling exceeds the EPA standard for human exposure for over one hundred years. Put in other terms, it takes only ½ gram of mercury (the amount in one filling) to contaminate all fish in a ten acre lake.

According to Dr. Joseph Mercola, *"A single dental amalgam filling ... is estimated to release as much as 15 micrograms of mercury per day primarily through mechanical wear and evaporation. The average individual has eight amalgam fillings and could absorb up to 120 micrograms of mercury per day from their amalgams. These levels are consistent with reports of 60 micrograms of mercury per day collected in human feces."* www.mercola.com/article/mercury/mercury_elimination.htm

You wouldn't take a leaky thermometer, put it in your mouth, and leave it there 24 hours a day, would you? But, according to Dr. Michael Ziff, executive director of the International Academy of Oral Medicine and Toxicology (*IAOMT*), that is *"exactly what happens when an amalgam filling is installed in your mouth."* Evidence now demonstrates that amalgam fillings are constantly being broken down and then are released into the mouth. These minute particles of mercury fillings are then acted upon by oral and intestinal bacteria to produce methyl mercury (an even more toxic form of mercury than elemental mercury) with target areas being primarily the pituitary gland, thyroid gland, and the brain. That's right, the brain!

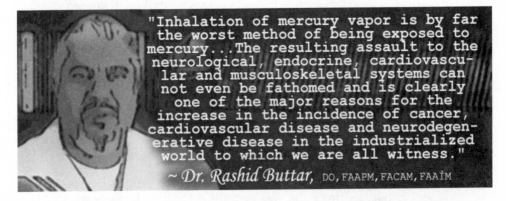

"Inhalation of mercury vapor is by far the worst method of being exposed to mercury...The resulting assault to the neurological, endocrine, cardiovascular and musculoskeletal systems can not even be fathomed and is clearly one of the major reasons for the increase in the incidence of cancer, cardiovascular disease and neurodegenerative disease in the industrialized world to which we are all witness."

~ *Dr. Rashid Buttar,* DO, FAAPM, FACAM, FAAIM

The late Dr. Patrick Störtebecker, world renowned neurologist and writer from Stockholm, Sweden, wrote in his book Mercury Poisoning from Dental Amalgam– a Hazard to Human Brain, *"Dental amalgam is a highly unstable metal that easily gives off mercury vapor. The most dangerous route for transport of mercury vapor, being released from dental amalgams, is from the mucous membranes of the upper nasal cavity and directly upwards to the brain where mercury vapor easily penetrates the dura mater (i.e., blood-brain barrier). Mercury (vapor) can act in a much stronger concentration straight on the brain cells."*

Recent studies of the effects of various toxic heavy metals on your brain (including aluminum, lead, arsenic, cadmium and mercury) reveal that mercury is by far the **most** toxic. No others even come close! This is because of mercury's interaction with sulfur-containing proteins that are critical to your brain function.

But this isn't surprising, in light of the fact that the mercury used by dentists to manufacture dental amalgam is shipped as a **hazardous material** to the dental office. When amalgams are removed, for whatever reason, they are considered to be a hazardous waste (according to the EPA) and are required to be disposed of in accordance with OSHA regulations. I guess your mouth is considered to be a safe "storage container" for this hazardous material. Yeah right!

Just to be crystal clear. If a dentist were to dump some mercury amalgam in a lake, he'd be breaking the law. He can't put it in the trash or bury it in the ground either. Nor can he put it in a landfill. But if this same dentist dumps some mercury in your mouth (via dental amalgam fillings), then it's completely legal and even becomes "good for your health." Apparently, Gandalf the Grey performs some serious magic and the poison becomes a nutrient. Voila!

Seriously folks! Are we living in the FDA/ADA's version of the "twilight zone" here?

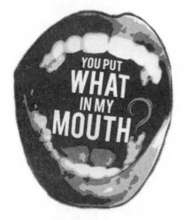

Don't get me wrong. The FDA isn't 100% corrupt. There are still some good things that happen there. For instance, in December of 2010, the FDA's advisory panel on dental amalgam warned against the use of amalgam in "vulnerable" populations (like pregnant women and children) and insisted that FDA had a duty to disclose amalgam's risks to parents and consumers. Panelist Dr. Suresh Kotagal (a pediatric neurologist at the Mayo Clinic) was dead on accurate when he stated that there is *"no place for mercury in children."*

But don't expect your dentist to jump on board with you if you ask to have your fillings removed. According to the ADA's code of ethics, a dentist who acknowledges that mercury amalgam fillings are toxic and recommends their removal has acted unethically. According to ADA Resolution 42H-1986, *"The removal of amalgam restorations from the non-allergic patient for the alleged purpose of removing toxic substances from the body when such treatment is performed solely at the recommendation of the dentist is **improper and unethical**...."*

What? It's **unethical** to remove toxic poison from your mouth? Yet more proof that the ADA is still in the Dark Ages...

If your dentist refuses to abandon his or her use of amalgam, you may want to consider consulting another dentist. There are a growing number of mercury-free dentists, and dentists who offer a more holistic or "biological" approach. And please do **not** have your amalgam fillings removed by a dentist who is not properly trained on this procedure. Quite honestly, there is nothing that has the potential to release more mercury vapor directly into your body than removing an amalgam filling without the requisite rubber dam, as well as vacuums in and around the mouth to capture mercury while the extraction is taking place. Once the mercury fillings have been removed, it's important to include chlorella and cilantro in your diet, since both of these have incredible abilities to bind to heavy metals and whisk them out of your body.

Is there a connection between autism and Alzheimer's? In the words of my good friend, Dr. Rashid Buttar, *"Children diagnosed with autism or autism spectrum disorders suffer from acute **mercury toxicity** secondary to huge exposure while in utero (maternal amalgam load, dietary factors, maternal inoculations, Rhogam injections, etc.) and early on in life (vaccinations preserved with thimerosal, etc.). Adults diagnosed with Alzheimer's suffer from chronic, insidious **mercury toxicity** secondary to exposure over a long time (amalgam load, inhalation of mercury vapors, combustion of fossil fuels, dietary factors, etc.). By addressing and eliminating the mercury 'spark,' the secondary 'fires' become far easier to manage clinically and the improvements realized from treatment of the resulting imbalances become easier to maintain."*

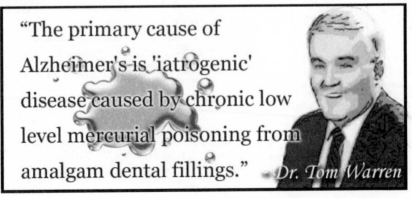

"The primary cause of Alzheimer's is 'iatrogenic' disease caused by chronic low level mercurial poisoning from amalgam dental fillings." — Dr. Tom Warren

Have you ever read <u>Alice in Wonderland</u>? Do you remember the "Mad Hatter?" Did you know that the term "mad as a hatter" originated from a disease peculiar to the hat making industry in the 1800s? A complicated set of processes was needed to turn the fur into a finished hat. With the cheaper sorts of fur, an early step was to brush a solution of a mercury compound on the fur to roughen the fibers. This caused the hatters to breathe in the fumes of this highly toxic metal, leading to an accumulation of mercury in the hatter's bodies. This resulted in symptoms such as trembling (known as "hatters' shakes"), anxiety, slurred speech, loss of coordination, personality changes, depression, and memory loss. This eventually became known as "Mad Hatter Syndrome" and is still used today to describe mercury poisoning.

Did you know that dentists have the highest rate of suicide of any profession? They also suffer a high incidence of depression and memory disorders. Two of the effects of mercury poisoning are loss of memory and depression. Do you think the high rate of suicide (due to depression) and memory disorders in dentists has anything to do with low-level mercury exposure over several years? This is mercury toxicity, plain and simple.

Here's a bit of trivia. The original "quacks" were actually dentists who advocated the use of mercury amalgam? "*Quacksalver*" is the old German word for "mercury."

RESOURCES

Websites
http://www.medicalrewind.com/autism-and-mercury-toxicity/
http://www.toxicteeth.org/
http://iaomt.org/
http://www.drbuttar.com

Video
"Smoking Teeth = Poison Gas" – IAOMT
http://www.youtube.com/watch?v=9ylnQ-T7oiA

Books
The 9 Steps to Keep the Doctor Away (Dr. Rashid Buttar)
Mercury Poisoning from Dental Amalgam – a Hazard to Human Brain (Dr. Patrick Störtebecker)

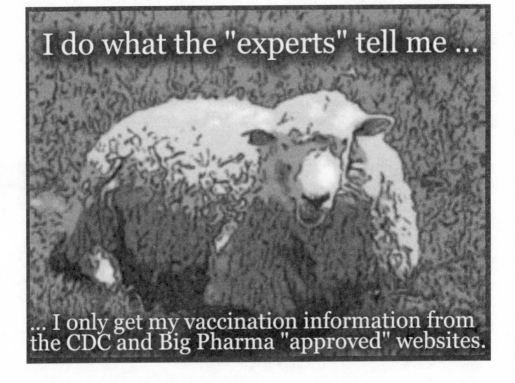

Chapter 10

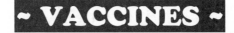

MONUMENTAL MYTH

Vaccines are safe, effective, and based on sound scientific studies and evidence. Vaccines work by injecting foreign antigens which cause the immune system to produce antibodies to fight the antigen. Vaccines save lives. Vaccines prevent disease. Vaccines are among medicine's greatest discoveries.

CAN YOU HANDLE THE TRUTH?

Are you ready to have your world rocked? Are you ready to dive head over heels down the rabbit hole? I hope so, because we're about to embark on an expedition that will inspire, astonish, and likely infuriate you. We'll take a ride down memory lane while exposing the modern Medical Mafia's "magnum opus" (when it comes to medical "quackery") **– vaccines.**

Vaccines are the sacred cow of modern medicine, or as my friend, Robert Scott Bell, often declares, *"The Church of Biological Mysticism."* The first vaccines (smallpox) were derived from pus and blood scraped from sores on cows and horses, then put on a lancet, scalpel, or needle, then jabbed into someone's arm. *"Blood and pus, anyone? How about some feces?"* Do you think that it's a good idea to inject our bodies with blood and pus from infected animals? That's not only disgusting, it borders on insane. But that's where the modern practice of vaccination came from. And it's only gotten more repulsive and more insane since the smallpox vaccine.

The fact is that vaccines have emerged as one of the most sinister monumental myths ever fabricated by the modern Medical Mafia. The absurd ideas that vaccines protect you from infectious diseases and increase immunity are blatantly false. Health "authorities" credit vaccines for disease declines and assure us of their safety and effectiveness, yet these assurances are directly contradicted by government statistics, published medical studies, FDA and CDC reports, and the opinions of credible research scientists from around the world.

Now, for the nasty stuff. Vaccines must be "grown" in a "substrate," which simply means that it takes living tissue to grow the microscopic vaccine ingredients. So where do they get the living tissue? Lots of places. Animal brains, kidneys, blood, pus, testicles, and the likes. Yummy. Oh yes, and here's a real favorite with my Christian brothers and sisters – tissue from aborted babies. That's right! The government is allowing Big Pharma companies to sell vaccines which contain aborted fetal tissue. Have you ever wondered why abortion is so widely accepted and often encouraged? The abortion industry gets paid by Big Pharma and the government in exchange for deceased human beings in a syringe! **Question:** in light of this fact, how can you be a Christian who is both "pro-life" and "pro-vaccine"? Hmmmmm...

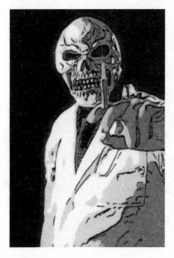

But that's not all. Vaccines also have lots of additives, preservatives, and adjuvants, which are supposed to increase the body's immune response to the vaccine. Substances like mercury, formaldehyde, MSG, squalene, and antifreeze. Medical research has well established that the direct injection of foreign proteins and other toxic materials (listed above) makes the recipient **more**, not less, easily affected by what he/she encounters in the future. This means they do the opposite of immunize, commonly even preventing immunity from developing after natural exposure. I have heard vaccinations described as "toxic cocktails" of the most noxious substances on earth.

In his book, <u>Official Stories</u>, my friend, Liam Scheff, asserts, *"Vaccines are not conjured at Hogwarts by honest wizards. Willy Wonka doesn't brew them in his chocolate factory. They are not magical and there is a reason, or many, why some people oppose them too strongly. Vaccines are toxic, by their very nature."*

What if I were to take some formaldehyde, antifreeze, aluminum, and mercury, along with a few live viruses cultured in dead animal brains and aborted fetal tissue, then mix them together with some mayonnaise and spread the resulting liquid on a piece of bread for my children to eat for a snack? Would you think I was a good parent? If I said, *"this will keep them from getting sick,"* would you question my sanity? The odds are that I would (and should) be arrested for child abuse. However, when doctors inject our children with the **exact same** toxic ingredients (minus the mayonnaise) and tell us *"this will keep them from getting sick,"* most of us don't even question them. You see, if you or I inject our child with mercury or formaldehyde, we are going to jail. But if a drug company and a doctor inject the same toxic poisons, then they are "perfectly safe." What's wrong with this picture? Unfortunately, most Americans follow the masses, believe what we're told, don't ask questions, and place blind faith in our doctors. Most Americans are "sheeple."

But where do doctors get their medical training? That's right...in medical school. Medical schools, which are largely subsidized by Big Pharma, brainwash students into believing that vaccinations are safe and prevent the spread of infectious diseases. Not surprisingly, there is a huge financial incentive for Big Pharma to "peddle" vaccinations, as they make a fortune on the sale of these toxic cocktails. Once these medical students graduate and become physicians, they are offered large commissions to sell more vaccinations to patients and continue their blind faith in the necessity of these poisons.

Then, most people acquiesce to the poisoning of their children because they simply cannot believe (or refuse to believe) that their "omniscient" physician could possibly be wrong. What we have is blind faith in doctors, who have blind faith in what they learned in medical school, which are governed by the AMA, which is "in bed" with Big Pharma, which is interested in shareholder profits, not in the safety of our children. Many parents vaccinate their children because they simply don't know all the facts, and they don't know about the financial connections. That's one of the reasons I wrote this book – to educate people with the truth.

Vaccines & Infant Death

An alarming medical study (recently published in a medical journal) has found a direct statistical link between higher vaccine doses and infant mortality rates. **Translation:** Vaccines Kill Infants! The study was conducted by Neil Z. Miller and Gary S. Goldman and was published in the reputable *Journal of Human and Experimental Toxicology*, which is indexed by the National Library of Medicine.

Who are the authors? According to his biography, *"Goldman has served as a reviewer for the Journal of the American Medical Association (JAMA), Vaccine, AJMC, ERV, ERD, JEADV,and British Medical Journal (BMJ). He is included on the Editorial Board of Research and Reviews in BioSciences."* Miller, a medical research journalist and the Director of the Thinktwice Global Vaccine Institute, has been studying the dangers of vaccines for 25 years.

The table on the top of the next page shows the countries with the lowest infant deaths at the top of the left side, while the countries with the lowest number of vaccines administered are at the top of the right side.

Table 1. 2009 Infant mortality rates, top 34 nations[a]

Rank	Country	IMR
1	Singapore	2.31
2	Sweden	2.75
3	Japan	2.79
4	Iceland	3.23
5	France	3.33
6	Finland	3.47
7	Norway	3.58
8	Malta	3.75
9	Andorra	3.76
10	Czech Republic	3.79
11	Germany	3.99
12	Switzerland	4.18
13	Spain	4.21
14	Israel	4.22
15	Liechtenstein	4.25
16	Slovenia	4.25
17	South Korea	4.26
18	Denmark	4.34
19	Austria	4.42
20	Belgium	4.44
21	Luxembourg	4.56
22	Netherlands	4.73
23	Australia	4.75
24	Portugal	4.78
25	United Kingdom	4.85
26	New Zealand	4.92
27	Monaco	5.00
28	Canada	5.04
29	Ireland	5.05
30	Greece	5.16
31	Italy	5.51
32	San Marino	5.53
33	Cuba	5.82
34	United States	6.22

Table 2. Summary of International Immunization Schedules: vaccines recommended/required prior 34 nations

Nation	Vaccines prior to one year of age	Total[a] doses
Sweden	DTaP (2), Polio (2), Hib (2), Pneumo (2)	12
Japan	DTaP (3), Polio (2), BCG	
Iceland	DTaP (2), Polio (2), Hib (2), MenC (2)	12
Norway	DTaP (2), Polio (2), Hib (2), Pneumo (2)	12
Denmark	DTaP (2), Polio (2), Hib (2), Pneumo (2)	12
Finland	DTaP (2), Polio (2), Hib (2), Rota (3)	13
Malta	DTaP (3), Polio (3), Hib (3)	15
Slovenia	DTaP (3), Polio (3), Hib (3)	15
South Korea	DTaP (3), Polio (3), HepB (3)	15
Singapore	DTaP (3), Polio (3), HepB (3), BCG, Flu	17
New Zealand	DTaP (3), Polio (3), Hib (2), HepB (3)	17
Germany	DTaP (3), Polio (3), Hib (3), Pneumo (3)	18
Switzerland	DTaP (3), Polio (3), Hib (3), Pneumo (3)	18
Israel	DTaP (3), Polio (3), Hib (3), HepB (3)	18
Liechtenstein[a]	DTaP (3), Polio (3), Hib (3), Pneumo (3)	18
Italy	DTaP (3), Polio (3), Hib (3), HepB (3)	18
San Marino[a]	DTaP (3), Polio (3), Hib (3), HepB (3)	18
France	DTaP (3), Polio (3), Hib (3), Pneumo (2), HepB (2)	19
Czech Republic	DTaP (3), Polio (3), Hib (3), HepB (3)	19
Belgium	DTaP (3), Polio (3), Hib (3), HepB (3), Pneumo (2)	19
United Kingdom	DTaP (3), Polio (3), Hib (3), Pneumo (2), MenC (2)	19
Spain	DTaP (3), Polio (3), Hib (3), HepB (3), MenC (2)	20
Portugal	DTaP (3), Polio (3), Hib (3), HepB (3), MenC (2), BCG	21
Luxembourg	DTaP (3), Polio (3), Hib (3), HepB (2), Pneumo (3), Rota (3)	22
Cuba	DTaP (3), Polio (3), Hib (3), HepB (4), MenBC (2), BCG	22
Andorra[a]	DTaP (3), Polio (3), Hib (3), HepB (3), Pneumo (3), MenC (2)	23
Austria	DTaP (3), Polio (3), Hib (3), HepB (3), Pneumo (3), Rota (2)	23
Ireland	DTaP (3), Polio (3), Hib (3), HepB (3), Pneumo (2), MenC (2), BCG	23
Greece	DTaP (3), Polio (3), Hib (3), HepB (3), Pneumo (3), MenC (2)	23
Monaco[a]	DTaP (3), Polio (3), Hib (3), HepB (3), Pneumo (3), HepA, BCG	23
Netherlands	DTaP (4), Polio (4), Hib (4), Pneumo (4)	24
Canada	DTaP (3), Polio (3), Hib (3), HepB (3), Pneumo (3), MenC (2), Flu	24
Australia	DTaP (3), Polio (3), Hib (3), HepB (4), Pneumo (3), Rota (2)	24
United States	DTaP (3), Polio (3), Hib (3), HepB (3), Pneumo (3), Rota (3), Flu (2)	26

Notice a pattern? The study showed that the USA, which administers **more** childhood vaccines than any other country in the developed world (26), also has the **highest** number of infant deaths per 1000 births in the developed world (6.22). It also showed that Japan and Sweden, which require the **fewest** vaccinations, have the **lowest** mortality rates. I have been preaching this message for years. In light of the voluminous amount of research which proves that vaccines are deadly, those who advocate vaccines are either ignorant or evil. There is no other choice.

"Didn't the smallpox vaccine eradicate the disease?"

Oh, if I had a nickel for each time I heard someone ask these questions! England's Edward Jenner, born in 1749, is credited with being the "Father of Vaccines." He believed the superstition among the dairymaids that a person who had suffered cowpox could not contract smallpox.

In 1786, for his initial "human guinea pig" test, Jenner scraped pus from the lesions from a dairymaid and injected this pus into James Phipps, an eight year old boy. A short time afterwards, he injected the boy with small-pox, and the small-pox did not take. Jenner believed that he had found the cure to smallpox. Over the next twelve years, Phipps was vaccinated over a dozen times and eventually died of tuberculosis at the age of twenty. Jenner's own son also served as one of his guinea pigs and also died of tuberculosis at the age of twenty-one. By the way, the smallpox vaccine has been linked to tuberculosis.

Over the next few years, Jenner gathered the "proof" that his smallpox vaccine worked, and then he presented it to Parliament. Much like Pasteur, he was sure to report only the data which supported his theory, and to never mention the multitudes of people who would disprove his theory (*i.e.*, those people who contracted cowpox and then contracted smallpox afterwards). He was careful to mention only the cases of a dozen old men who had cowpox and did not contract smallpox afterwards, while conveniently omitting the hundreds of cases who had had both. Eventually, after years of manipulating data and "tweaking" his smallpox vaccination formula, he "sold" his theory of vaccinations to the intellectual elite and governmental officials alike.

Despite Jenner's efforts, widespread vaccination did not really catch on. As of 1807, only 1.5% of the Brits had been vaccinated. Up until 1823, the year that Jenner died, there were only regional outbreaks of smallpox in England, nothing that would be considered an epidemic. For the next thirty years, smallpox was under control. However, vaccinations became mandatory in England in 1853, and by 1857, fines and imprisonment awaited people who refused to be vaccinated against smallpox.

Once smallpox vaccination became mandatory in England, massive epidemics began to occur. Between 1857 and 1859, there were over 14,000 deaths from smallpox. Then, between 1863 and 1865, there were over 20,000 smallpox deaths. A few years later, there were almost 45,000 smallpox deaths between 1870 and 1872. According to official estimates, as recorded by Anne Riley Hale in her book, <u>The Medical VooDoo</u>, over 97% of the population had been vaccinated. Official British government documents from the early 1900s indicate that as more people were vaccinated against smallpox, more people died.

Japan introduced compulsory vaccinations in 1872. In 1892 there were over 165,000 cases of smallpox with almost 30,000 deaths despite the vaccination program. However, in the 1800s, when Australia banned the smallpox vaccine, miraculously the disease vanished.

What's the bottom line?

At *best*, the smallpox vaccine does **not** work.

At *worst*, it actually **causes** the disease.

"But what about pertussis? Didn't vaccines wipe it out?"

Think again, my friend. If you look at the graph below, it will be crystal clear that the decline in deaths from pertussis ("whooping cough") occurred **before** the introduction of the related vaccine. According to the *British Association for the Advancement of Science*, childhood diseases decreased 90% between 1850 and 1940, paralleling improved sanitation and hygienic practices, well before mandatory vaccination programs. Deaths from infectious disease in the USA, Canada, and England declined steadily by an average of about 80% during the same period.

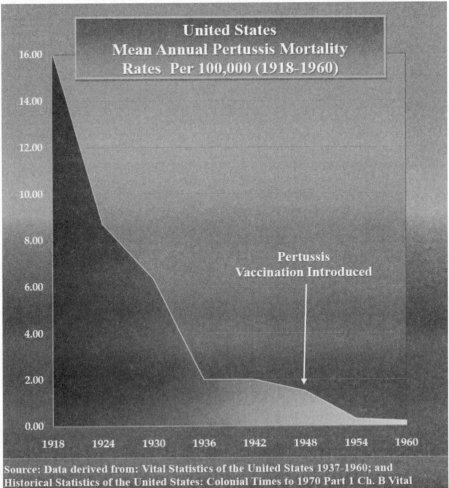

United States
Mean Annual Pertussis Mortality
Rates Per 100,000 (1918-1960)

Pertussis
Vaccination Introduced

Source: Data derived from: Vital Statistics of the United States 1937-1960; and Historical Statistics of the United States: Colonial Times to 1970 Part 1 Ch. B Vital Statistics and Health and Medical Care, pp. 44-86H.

The pertussis vaccine has also been implicated in sudden in[f]
syndrome ("SIDS"). So, I took a close look at the Sanofi Past[eur]
vaccine (Diphtheria, Tetanus, Pertussis). See the image below.

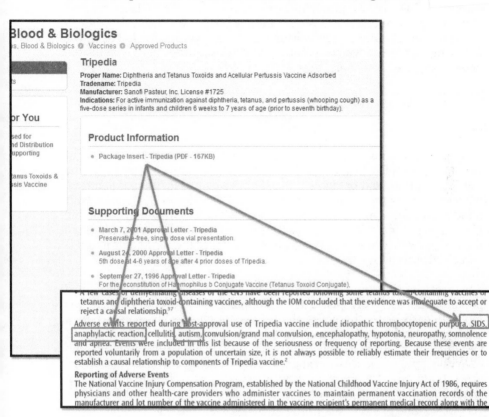

I was astonished to discover that **anaphylactic reaction, autism,** and **SIDS** are listed as "*adverse events reported during post-approval use ... Events were included in this list because of the seriousness or frequency of reporting.*" Wow!

The CDC, the FDA, Paul Offit, and every Medical Mafia "flunky" swear up and down the aisle that vaccines are perfectly safe and don't cause autism or SIDS. Yet those conditions are **actually** listed on the DTaP package insert with the statement that they are included because such vaccine adverse reactions are serious and frequent. Despite these facts, the mainstream media bobble-heads are making a full court press with news stories everywhere to convince the public that vaccines are totally safe and it is our moral obligation to accept them.

They are so far down the road of denial and dishonesty that they are incapable or unwilling to acknowledge the fact prominently displayed on the DTaP package insert: **Autism** and **SIDS** are associated with this vaccine. This is a powerful indictment of the CDC, vaccine manufacturers, and Medical Mafia "talking heads" like Offit. As you can see from the DTaP package warning insert above, it also includes the following serious adverse events: convulsion/grand mal convulsion, neuropathy, and encephalopathy.

"Outbreaks always occur in non-vaccinated people, right?"

You see, we're constantly inundated with false information (lies) about vaccines. One tidbit of information that is conveniently swept under the rug is how often (and badly) vaccines fail. Ask yourself, *"Why don't these vaccine failures regularly make the news?"* If you can imagine in your mind's eye, for a moment, the cash register "ka-chinging" while Big Pharma is pulling out a wad of cash, I think you may be getting close to the real answer. There's big money in making sure the vaccine program is perceived as a success by you.

The fact is that most outbreaks of disease occur in vaccinated populations. Here are just a few examples. There are literally dozens more. In early 2010, there was an outbreak of mumps among more than 1,000 people in New York and New Jersey. What's interesting is that in Ocean County, New Jersey, county spokeswoman Leslie Terjesen told *CNN* that 77% of those who caught mumps had already been vaccinated against mumps. If mumps vaccines actually worked, then what you should see instead is mumps spreading among those who refused the vaccines, right? That is logical, isn't it? But, in this case, reality tells a different story.

An objective analysis must conclude that it is the vaccinated people who caused this outbreak of mumps. In 1967, the WHO declared Ghana to be "measles free" after 96% of its population was vaccinated. However, in 1972, Ghana experienced one of its worst measles outbreaks with its highest ever mortality rate. The November 21, 1990, issue of the *Journal of the American Medical Association* stated, *"Although more than 95% of school-aged children in the US are vaccinated against measles, large measles outbreaks continue to occur in schools, and most cases in this setting occur among previously vaccinated children."*

An article published in the March 1987 issue of the *New England Journal of Medicine* (*NEJM*) indicated that an outbreak of measles occurred in a 99% vaccinated school population in Corpus Christi, Texas. Check out the graph on the top of the next page.

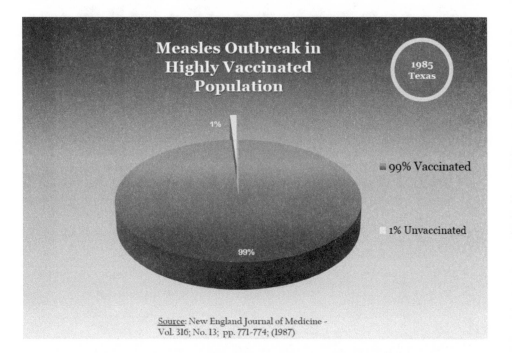

Here are a few more examples represented by the following graphs.

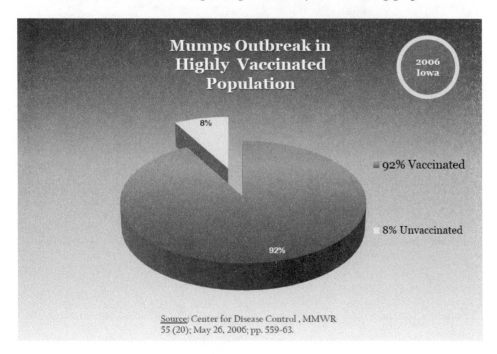

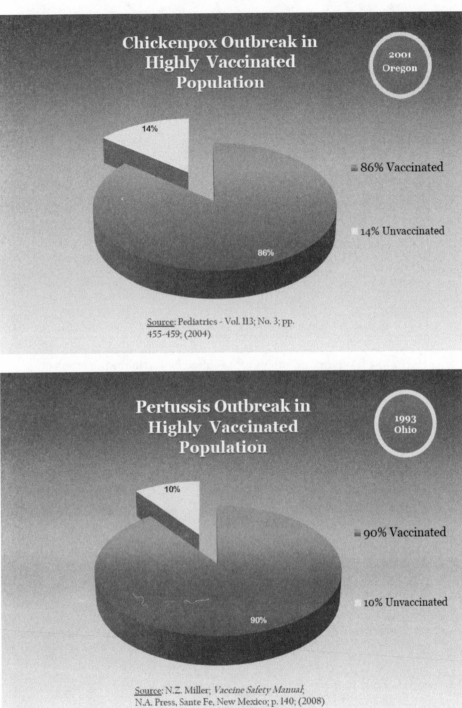

Chickenpox Outbreak in Highly Vaccinated Population

2001 Oregon

14%

86%

◼ 86% Vaccinated

◼ 14% Unvaccinated

Source: Pediatrics - Vol. 113; No. 3; pp. 455-459; (2004)

Pertussis Outbreak in Highly Vaccinated Population

1993 Ohio

10%

90%

◼ 90% Vaccinated

◼ 10% Unvaccinated

Source: N.Z. Miller; *Vaccine Safety Manual*; N.A. Press, Sante Fe, New Mexico; p. 140; (2008) (Refers to CDC & Official Surveillance data)

"At least we know that the flu shot is safe and effective!"

Well, not exactly. But before we debunk the myths surrounding the flu shot, first let's learn how they make the flu shot. In January or February of each year, health "authorities" travel to Asia to determine which strains of the flu are currently active. Based on their findings in Asia, they assume that the same strains of viruses will spread to the USA by fall. In other words, they guess at the strain of flu that will hit the USA. If the viral strains circulating in the USA are not identical to those in Asia (which they never are since the flu virus mutates), then the vaccine you receive will be a complete dud (at best).

According to the CDC, the majority of flu vaccines contain thimerosal. Some contain as much as 25 micrograms of mercury per dose. This means that it may contain more than **250 times** the Environmental Protection Agency's safety limit for mercury. That's one good reason to avoid the flu shot, isn't it?

For those of you, who are still unconvinced, know that there's plenty of scientific evidence available to back up the recommendation to avoid flu vaccines. A study published in the October 2008 issue of the *Archives of Pediatric & Adolescent Medicine* found that vaccinating young children against the flu had **no impact** on flu-related hospitalizations or doctor visits during two recent flu seasons. The researchers concluded that *"significant influenza vaccine effectiveness could not be demonstrated for any season, age, or setting."* Research published in the September 2008 issue of the *American Journal of Respiratory and Critical Care Medicine* also confirms that there has been **no decrease** in deaths from influenza and pneumonia in the elderly, despite the fact that vaccination coverage among the elderly has increased from 15% in 1980 to 65% now.

In 2007, researchers with the National Institute of Allergy and Infectious Diseases, and the National Institutes of Health published this conclusion in the *Lancet Infectious Diseases*: *"We conclude that frailty selection bias and use of non-specific endpoints such as all-cause mortality, have led cohort studies to greatly exaggerate vaccine benefits."* Did you get that? Please allow me to translate. *"We conclude that the tests are rigged and that the flu vaccine is worthless."*

Still not convinced? Check this out. A large-scale, systematic review of 51 studies involving over 260,000 children, published in the Cochrane Database of Systematic Reviews in 2006, found **no evidence** that the flu vaccine is any more effective than a placebo in children between the ages of 6 months and two years. **Zero percent effective!** In a review of 64 studies covering over 40 years, the Cochrane Database also reported that, for elderly living in nursing homes, flu shots provided "**little or no effectiveness**" at preventing the flu.

But it's good for pregnant women, right? The CDC even states on their own website (www.cdc.gov): "*If you're pregnant, a flu shot is your best protection against serious illnesses caused by the flu ... A flu shot can protect pregnant women, their unborn babies, and even the baby after birth.*" **Au contraire!** Documentation from the National Coalition of Organized Women (NCOW) demonstrated that between 2009 and 2010 the mercury-laden flu vaccines increased Vaccine Adverse Events Reporting Systems (VAERS) fetal death reports by **4,250%** in pregnant women. The director of NCOW, Eileen Dannemann, indicated that despite these figures being known to the CDC, they still recommend the flu vaccine containing mercury (Thimerosal) to pregnant women as a "safe" vaccine.

Want more? OK. There was the 2012 study published in *The Lancet*, which (according to the vaccine-pushing CDC bureaucrats) established that the flu vaccine is 60% effective. But, is it really? My friend, Mike Adams (aka the "Health Ranger") had the audacity to actually read the *Lancet* study and crunch the actual numbers. How dare he! What did he determine about the study? The "60% effectiveness" claim is a total lie.

In his own words, "*What we found is that the '60% effectiveness' claim is utterly absurd and highly misleading. For starters, most people think that '60% effectiveness' means that for every 100 people injected with the flu shot, 60 of them won't get the flu! Thus, the '60% effectiveness' claim implies that getting a flu shot has about a 6 in 10 chance of preventing you from getting the flu. This is utterly false. In reality ... only about 2.7 in 100 adults get the flu in the first place! ... The 'control group' of adults consisted of 13,095 non-vaccinated adults who were monitored to see if they caught influenza. Over 97% of them did not. Only 357 of them caught influenza, which means only 2.7% of these adults caught the flu in the first place.*"

Mike continues, "*The 'treatment group' consisted of adults who were vaccinated with a trivalent inactivated influenza vaccine. Out of this group, according to the study, only 1.2% did not catch the flu. The difference between these two groups is 1.5 people out of 100. So even if you believe this study, and even if you believe all the pro-vaccine hype behind it, the truly 'scientific' conclusion from this is rather astonishing: Flu vaccines only prevent the flu in 1.5 out of every 100 adults injected with the vaccine!*" www.NaturalNews.com

Honestly folks, this is **truly** amazing. Flu shots are **1.5%** effective? Are you kidding me? That means that they have approximately the same efficacy as waving a magic wand, wearing a lucky hat, wishing on a four-leaf clover, or rubbing a rabbit's foot.

Hey, let's not forget to pick up that lucky penny ... and maybe toss some salt over our shoulder.

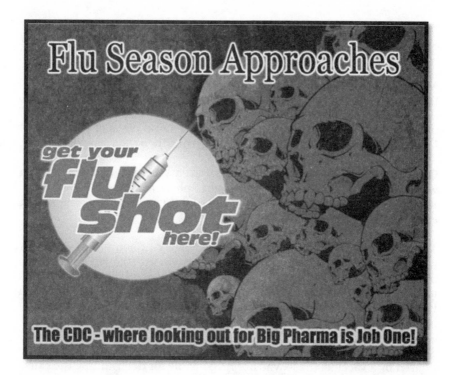

What many people do not know is that death caused directly by the flu virus is very rare, despite the fact that the CDC has been telling the public for a decade that there are more than 200,000 estimated hospitalizations and 36,000 estimated deaths from influenza in the USA each and every year.

Here's how it happened. In 2003, CDC employees used a convoluted statistical modeling scheme to "guesstimate" that 36,000 people die from influenza in the USA every year. The problem was that they counted not just deaths from influenza, but also threw in other respiratory, circulatory, cardiac, and pulmonary deaths they thought **might** have been associated with influenza.

Barbara Fisher, Co-Founder and President of the National Vaccine Information Center (NVIC), analyzed the vital statistics data and concluded flu deaths peaked in 1941 at 21,047 and have been dropping ever since. Over the past decade, deaths from influenza ranged from a low of 494 (in 2010) to a high of 1,722 (in 2008).

Meanwhile, on their own website, doctors at the CDC now sheepishly admit that the *"CDC does not know exactly how many people die from seasonal flu each year."* Having gotten that cradle to the grave flu shot recommendation firmly in place, they are backing away from the 36,000 influenza annual death figure. CDC now says that *"only 8.5% of all pneumonia and influenza deaths and only 2.1% of all respiratory and circulatory deaths"* are influenza related.

Now compare those statistics to the following facts. As of the end of 2012, there were more than 84,000 reports of reactions, hospitalizations, injuries and deaths following influenza vaccinations made to the VAERS, including over 1,000 related deaths and over 1,600 cases of GBS. **Wow**! Looks like the vaccine is much more dangerous than the virus, doesn't it?

Case in point: On December 2, 2011, seven year-old Kaylynne Matten was taken by her parents for her annual physical. During the physical Kaylynne was given a flu shot. Four days later she was dead. She wasn't even sick when she went to the doctor!

The state health commissioner, Dr. Harry Chen (no, I'm not kidding...this is his real name), was "not convinced" the girl's death was from the flu vaccine, citing the "very rare" incidence of serious reactions to the flu shot and the huge numbers of people who receive them each year. Apparently Dr. Chen is not familiar with the VAERS statistics cited in the previous paragraphs.

That's the problem! Every time a healthy child dies or is seriously injured by a vaccine, those who are responsible for determining the cause of death immediately rule out vaccines because they are "so safe" and serious reactions are "so rare," being completely ignorant of the thousands of injuries and deaths caused by the vaccine. And can we say "conflict of interest"? Dr. Chen's job is dependent on the sale of vaccines. That's what he does. He ensures that all of the people in his state are fully vaccinated. Without vaccines, Dr. Chen would be unemployed, and so would a whole heap of doctors!

In the 2011 report, Dr. Chen was worried that people would "over-react" to Kaylynne's death, and he cautioned about "alarmist" reactions. Excuse me? We are not supposed to be **alarmed**? Clearly, Dr. Chen has become condescending and self-righteous when it comes to young children dropping dead for "no apparent reason."

Dr. Chen is worried that if people become "alarmed" their concerns may lead them to avoid getting a flu shot. If they start looking into the dangers of flu shots, it's a very slippery slope. You know how it goes. Flu shot research is like "the gateway drug" that causes "investigative" parents to become "fanatics." We research the flu vaccine and the true dangers of the flu, and before you know it we start to realize we've been lied to about influenza. From there it's all downhill for Dr. Chen and his cronies. As we become "hooked" on research we learn more and more about vaccines and the more we learn the more we realize that vaccines are dangerous and the risks of infectious diseases are small in comparison.

Heavens! That would be a real tragedy for Dr. Chen, who is another example of the fox guarding the henhouse. How in the world can this vaccine-related death even be questioned? It's like saying *"Jane Doe was crossing the interstate when she was hit by a taxi. Ms. Doe was taken to the hospital where she lapsed into a coma and died 4 days later. Her husband, John Doe, believes that it was the impact from the taxi that killed his wife. However, the coroner (who just happens to be married to the taxi driver) is not quite sure about the cause of death. Autopsy results are pending..."*

According to Hugh Fudenberg, MD, the world's leading immune-geneticist and 13th most quoted biologist of our time (with nearly 850 papers in peer reviewed journals): If an individual has had 5 consecutive flu shots between 1970 and 1980 (the years studied) his/her chances of getting Alzheimer's Disease is **10 times higher** than if he/she had one, two or no shots. As I mentioned earlier, flu shots contain 25 micrograms of mercury. One microgram is considered toxic.

"What about the HPV vaccine?"

A March 2013 publication in the *Annals of Medicine* exposed the "monumental mythical" nature of Human papillomavirus (HPV) vaccines such as Gardasil (from Merck) and Cervarix (from GlaxoSmithKline). The researchers reported that there is a lack of evidence that HPV vaccines prevent cervical cancer and there has been no evaluation of health risks associated with the vaccines. The researchers concluded that due to the presentation of "partial and non-factual information" regarding cervical cancer risks and the usefulness (or lack thereof) of HPV vaccines, the current research on HPV is **neither** scientific **nor** ethical.

But this isn't the first study to indicate that, at best, the HPV vaccine is virtually worthless. Research published in the August 2007 *JAMA* sought to determine the usefulness of the HPV vaccine among women who already carry HPV (which includes virtually all women who are sexually active, regardless of their age). This document revealed startling information about the ineffectiveness of the Gardasil vaccine. It revealed that the HPV vaccine often caused an increase in the presence of HPV strains while utterly failing to clear the viruses in most women. The fact of the matter is that Merck's Gardasil vaccine was studied for less than 3 years in about 12,000 healthy girls and 14,000 healthy boys under age 16 before it was licensed in 2006. Gardasil was **not** studied in children with health problems or in combination with all other vaccines routinely given to American adolescents. Clinical trials did **not** use a true placebo to study safety but compared Gardasil against the reactive aluminum adjuvant in Gardasil.

One major problem is that there are over 100 strains of HPV, yet only 30 of them are even theoretically linked with cervical cancer. In addition, HPV is present in at least half the normal population, yet it almost never causes any disease or problems whatsoever. Truth be told, HPV has never been proven as a pathogen for any disease. As a matter of fact, studies show that over 90% of women have some form of HPV and in almost all those cases, **it goes away by itself**. Heck, even the CDC's own website states, *"In most cases HPV goes away by itself before it causes any health problems."*

Another major problem is the side effects of the HPV vaccines. According to the National Vaccine Information Center (www.NVIC.org), *"after Gardasil was licensed and three doses recommended for 11-12 year old girls and teenagers, there were thousands of reports of sudden collapse with unconsciousness within 24 hours, seizures, muscle pain and weakness, disabling fatigue, Guillain Barre Syndrome, facial paralysis, brain inflammation, rheumatoid arthritis, lupus, blood clots, optic neuritis, multiple sclerosis, strokes, heart and other serious health problems, including death, following receipt of Gardasil vaccine."*

And they want to inject this unproven, uninsurable brew into our children first to *"wait and see if there aren't too many adverse events"*? I say, *"Over our collective cold, dead bodies!"* Let's put on our "math hats." As of the middle of 2013, there have been almost 30,000 reports made to the federal Vaccine Adverse Events Reporting System (VAERS) associated with Gardasil or Cervarix vaccines, including 118 deaths. It is estimated that 90% of adverse events are not reported, so if we extrapolate the total numbers, it's likely that there have been close to 300,000 adverse reactions and over 1,000 deaths!

It turns out that studies actually show that not only does HPV **not** cause cervical cancer, the HPV vaccine itself **does**. Are you ready for this? Gardasil appears to *increase* cancer by 44.6% in folks who were already carriers of the same HPV strains used in the vaccine. The FDA actually had this information on its own website, but they removed it. Surprise surprise. But fortunately, Mike Adams (the "Health Ranger") anticipated this and saved a copy here: http://www.naturalnews.com/downloads/FDA-Gardasil.pdf.

In other words, it appears that if the vaccine is given to a young woman who already carries HPV in a "harmless" state, it may "activate" the infection and directly cause precancerous lesions to appear. The vaccine, in other words, may accelerate the development of cancer!

In an ABC News interview in September of 2009, Dr. Diane Harper (the leading international developer of the HPV vaccines) admitted that *"the rate of serious adverse events is greater than the incidence rate of cervical cancer. The incidence of cervical cancer in the US is so low that* *if we get the vaccine and continue PAP screening, **we will not lower the rate of cervical cancer** in the US ... if you vaccinate a child, she won't keep immunity in puberty and **you do nothing to prevent cervical cancer**.*" http://abcnews.go.com/m/story?id=8356717

What exactly is "Herd Immunity"?

The "herd immunity" theory was originally coined in the 1930s by a researcher named A.W. Hedrich. He had been studying measles patterns in the USA since 1900 (before any vaccine was ever invented for measles) and he observed that epidemics of the illness only occurred when less than 68% of children had developed a **natural immunity** to it. Hedrich's "herd immunity" theory was, in fact, about natural disease processes and had nothing to do with vaccinations.

Over the next half century, some of those who worship at the altar of "modern medical mysticism" (vaccinologists) adopted the phrase and magically increased the figure from 68% to 95% (with no scientific justification as to why) and then stated that there had to be 95% **vaccine coverage** to achieve immunity. Essentially, they took Hedrich's study and manipulated it to promote their own vaccination programs.

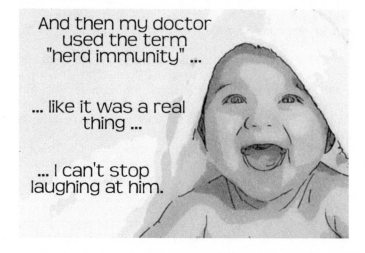

And then my doctor used the term "herd immunity" ...

... like it was a real thing ...

... I can't stop laughing at him.

Now, over 80 years since Hedrich developed his theory, the mainstream media and Medical Mafia are attempting to keep vaccination rates high by **mis**using his concept of "herd immunity" and pitting parent against parent. What better way to keep Mr. and Mrs. Jones vaccinating "Junior" than through good old fashioned peer pressure and the fear that their next door neighbor won't let Johnny come over and play because Junior isn't vaccinated. A very powerful influence of behavior is it not?

The "guilt trip" method is a common vaccine marketing technique. If a parent is concerned, say about the ingredients in the shot for their child, they are told that they "have to" vaccinate for the greater good of all other children to prevent the spread of disease in the community. What a bunch of bunk. As I have showed with numerous graphs and charts in this chapter, much to the dismay of vaccination proponents, outbreaks still occur in groups of children who have been fully vaccinated.

My friend, Dr. Russell Blaylock MD, a retired neurosurgeon, says the fact that vaccine-induced herd immunity is mostly myth can be proven quite simply. According to Dr. Blaylock, *"When I was in medical school, we were taught that all of the childhood vaccines lasted a lifetime. This thinking existed for over 70 years. It was not until relatively recently that it was discovered that most of these vaccines lost their effectiveness 2 to 10 years after being given. What this means is that at least half the population, that is the baby boomers, have had no vaccine-induced immunity against any of these diseases for which they had been vaccinated very early in life. In essence, at least 50% or more of the population was unprotected for decades. If we listen to present-day wisdom, we are all at risk of resurgent massive epidemics should the vaccination rate fall below 95%. Yet, we have all lived for at least 30 to 40 years with 50% or less of the population having vaccine protection. That is, herd immunity has not existed in this country for many decades and no resurgent epidemics have occurred. **Vaccine-induced herd immunity is a lie used to frighten** doctors, public-health officials, other medical personnel, and the public into accepting vaccinations."*

We have an ever growing (and desperate) propaganda campaign based upon smearing those who refuse to inject themselves or their precious children with toxic (and potentially deadly) poison and blaming every failure on their unwillingness to submit to the needle. Folks who are critical thinkers and thus opposed to vaccinations are referred to as "denialists," "kooks," "quacks," "uneducated," "confused," and "enemies of public safety." This desperation is based upon their fear that the public might soon catch on to the fact that the entire vaccine program is based upon unscientific drivel, nonsense, fear, and concocted fairytales.

If you are a parent who chooses to vaccinate, note that the concept of herd immunity as it is erroneously applied to vaccines is being used to manipulate you into using scorn and fear to pressure family and friends within your circle of influence into accepting vaccination against their will. Without the mantra of "herd immunity," the Medical Mafia dons wouldn't be able to justify forced mass vaccinations.

Please remember: Scientific fraud isn't the exception in modern medicine; **it is the rule.** Most of the "science" you read in today's medical journals is really just corporate-funded "quackery" dressed up in the language of pseudoscience. The fact of the matter is that, in classic

Orwellian maneuvering, the journals of the Medical Mafia are actually rewriting history to remove any studies that document the harm caused by vaccines.

But they won't succeed. The truth is slowly trickling out, and doctors across the globe are admitting that vaccines are responsible for a whole host of ailments, diseases, and even death. In a shocking report, the *Global Times* reported that an expert from the Chinese CDC, Dr. Wang Yu, has openly admitted that vaccines can cause severe adverse reactions, swollen organs, epilepsy, the diseases that they were supposed to prevent, and even death! As they say in New Zealand, "*Good on you*," Dr. Yu. The truth shall set you free!

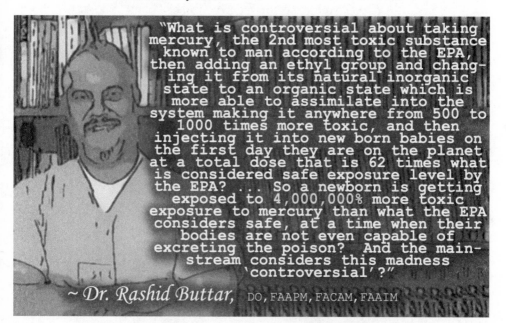

"What is controversial about taking mercury, the 2nd most toxic substance known to man according to the EPA, then adding an ethyl group and changing it from its natural inorganic state to an organic state which is more able to assimilate into the system making it anywhere from 500 to 1000 times more toxic, and then injecting it into new born babies on the first day they are on the planet at a total dose that is 62 times what is considered safe exposure level by the EPA? ... So a newborn is getting exposed to 4,000,000% more toxic exposure to mercury than what the EPA considers safe, at a time when their bodies are not even capable of excreting the poison? And the mainstream considers this madness 'controversial'?"

~ *Dr. Rashid Buttar*, DO, FAAPM, FACAM, FAAIM

Bottom line: Vaccine mythology is medical fascism based on "voodoo" science and fraudulent data. It is a "medical house of cards" that is collapsing right before our very eyes. Vaccines cause disease, disability, and even death. Hygiene and sanitation, **not** vaccinations, have resulted in the decrease of nearly every infectious disease over the past century.

Hey, what's that chuckling noise I hear? It must be those "liability-free" Big Pharma companies and vaccine-pushing "ne'er-do-well" doctors laughing all the way to the bank.

Don't dare get in the way of their gravy train or prepare to be run over. **Honk! Honk!**

RESOURCES

Websites
http://www.nvic.org/
http://www.vaccinationcouncil.org/
http://www.naturalnews.com/vaccines.html

Videos
"The Vaccine Safety Conference" – Dr. Russell Blaylock, M.D.
http://www.youtube.com/watch?v=4zJrkPJXAh0
"The Vaccine-Autism Connection" – Dr. Rashid Buttar
http://www.youtube.com/watch?v=4zJrkPJXAh0
"Vaccines: Armed and Dangerous" – Robert Scott Bell & John Rappoport

Books
Official Stories (Liam Scheff)
The Medical VooDoo (Anne Riley Hale)
Vaccination: A Mythical History
(Roman Bystrianyk and Dr. Suzanne Humphries, M.D.)

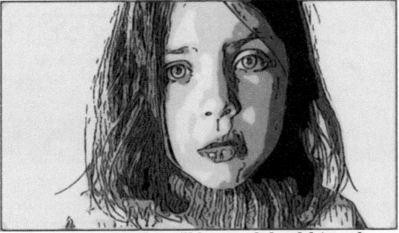

The nurse says that I'll be much healthier after you inject me with mercury, aluminum, embalming fluid, neurotoxins, anti-freeze, and other carcinogens. Thank you doctor. I trust you.

Chapter 11

~ CHEMOTHERAPY ~

MONUMENTAL MYTH

Chemotherapy is the most effective treatment for cancer, with its main purpose being to kill cancer cells. It can be used as the primary form of treatment or as a supplement to other treatments. Chemotherapy is often used to treat patients with cancer that has spread from the place in the body where it started (metastasized), but it may also be used the keep cancer from coming back (adjuvant therapy). Chemotherapy destroys cancer cells anywhere in the body. It even kills cells that have broken off from the main tumor and traveled through the blood or lymph systems to other parts of the body. Chemotherapy cures many types of cancer.

CAN YOU HANDLE THE TRUTH?

Chemotherapy is the cornerstone of modern conventional treatments for cancer. Unfortunately for millions of cancer patients, chemotherapy is one of the most monumental myths in the history of the Medical Mafia. For over half a century, the dark brigade of medieval mainstream medical oncology has known that chemotherapy is extremely poisonous and fundamentally worthless in the management of most malignancies. This information is carefully covered up by the controlled mainstream media so that non-doctors typically believe that chemo is a proven therapy for cancer. Like lemmings going over a cliff, the general public lines up for round after round of chemo. Sadly, most folks who undergo multiple rounds of chemotherapy proceed to die.

Chemotherapy is a barbaric and pointless procedure. It is, admittedly, effective at reducing tumors because it's a highly effective and toxic poison. It's designed to kill cells and it does its job very well. It's also very effective at hampering the immune system, damaging the gastrointestinal system and, effectively, causing a great deal of damage to the human body. While this extreme treatment has been called "effective" against testicular cancers and lymphocytic leukemia, in many cases it's hard to tell which the supposed "therapy" will kill first – the cancer or the patient.

Aside from the customary headaches, hair loss, dizziness, nausea, and vomiting, many chemotherapy drugs have other severe side effects. Most have an immediate suppressive effect on bone marrow, which is where new blood cells are typically being produced. In other words, it destroys the immune system at the one time in your life you need it the most. I'm not a rocket scientist, but it certainly seems strange to treat cancer (which is a result of a compromised immune system) with a set of chemotherapy drugs that further compromise the immune system. That makes about as much sense as treating alcoholism by sending the person to a bar or treating obesity by sending the person to a buffet or treating diabetes by sending the person to a candy shop.

Suppose you have a termite infestation in your home. The exterminator (someone you really trust) tells you that the best course of action will be to use a chemical that will kill the termites, but which is also known to eat away at both the wood and the foundation of homes, as well as causing irreparable damage to furniture and windows. After all, you really do want to get rid of those termites, right? Well, maybe not. Isn't that sort of like using a sledgehammer to open a peanut? Or using a sword to trim your fingernails?

So why does chemotherapy continue to be shoved down our throats, metaphorically speaking? The answer is simple. Follow the money. Treating cancer is **big** business. In fact, it's a $200 billion business each and every year, with revenues continuing to grow. Oncologists frequently make in excess of $1000 from every injection administered to a patient. As a matter of fact, most oncologists don't make their money by treating patients, but by selling cancer drugs. In fact, according to the *Journal of the American Medical Association*, as much as 75% of the average oncologist's earnings come from selling chemotherapy drugs in his or her office – at a substantially marked-up price.

One of the problems is that we're being duped by the Medical Mafia and the Cancer Industry with phony statistics, bad science, and fraudulent studies. However, once you "slice and dice" the phony statistics of the Cancer Industry, you will learn that the true cure rate (*i.e.,* 5-year survival) for chemotherapy is barely over 2%. As a matter of fact, according to a study conducted by the Department of Radiation Oncology at Northern Sydney Cancer Centre and published in the December 2004 issue of *Clinical Oncology*, the actual impact of chemotherapy on 5-year survival in American adults is a paltry 2.1%.
www.ncbi.nlm.nih.gov/pubmed/15630849

In the 1980s, Dr. Ulrich Abel, a German epidemiologist from the Heidelberg/Mannheim Tumor Clinic, did a comprehensive analysis of every major study and clinical trial of chemotherapy that has ever been done. To insure that he didn't leave anyone out, he contacted over 350 medical centers worldwide requesting them to furnish him with anything they had published on the subject of cancer. By the time he published his report, it is likely that he knew more about chemotherapy than any person in the world.

The results were amazing! In his report, published in the August 1991 issue of *The Lancet*, Dr. Abel stated, *"Success of most chemotherapies is appalling...There is* **no scientific evidence** *for its ability to extend in any appreciable way the lives of patients suffering from the most common organic cancer...Chemotherapy for malignancies too advanced for surgery, which accounts for 80% of all cancers, is a scientific wasteland."* The "cancer emperor" has no clothes! Of course, the Medical Mafia immediately attacked Dr. Abel's character since they couldn't attack his science. This is standard operating procedure. Not surprisingly, no mainstream media outlet ever mentioned Abel's comprehensive study: it was totally buried.

"Success of most chemotherapy is appalling . . . (chemotherapy) is a scientific wasteland."

Dr. Ulrich Abel, MD

I know a medical examiner named Dr. Larry Smith who has performed dozens of autopsies on cancer patients. I was dumbfounded to learn that, according to Dr. Smith, he never performed an autopsy on a cancer patient that died from "cancer," *per se*. He expressed to me that every cancer patient that he autopsied had actually died from **toxicity** from either chemotherapy or radiation!

Chemotherapy drugs have always been developed from toxic poisonous chemicals, right? So, if we think about it logically, there has always been a fine line between administering a "therapeutic dose" and killing the cancer patient. Many doctors step over that line. In his book, <u>When</u>

Healing Becomes a Crime, Kenny Ausubel noted that in a trial on a chemotherapy drug tested for leukemia, a whopping 42% of the patients died directly from the toxicity of the chemotherapy drug!

It's interesting to note that chemotherapy drugs were initially derived from the nitrogen mustard gas experiments during World Wars I and II (which were eventually banned by the Geneva Conventions). It was noticed that exposure to mustard gas caused destruction of fast growing tissues, thus it was surmised that since cancer grew quickly, these poisons could kill cancer tissue. Well, they were right ... exposure to these gases did kill cancerous tissue. Make no mistake about it, chemotherapy **does** shrink the size of tumors and kills cancer cells. But is shrinking a tumor equivalent to curing cancer? Is there a direct correlation? The answer is "no."

According to Dr. Ralph Moss, "*If you can shrink the tumour 50% or more for 28 days you have got the FDA's definition of an active drug. That is called a response rate, so you have a response...(but) when you look to see if there is any life prolongation from taking this treatment what you find is all kinds of hocus pocus and song and dance about the disease free survival, and this and that. In the end there is no proof that chemotherapy in the vast majority of cases actually extends life, and this is the great lie about chemotherapy, that somehow there is a correlation between shrinking a tumour and extending the life of the patient.*"

Here are the facts. In 1942, Memorial Sloan-Kettering Cancer Center quietly began to treat breast cancer with these mustard gas derivatives. **No one was cured**. Chemotherapy trials were also conducted at Yale around 1943 where 160 patients were treated. Again, **no one was cured.** But, since the chemotherapy **did shrink tumors**, researchers were so excited that they proclaimed the chemotherapy trials to be a "success." I suppose that we need to define exactly what "success" means, don't we?

In a courageous letter dated 4/20/1973 written to Dr. Frank Rauscher (his boss at the National Cancer Institute), Dr. Dean Burk condemned the Institute's policy of continuing to endorse chemotherapy drugs when everyone knew that they caused cancer. In his own words, he stated: "*Ironically, virtually all of the chemotherapeutic anti-cancer agents now approved by the Food and Drug Administration for use or testing in human cancer patients are (1) highly or variously toxic at applied dosages; (2) markedly immunosuppressive, that is, destructive of the patient's native resistance to a variety of diseases, including cancer; and (3) usually highly carcinogenic ... These now well established facts have been reported in numerous publications from the National Cancer Institute itself, as well as from throughout the United States and, indeed, the world.*"

It's a word game. One of the problems with the Cancer Industry is that their lexicon is entrenched amongst a labyrinth of lies and couched in ambiguous phrases. Like *"response rate."* If a dying patient's condition changes even for a week or a month, especially if the tumor shrinks temporarily, the patient is listed as having "responded to" chemotherapy. No joke! The fact that the tumor comes back stronger and more viciously soon after chemo is stopped is not figured into the equation. The fact that the patient has to endure ghastly side effects in order to momentarily shrink the tumor is not considered. That fact that the patient soon dies is not figured into the equation. The idea is to sell, sell, and sell. Sell chemotherapy. Period. It's a business.

If you listen to the boisterous, blabbermouth, bobble-head bleached blondes of the controlled mainstream media, you will hear stories about the amazing success that chemotherapy has had on certain rare types of cancer, like childhood leukemia and Hodgkin's lymphoma. But what you don't hear is that even with Hodgkin's disease, one of chemo's purported "triumphs," the treatment is deemed to be a success even though the patient dies. Just not from Hodgkin's disease, that's all.

In the 1987 *Journal of the National Cancer Institute*, Dr. John Diamond asserted: *"A study of over 10,000 patients shows clearly that chemo's supposedly strong track record with Hodgkin's disease (lymphoma) is actually a lie. Patients who underwent chemo were **14 times** more likely to develop leukemia and **6 times** more likely to develop cancers of the bones, joints, and soft tissues than those patients who did not undergo chemotherapy."*

The March 21, 1996, issue of the *New England Journal of Medicine* reported that children who are successfully treated for Hodgkin's disease are **18 times** more likely later to develop secondary malignant tumors. So, when the patient eventually died from leukemia or another type of cancer, he or she was deemed to be "cured" of Hodgkin's lymphoma and the chemotherapy was acclaimed to be a huge success. Even though the patient was six feet under.

What a load of hooey!

It's an epidemic. Seriously. There are about 600,000 new cancer patients each year ... over 1,500 a day. Enough people to fill four fully loaded jet planes! Millions have died along the way. You may have a personal story, or perhaps you've heard the stories of Patrick Swayze, Farrah Fawcett, Peter Jennings, Sydney Pollack, Gary Cooper, and Tony Snow. All were "celebrities." All had cancer. All received chemotherapy. And soon ... they all died.

It's no coincidence. **Chemo kills.**

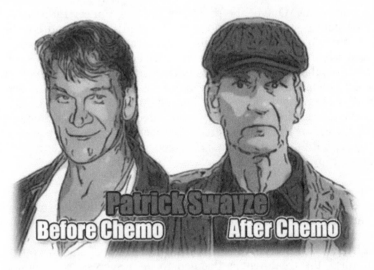

Patrick Swayze
Before Chemo   After Chemo

Since chemotherapy drugs are some of the most toxic substances ever designed to enter a human body, their effects are exceptionally severe, and, as I mentioned previously, are often the direct cause of death. Like the case of Jackie Kennedy Onassis, who underwent chemotherapy for non-Hodgkin's lymphoma. She went into the hospital on Friday and was dead by Tuesday. What happened? Some sources speculated that since this was such a high profile patient, they gave her an "extra strong" dose to "kill the cancer" faster. Unfortunately they miscalculated: there was a patient attached. She was only 64.

Do you think that your oncologist would submit himself to chemo if he were diagnosed with cancer? The McGill Cancer Center in Montreal, one of the largest and most esteemed cancer treatment centers in the world, surveyed 64 oncologists to see how they would respond to a diagnosis of cancer. The results will blow your mind. Are you sitting down? Fifty-eight (58) said that chemotherapy was unacceptable to them and their family members due to the fact that the drugs don't work and are toxic to one's system. (Philip Day, Cancer: Why We're Still Dying to Know the Truth) That means 91% of the oncologists would **not** take chemo themselves!

So why do they keep giving it to cancer patients? When President Nixon declared the "war on cancer," researchers were given access to **billions** of dollars of research money earmarked for cancer drug research. So, if you are a medical doctor who makes money through publishing cancer research, you better not challenge the status quo (*i.e.*, the "Big 3"), because if you do, then you are likely to have your funding pulled. For example, in 1966, Dr. Irwin D. Bross and four colleagues published a series of pioneering articles entitled *"Is Toxicity Really Necessary."* In these articles, they merely questioned whether it was possible to find an alternative to chemotherapy and radiation, since chemo and radiation are both so toxic. **The result:** They promptly lost their government support for drug testing studies.

Preventing unfavorable chemotherapy results from being seen by the public in TV, radio, and newspaper reporting is combined with malicious quackery charges and actual death threats to practitioners who have legitimate cancer cures. I am aware of several dozen cancer cures since 1900 that have been ignored or suppressed. Several persons with bona fide cancer cures have been so vilified they died alcoholics or committed suicide. Prominent physician Dr. Milbrook Johnson was poisoned the night before he was scheduled to speak on a national radio network in the 1940s about the ability of Dr. Royal Rife's electronic equipment to cure cancer and infections.

Yes, the propaganda machine is in full swing when it comes to cancer treatments. Big Pharma companies not only hire charismatic people to charm doctors, exaggerate drug benefits, and underplay side effects, but they also pay oncologists kickbacks to push their drugs. For example, AstraZeneca, Inc. had to pay $280 million in civil penalties and $63 million in criminal penalties to the federal government after it paid kickbacks to doctors for promoting its prostate cancer drug. Oncologists not only bully patients into taking these dangerous chemotherapy drugs, but they also do **not** tell their patients the whole truth about the fact that they actually might die from the drugs rather than the disease.

The very failure of the entire cancer industry to slow the death rate over the past fifty years indicates that it's time to look for another paradigm. They have failed, but they can't admit it because the whole thing is market-driven. It's imponderable that doctors continue to prescribe a volatile poison which they **know** will kill the patient, simply because it's their only tool! This can't be an acceptable excuse! It's almost like the oncologists that prescribe chemo are either on a really, really bad "acid trip" or they've caught a really, really bad case of "greed." You decide.

In my opinion one of the most important verses in the Bible is Proverbs 14:12 – "*There is way that seems right unto man but its end is the way of death.*" Many doctors (specifically oncologists), Big Pharma sales reps and executives, politicians, world leaders, and mainstream media owners have unbelievable wealth and power in this world. However, they may face a tortured eternity following death. This seems to be a very unwise tradeoff.

Chemotherapy is almost a "self-fulfilling prophecy" when it comes to "treating" cancer, actually causing additional long-term and potentially lethal cancers. And if you are unfortunate enough to have been **mis**diagnosed with cancer (which the NCI recently admitted has occurred over 1.3 million times over the past few decades) and opt for chemo, it's likely that the treatment will, in fact, **cause** the disease that it purportedly prevents. It's the equivalent of a "medical false flag." You see, the Medical Mafia and the cancer industry operate much like the government does: They cause the problem and then they swoop down and provide a solution (which doesn't really solve anything), reminding you all the while of how "lucky" you are to have them, even though they created the problem in the first place.

Stay away from chemotherapy. Build your immune system.

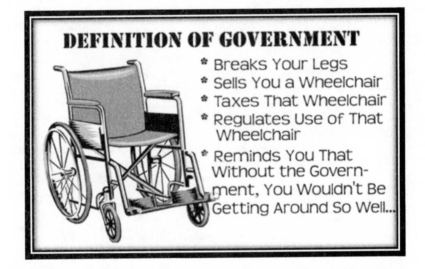

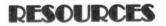

RESOURCES

Websites
http://www.chrisbeatcancer.com/why-i-didnt-do-chemo/
http://www.naturalnews.com/chemotherapy.html
http://www.cancertutor.com/

Books
Cancer: Why We're Still Dying to Know the Truth (Philip Day)
Cancer – Step Outside the Box (Ty Bollinger)
Questioning Chemotherapy (Dr. Ralph Moss)
Chemotherapy Heals Cancer and the World is Flat (Lothar Hirneise)

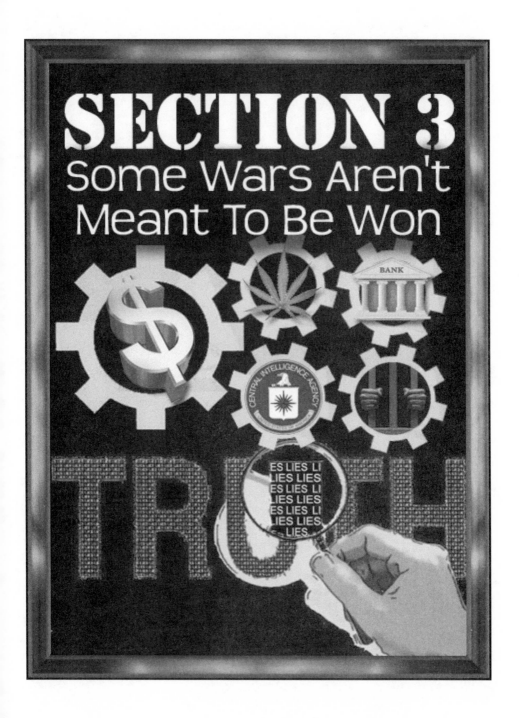

SECTION 3
Some Wars Aren't Meant To Be Won

Chapter 12

~ THE WAR ON CANCER ~

MONUMENTAL MYTH

The "war on cancer" was officially declared by the Federal Government in 1971, and enthusiastically signed into law by President Richard Nixon. Since then, we have made huge strides in combating the disease. Cancer death rates have been falling steadily and we will soon eradicate the "C" word. One day, we will find "the cure."

CAN YOU HANDLE THE TRUTH?

The so-called "war on cancer" is not only a miserable failure but has also become a monumental myth perpetuated by the Medical Mafia. The "war on cancer" was an effort to create a perpetual income stream for the Cancer Industry while concurrently deflecting attention from Nixon's failed presidency and extracurricular exploits. In 1971-1972, the US government quickly tossed a gargantuan gigantic gob of cash (around $100 million) into this new project. And remember those "germ hunters" I mentioned in Chapter 6? Well, they quickly dispatched in full force to prove that cancer was caused by a germ or virus, because a contagious cancer (*"Achoo!"*) would result in the development of new drugs and vaccines that folks would want ... **forever**. Ka-ching! They could hear the jingle of coins in their piggy banks!

But money doesn't necessarily equal results. In the past four decades, we've thrown trillions of dollars at this phony war. One would think that after four decades of zealous research and trillions of dollars spent, we would have this dreadful disease under control. Just think of the rapid explosion of ideas and innovations within other technology areas. For example, your iPhone is now more powerful than the largest super-computers of the 1980s. However, after trillions of dollars spent and billions of doses of lucrative drugs and vaccines, not only are more people dying of cancer than ever before but more people are getting cancer at earlier ages than ever before.

Alas, over the past forty years, the "war on cancer" has, in reality, become a quagmire, a "medical Vietnam," an endless, calculated "no-win" war on cancer, since countless billions of dollars are being made each year by its perpetuation. Nevertheless, the Cancer Industry remains largely closed to innovative ideas in the realm of alternative cancer treatments. According to Dr. John Bailer, who spent twenty years on the staff of the NCI and was editor of its journal, speaking at the Annual Meeting of the American Association for the Advancement of Science in May 1985, *"My overall assessment is that the national cancer program must be judged a qualified failure."*

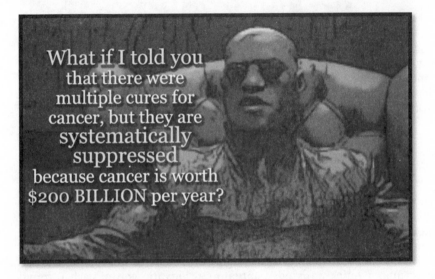

As a matter of fact, the Cancer Industry (led by their "mafia dons") has waged another war – a war **against** those who advocate the use of alternative cancer treatments. At the root of this new war is the almighty dollar. The truth is that since conventional treatments pay the best, they are touted as the most effective treatments. It's all about the economics of cancer, not finding a cure.

Being a CPA, I tend to look at things from an "economic" perspective. And I must tell you that from an economic perspective, the Cancer Industry has the perfect business model. Big Pharma and the other chemical companies make huge profits from selling carcinogenic chemicals that are dumped (oftentimes intentionally) in our food, water, and air. Then, they make even more profits by manufacturing and selling expensive, ineffective, toxic drugs to treat the cancers and other diseases caused by their own products. Then, in baseball lingo, they complete the "triple play" by selling additional drugs to make the side-effects of the primary drugs more bearable. In business lingo, the Cancer Industry is sitting on a "cash cow." Unfortunately, this cash cow is a scam at the expense of cancer patients.

Adding insult to injury, they let John and Jane Taxpayer (i.e., you and me) fund their research into more ways to **not** cure cancer while still pushing their drugs at obscene profits. To ensure that the public remains blissfully unaware of the true facts about cancer, they have set up front group "cheerleaders" (like the National Cancer Institute and the American Cancer Society) to spread disinformation in the name of cancer education, while the rest of the Medical Mafia is busy fighting a hostile turf war to make sure that alternative cancer treatments remain suppressed and the doctors that use these treatments are persecuted and run out of the county.

One of the ways that this turf war is fought is through advertising. Not only does Big Pharma make billions of dollars annually on the sale of drugs, but they also dump billions of dollars into the advertising of prescription drugs each year. And, since people in America typically make their key decisions based solely on what they see on TV and what they hear on the radio, is it any wonder that we are largely uninformed concerning alternative cancer treatments? The Medical Mafia has done everything in its power to make sure you do **not** know the truth about alternative cancer treatments. The TV stations and other media don't dare broadcast anything which may hurt one of their biggest advertisers – Big Pharma.

You see, the citizens of the world (especially in the USA) are hypnotically programmed and enthralled by the anesthetizing effects of a corrupt, monopolistic global mainstream media bought and paid for by Wall Street, Big Pharma, and the Medical Mafia. The US government is the head of the global government snake. From cradle to grave we are distracted by TV, impoverished by consumerism, and indebted by cancer. As a result, everyone is too mesmerized by Madison Avenue propaganda to see that the war on cancer is as phony as both the war on drugs and the war on terror, both of which we will "debunk" in the following chapters.

No matter how many people shave their heads or run for the cure or cycle all over the place, as long as the Medical Mafia is in control, the "cancer war" will never be won. According to Dr. Linus Pauling, (two-time Nobel Prize winner), "*Most cancer research is largely a fraud and the major cancer research organizations are derelict in their duties to the people who support them.*" This cancer war is one of the most costly frauds (in terms of money and human suffering) that have ever been perpetrated on the American public. Staggering amounts of money have been spent in its pursuit, but the "cancer emperor" is naked.

Rampant greed bordering on the grotesque has been allowed to call the shots in this 40+ yearlong "cancer war," with the primary beneficiaries being Big Pharma companies and the tremendously profitable cancer industry as a whole, including so-called "non-profit" organizations like the American Cancer Society. You see, finding the "cure" for cancer might just put Big Pharma out of business and would certainly end the careers of countless doctors and so called "researchers." Meanwhile, cancer charities and hospitals still confidently promise to "outrun cancer" while exhorting donors to walk, cycle or even play road hockey "for the cure." Heck, in 2010, you could have *"pigged out on cancer-causing Kentucky Fried Chicken for the cure,"* as KFC was one of the sponsors for breast cancer awareness month. Give me a break.

It's a simple economic equation, folks. Keeping the public ignorant about the **real** causes of cancer and **effective** treatments for cancer results in more cancer patients. More cancer patients results in more sales of chemotherapy drugs, more radiation, and more surgery.

You see, **money**, rather than moral ethics, is the deciding factor for the Cancer Industry and the Medical Mafia. To be honest, their goal is to provide temporary relief by treating the symptoms of cancer with drugs, while never addressing the cause of the cancer. This insures regular visits to the doctor's office and requires the patient to routinely return to the pharmacy to refill his prescriptions. This is what the game is all about folks, plain and simple.

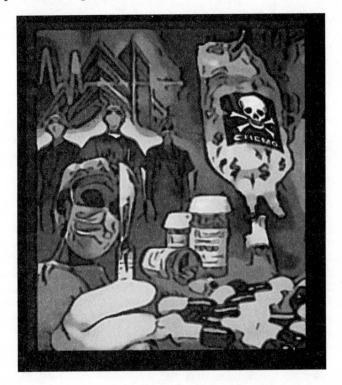

The survival of the Medical Mafia and Big Pharma is dependent upon the elimination (by any means) of effective natural cancer treatments and the perpetuation of the pretentious "war on cancer." By making it more difficult to access natural health remedies, these "medical gangsters" are protecting their monopoly while simultaneously feeding their own megalomania. Truth be told, especially relating to cancer treatments, the Medical Mafia and their Big Pharma buddies are running a huge extortion scheme, and their tactics make Pol Pot look like a choir boy!

In the words of Devra Davis, author of <u>The Secret History of the War on Cancer,</u> "*The war on cancer set out to find, treat, and cure a disease. Left untouched were many of the things known to cause cancer, including tobacco, the workplace, radiation, or the global environment. Proof of how the world in which we live and work affects whether we get cancer was either overlooked or suppressed. This has been no accident. The 'war on cancer' was run by leaders of industries that made cancer-causing products and sometimes also profited from drugs and technologies for finding and treating the disease.*"

Let's be honest. No profitable business will ever try to eliminate itself. The Cancer Industry (a cartel consisting of the NIH, the NCI, the ACS, the FDA, the AMA, and Big Pharma) survives and thrives by perpetually searching for "the cure" but never finding it. This multi-billion dollar juggernaut is simply not interested in finding a cure. The goal is to develop a continuous stream of cancer patients who are duped into thinking that they need to buy expensive "cancer drugs" for the rest of their life. The competition (effective non-toxic, natural cancer treatments) must be squelched ... regardless of the cost.

According to C.S. Lewis in The Screwtape Letters: "*The greatest evil is not now done in those sordid 'dens of crime' that Dickens loved to paint. It is not done even in concentration camps and labour camps. In those we see its final result. But it is conceived and ordered (moved, seconded, carried and minuted) in clean, carpeted, warmed and well-lighted offices, by quiet men with white collars and cut fingernails, and smooth-shaven cheeks who do not need to raise their voices. Hence, naturally enough, my symbol for Hell is something like...the offices of a thoroughly nasty business concern.*"

The next time you are asked to donate to a cancer organization, bear in mind that your money will be used to sustain an industry which has been deemed by many eminent scientists as a qualified failure, by many doctors as a complete fraud, and by others (including myself) as comparable to the Cosa Nostra.

I leave you with a quote from James Watson, the discoverer of DNA, and Nobel Laureate: "*The war on cancer is a bunch of sh*t.*"

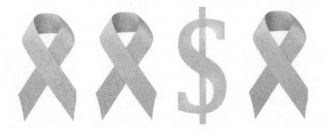

RESOURCES

Websites
http://rense.com/general9/cre.htm
www.peopleagainstcancer.com/pdfs/news/20080916n2.pdf
http://www.issues.org/19.4/updated/bailar.html

Books
The War on Cancer: An Anatomy of Failure –
A Blueprint for the Future (Dr. Guy Faguet)
The Secret History of the War on Cancer (Devra Davis)

Chapter 13

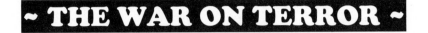
~ THE WAR ON TERROR ~

MONUMENTAL MYTH

The "war on terror" was officially declared by President George W. Bush on September 20, 2011 after the 9/11 "terrorist" attacks. This "war" involves open and covert military operations, new security legislation, efforts to block the financing of terrorism, and more. Bush called on other states to join in the fight against terrorism asserting that *either you are with us, or you are with the terrorists.*" The "war on terror" typically has a particular focus on countries supporting militant Islamists, al-Qaeda, and other jihadi groups.

CAN YOU HANDLE THE TRUTH?

Remember the bomb that went off at the Dallas Cowboys football game in 2002 that killed 50,000 fans? Remember the nerve gas that killed thousands of shoppers in Seattle in 2007? Remember the bomb that killed over 100,000 people celebrating in Times Square on New Year's Eve 2009? Remember the suicide bomber that killed hundreds of children at Disneyworld in 2012? Remember? Remember?

I don't remember those either ... because they **never** happened. Honestly, these fictional events would have been easy to perpetrate if there were well-organized terror groups that had infiltrated the USA. Seriously, try to clear the cobwebs out of your head and try to think outside the box.

What if there weren't any real terrorists threatening the USA and the entire "war on terror" was a monumental myth created to justify an imperialistic military agenda coupled with rampant obliteration of the Constitutional rights of US citizens?

Go outside. Do you see any suicide bombers walking around with a vest full of explosives? **Nope.** Any "terrorists" with automatic weapons and grenades? **Nope.** Ever seen a TSA agent catch a terrorist at the airport?

Nope. Any scary hobgoblins setting off explosives at sporting events or malls? **Nope.**

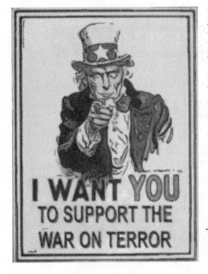

If we are going to forfeit our rights and have checkpoints at every corner to protect us from the "boogeyman" terrorists, then a "thinking" person would require that there be **actual evidence** that America has been infiltrated with terrorists, right? Other than the ones they fabricate, plan, and carry out, have you ever heard of the FBI stopping a terrorist plot?

In an April 28, 2012 article in the *New York Times*, David Shipler writes, "*The United States has been narrowly saved from lethal terrorist plots in recent years — or so it has seemed. A would-be suicide bomber was intercepted on his way to the Capitol; a scheme to bomb synagogues and shoot Stinger missiles at military aircraft was developed by men in Newburgh, N.Y.; and a fanciful idea to fly explosive-laden model planes into the Pentagon and the Capitol was hatched in Massachusetts. But all these dramas were facilitated by the F.B.I., whose undercover agents and informers posed as terrorists offering a dummy missile, fake C-4 explosives, a disarmed suicide vest and rudimentary training. Suspects naïvely played their parts until they were arrested.*"

Of course, the government does (from time to time) stage some sort of terrorist event (like 9/11) to remind everyone to be "very very afraid." That's a given. Speaking of 9/11, let's take a brief look at what has happened in the USA since President Bush declared the war on terror on September 20, 2011. Much of the information below was gleaned from Steve Nolan and M.S. Wall's "timeline to tyranny" on www.infowars.com.

On October 23, 2011, just weeks after the tragic events of 9/11, the first draft of the USA PATRIOT Act, which stands for "*Uniting (and) Strengthening America (by) Providing Appropriate Tools Required (to) Intercept (and) Obstruct Terrorism.*" No member of Congress was even allowed to read the first USA PATRIOT Act. Writing for the *New York Times*, William Safire described the first USA PATRIOT Act's powers by saying that President Bush was "*seizing dictatorial control.*" The USA PATRIOT Act and its 300 pages were printed at 3:00 AM for a vote that took place at 11:00 AM that same morning. With the passage of this act, the US federal government was given the ability to wiretap, conduct electronic surveillance, pry into private medical records, and to access financial records such as bank and credit card statements. They were even given the power to look into public library records. On October 26, 2001, President Bush signed the USA PATRIOT Act into law.

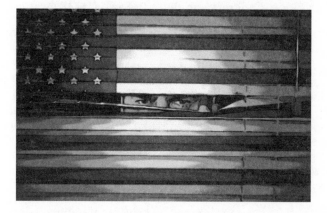

On November 25, 2001, President Bush created the Department of Homeland Security (DHS) in response to the 9/11 attacks. Since then, DHS has become the employer to more than 200,000 employees and is now the third largest Cabinet department after the Department of Defense and the Department of Veterans Affairs. On January 14, 2005, The Department of the Army published *Army Regulation 210-35: Civilian Inmate Labor Program*, which provided Army policy and guidance for establishing civilian inmate labor programs and civilian prison camps on Army installations.

On October 17, 2006, President Bush signed into law the *John Warner Defense Authorization Act* which expanded the President's power to declare martial law under revisions to the Insurrection Act, and take charge of United States National Guard troops without state governor authorization. That same day, President Bush also signed into law *The United States Military Commissions Act of 2006* with stated purpose *"To authorize trial by military commission for violations of the law of war and for other purposes."*

On May 9, 2007, President Bush signed National Security Presidential Directive 51 (NSPD51) and the Homeland Security Presidential Directive (HSPD-20). These directives essentially say that when the president determines a national "catastrophic emergency" has occurred, he can assume dictatorial powers to direct any and all government and business activities. They loosely define *"catastrophic emergency"* as *"any incident, regardless of location, that results in extraordinary levels of mass casualties, damage, or disruption severely affecting the US population, infrastructure, environment, economy or government functions."* It should be noted that neither NSPD-51 nor HSPD-20 has any reference to Congress. This Executive Order ensures a continuity of governmental program can be implemented without any Congressional approval or oversight.

On July 20, 2007, Congressman Peter DeFazio (D-OR) was asked by his constituents to see what was contained in the classified portion of the White House's plan for operating the government after a terrorist attack. DeFazio, who sat on the Homeland Security Committee and had clearance to view classified material, was **denied** access to view the documents, and he was not given a reason why. He stated, *"I just can't believe they're going to deny a member of Congress the right of reviewing how they plan to conduct the government of the United States after a significant terrorist attack. We're talking about the continuity of the government of the United States of America. I would think that would be relevant to any member of Congress, let alone a member of the Homeland Security Committee. Maybe the people who think there's a conspiracy out there are right."*

On November 4, 2008, The US Army War College's Strategic Institute publishes *Known Unknowns: Unconventional "Strategic Shocks" in Defense Strategy Development* warning that the United States may experience massive civil unrest in the wake of a series of crises which it has termed "strategic shock."

According to Michael Chossudovsky in his book <u>The 9/11 Reader</u>, *"The myth of the 'outside enemy' and the threat of 'Islamic terrorists' was the cornerstone of the Bush administration's military doctrine, used as a pretext to invade Afghanistan and Iraq, not to mention America's 'War on Terrorism' mention the repeal of civil liberties and constitutional government in America . . . without an 'outside enemy,' there could be no 'war on terrorism.' The entire national security agenda would collapse like a deck of cards. The war criminals in high office would have no leg to stand on."*

Second verse ... same as the first ...

Enter Obama with his promises of "hope and change" and an end to the Bush era. All these unprecedented powers were handed over to President Obama, allowing him the ability to declare martial law without any Congressional oversight or approval. On January 11, 2010, President Barack Hussein Obama signed an Executive Order creating a "Council of Governors." This body of ten state governors (directly appointed by Obama) works with the US federal government to help advance the *"synchronization and integration of State and Federal military activities in the United States."* This group of non-elected governors liaises with the Pentagon's Northcom, DHS, the National Guard, as well as Department of Defense (DOD) officials from the Pentagon.

In 2010, the Department of the Army published *Regulation: FM 3-39.40, Internment and Resettlement Operations Manual.* This US Army document was prepared for the DOD and *"was not meant for public consumption."* It contained shocking plans for "political activists" to be pacified by "PSYOP officers" into developing an "an appreciation of US policies" while detained in prison camps **inside the USA**. Both the UN and Red Cross are named as partners including federal agencies such as the DHS and FEMA. If this doesn't bother you, perhaps you should apply.

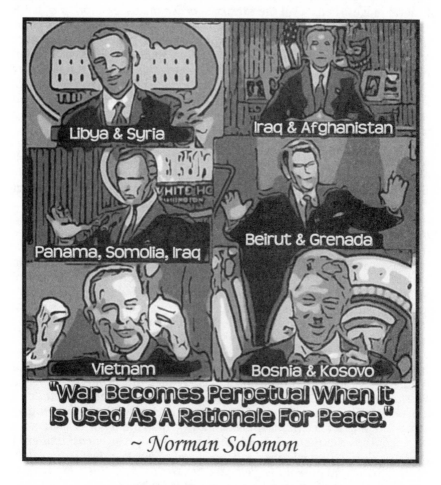

Libya & Syria

Iraq & Afghanistan

Panama, Somolia, Iraq

Beirut & Grenada

Vietnam

Bosnia & Kosovo

"War Becomes Perpetual When It Is Used As A Rationale For Peace."

~ *Norman Solomon*

On Feb. 11, 2011, Obama created a "Continental Perimeter" described as a key step in advance of the North American Union. Obama and Canadian Prime Minister Stephen Harper quietly bypassed Congress to sign on the basis of their executive authority a declaration that put in place a new national security vision defined not by the US national borders, but by a continental view of a "North American perimeter."

On May 26, 2011, Obama signed a four-year extension of three key provisions in the USA PATRIOT Act allowing for roving wiretaps, searches of business records and conducting surveillance of "lone wolves" – individuals suspected of terrorist-related activities not linked to terrorist groups.

On September 30, 2011, Anwar al-Awlaki (an American citizen) and his teenage son were assassinated under orders of President Obama without regard for a previous executive order that forbids assassinations. A US Federal judge asked: *"Can the executive order the assassination of a US citizen without first affording him any form of judicial process whatsoever, based on the mere assertion that he is a dangerous member of a terrorist organization?"* Keep in mind this took place in Yemen. Now we have drones flying over the USA. According to the a statement by the ACLU on December 31, 2011, *"The Obama administration and its enablers have established, legitimized, and normalized a national security state apparatus that removes any doubt that domestic policing is a prelude to a totalitarian police state."*

Also on December 31, 2011, under the cloak of darkness when most Americans were celebrating New Year's Eve, Obama surreptitiously signed the highly controversial The National Defense Authorization Act (NDAA) which is unprecedented, unconstitutional, and gives the office of the president unchecked dictatorial powers in the name of *"protecting the security of the homeland."* This treasonous piece of legislation gives the President dictatorial authority to arrest any American citizen, or anyone for that matter, without warrant and "indefinitely detain" them in offshore prisons without charge and keep them there until "the end of hostilities." Obama lied to the public and said he would veto the NDAA's indefinite detention clauses. He didn't. He gave himself the right to "disappear" people in the middle of the night who dissent against his regime.

My former pastor, Chuck Baldwin, warns us in an essay entitled "Bill Of Rights Is No More": *"Americans should realize that, coupled with the Patriot Act, the NDAA, for all intents and purposes, completely nullifies a good portion of the Bill of Rights, turns the United States into a war zone, and places US citizens under military rule. And what is even more astonishing is the manner in which the national press corps, and even the so-called 'conservative' talking heads, have either completely ignored it, or have actually defended it. The likes of Rush Limbaugh, Sean Hannity, et al., should be ashamed of themselves!"*

On March 10, 2012, Obama signed The Federal Restricted Buildings and Grounds Improvement Act of 2011 commonly known as the anti-protest "Trespass Bill." This bill makes the simple trespass in an area under Secret Service protection (such as a campaign event) a federal offense punishable for up to 10 years. Federal agents now have sweeping powers to arrest protestors and charge them with a felony, effectively killing the First Amendment!

On March 16, 2012, Obama issued another unconstitutional executive order. The National Defense Resources Preparedness Executive Order allows the government to confiscate your property without due process under the direction of Janet Napolitano and the DHS. This Executive Order underscores Bill Clinton's Executive Order 12919 which he signed on June 6, 1994. Once again, this Executive Order violates our Constitution, specifically Article 1, Section 1, which states: "*All legislative Powers herein granted shall be vested in a Congress of the United States, which shall consist of a Senate and House of Representatives.*" Any enactment of law by the executive that is made in excess of jurisdiction is by definition **treason**. Is this a means to allow the federal government to steal private party similar to Mussolini's fascist corporatism?

As of the writing of this book (fall of 2013) Obama wants to strike Syria. "Cui bono" is an old Latin phrase that is still commonly used, and it roughly means "to whose benefit?" The key to figuring out who is really behind the push for war is to look at who will benefit from that war. Look no further than the "military industrial complex." According to George Washington University, the Pentagon has paid over **$3.3 trillion** to defense contractors since 9/11, and a war with Syria would add another trillion dollars to this number, according to some estimates.

And what about the private contractors and government agencies whose existence depends on a thriving "war on terror"? Where once we only had the CIA (foreign) and the FBI (domestic), the *Washington Post* reported that in 2010 there were, "*some 1,271 government organizations and 1,931 private companies work on programs related to counterterrorism, homeland security and intelligence in about 10,000 locations across the United States.*" Ka-ching!! Follow the money!

Unfortunately, it appears that the phony "war on terror" will go on forever, since they can always claim someone else is "a terroristic threat" and that there is a new "boogeyman" when it serves their best interests. That's why it's now patently obvious that this "war on terror" has been a monumental myth fabricated to achieve specific political and social agendas. For instance, the American people have been conditioned to worry and be scared whenever the word "terrorism" is mentioned. So effective has been this fear tactic we have spent trillions, employed millions, militarized the "homeland," surrendered our constitutional rights, and allowed many of our citizens to slide into a state of irrational paranoia, economic despair, and poverty as a result.

Oh yes, I almost forgot another result of this "war on terror" – the Transportation Security Administration (TSA). Remember when you could actually go to the airport and greet the people who got off the plane as soon as they came through the tunnel? Those days of yesteryear are long gone. Now, when you go to the airport, you are faced with two disgusting choices. You can either be photographed in your birthday suit by the full-body porno scanning "nudie nuker" machine. Or, if you prefer, you can be gate raped and have your crotch groped by a TSA pervert in an act that, anywhere else, would constitute sexual assault.

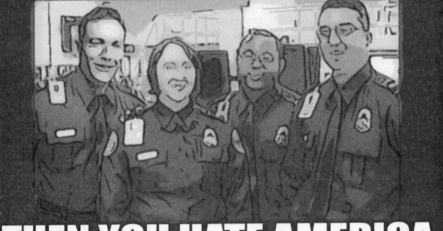

You see, the TSA does **not** provide security. It merely provides "security theater." Just check out the items that they confiscate. Are nail clippers and aftershave the tools of terrorists? What about the bottle of water I was relieved of at the Pittsburgh airport? What about my cup of coffee that the TSA goon said "might contain explosives"? And for goodness sake, why in the world do the TSA's sweaty oinkers insist on doing full body pat downs on children and grandmothers? People are in prison doing 20 years on the mere **accusation** they touched a child improperly. Yet these goons from the TSA can molest you and your children, and there is nothing you can say about it, unless you want to end up tasered, in Gitmo, or on a "no fly" list. Do you really think that the ruling class gives a hoot about the safety of the peasants? Or is it all about controlling the slaves?

One of the grievances articulated in the Declaration of Independence (and the basis for the Third Amendment) was *"quartering large bodies of armed troops among us."* I doubt that King George III ever dreamt of authorizing the redcoats to grope the crotches of the colonists; if he had, the "shot heard round the world" would have been fired much sooner than April 19, 1775. If you quietly accept the TSA's sexual humiliation, what will you **not** accept? Where **will** you draw the line? Personally, I would rather live in a free society with the **very remote** chance of being a victim of terrorism than in a place such as Cuba or North Korea, with a ubiquitous "national security" apparatus and no liberty whatsoever.

Do you know who is carrying out the real terror in America today? It's not Al Qaeda and it's not the Muslims. No, it's the beer-bellied, porker, fascist, overpaid, incompetent, lazy, child-molesting, worthless Gestapo deviants at the TSA who terrorize thousands of innocent air travelers every single day by stripping them down in those secret little rooms behind the security checkpoint and sexually molesting them. Of course, you better not say that in an airport, or you might be arrested. That's right. Recent "warnings" in airports across the USA indicate that if an air traveler is overheard "joking" about the TSA, they may be detained! I don't know about you, but that just makes me want to be even louder and more "in your face" to the TSA goons.

Lastly, I mustn't forget to mention Michael Chertoff. While he was the "Head of Homeland Security" under Bush, Chertoff advocated and pushed for installation and implementation of the full-body porno scanning "nudie nuker" machines at all USA airports. Once he was out of "public service," Chertoff's consulting company landed Rapiscan (the company that makes the scanners) as a client. **Surprise, surprise!** Chertoff also holds seats on the boards of giant defense and security firms and literally sits at the heart of the giant security nexus created in the wake of 9/11, in effect creating a "shadow" homeland security agency.

Bottom line: TSA does not keep you safe. It never has. It never will.

The best article yet written on this subject was penned by none other than Paul Craig Roberts, former Assistant Secretary of the US Treasury and former associate editor of the *Wall Street Journal*. As Roberts explains: *"The US government creates whatever new bogeymen and incidents are necessary to further the neoconservative agenda of world hegemony and higher profits for the armaments industry ... If we look around for the terror that the police state and a decade of war has allegedly protected us from, the terror is hard to find. Except for 9/11 itself, assuming we accept the government's improbable conspiracy theory explanation, there have been no terror attacks on the US. Indeed, as RT pointed out on August 23, 2011, an investigative program at the University of California discovered that the domestic 'terror plots' hyped in the media were plotted by FBI agents."*

He goes on to explain the real motivation behind the war on terror. It's not to fight terrorism (as claimed by the bobble-head bleached blondes in the mainstream media) but rather to scare Americans into a state of blind obedience to a police state government: *"When I observe the gullibility of my fellow citizens at the absurd 'terror plots' that the US government manufactures, it causes me to realize that fear is the most powerful weapon any government has for advancing an undeclared agenda. Apparently, Americans, or most of them, are so ruled by fear that they suffer no remorse from "their" government's murder and dislocation of millions of innocent people. In the American mind, one billion 'towel-heads' have been reduced to terrorists who deserve to be exterminated."*

What's really amazing in all this is how easily the American "sheeple" are sucked into believing all the imaginary fairytale terrorists. But many folks are really waking up, there's no doubt about that, so watch out for more engineered "false flags" which will be blamed on the "terrorists." The mainstream media will then declare that we're "losing the war on terror" and therefore we need police checkpoints at every street corner, TSA in the streets of US cities, and more illegal NSA wiretapping. For our good, of course...

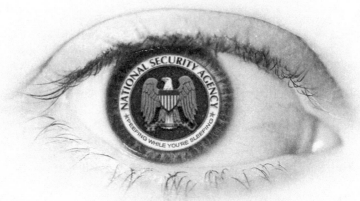

Oh yes, and we need to eliminate cash from society so that we can track everybody's purchases so the "terrorists" can't fund their operations. Heck, we need to get rid of the entire Bill of Rights! Who needs "rights" when all these police are everywhere to protect us, right?

According to Mike Adams (the "Health Ranger"), *"You who have bought into all this fabricated terror nonsense are the worst 'doom-and-gloomers' of our time, living your lives in a constant state of fear and despair, fretting about invisible imaginary terrorists who you think are going to magically leap out of your luggage and blow up an airplane. You've been indoctrinated by the 'if you see something, say something' paranoia, and you've been hoodwinked by a bunch of social engineers who know how to manipulate fear to achieve their desired political (and military) agendas. It's pathetic. And it's the oldest trick in the* *government book, of course: Use the **fear of terror** to manipulate the public into supporting a police state agenda which concentrates power in the hands of the executive branch, which quickly becomes a military dictatorship. Read your history, folks, or you will stupidly repeat it. It might also be worth your time to read George Orwell's 1984 novel, as it's very nearly a blueprint for the Department of Homeland Security's 'perpetual war' fraud.*" http://www.naturalnews.com

The "war on terror" is a carefully orchestrated, on-going, pre-emptive war of aggression which is unique in scope and ambition compared to anything before or since World War II. There is no doubt that the chief purpose of the "war on terror" has been to erect a control grid around the American people in our own homes.

Benjamin Franklin warned us that giving up our liberty to secure a little temporary safety, leaves us vulnerable to losing both. Mr. Franklin's quote was right in the middle of the true course of rectitude, wasn't it?

In the world of Dystopia: "*War is peace. Freedom is slavery. Ignorance is strength.*" ~ George Orwell in 1984.

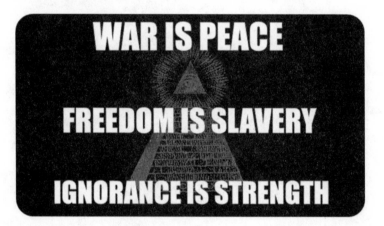

"*Terror is theatre ... Theatre's a con trick. Do you know what that means? Con trick? You've been deceived.*" ~ John Le Carré in The Little Drummer Girl.

RESOURCES

Websites
http://www.infowars.com/timeline-to-tyranny/
http://landdestroyer.blogspot.com/2011/09/war-on-terror-is-fraud.html
http://www.bollyn.com/the-fraudulent-war-on-terror/
http://www.infowars.com/?p=62008

Books
The War on Terror Fraud (Jose M. Paulino)
The Tyranny of Good Intentions (Paul Craig Roberts)

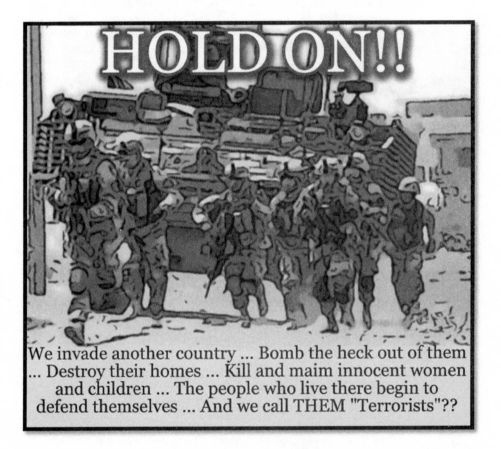

Chapter 14

~ THE WAR ON DRUGS ~

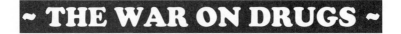

MONUMENTAL MYTH

The "war on drugs" is a term initially coined by President Nixon and commonly applied to an overt campaign of prohibition, military aid, and military intervention, with the stated aim being to define and reduce the illegal drug trade.

CAN YOU HANDLE THE TRUTH?

It's been almost 40 years since President Nixon ramped up the "war on drugs." The cost has been over **$1 TRILLION**, yet the USA continues to lead the world in drug use and we currently have 500,000 non-violent drug offenders living behind bars. In the past two chapters, I've presented the case that the "war on cancer" and the "war on terror" are both frauds. In this chapter, I will make the case that the Orwellian-named "war on drugs" is much the same. **A joke ... a farce ... a sham ... a charade**. You get the picture, right?

The "war on drugs" has resulted in one of largest bureaucracies in the District of Criminals (Washington DC). Of course, I'm talking about the Drug Enforcement Administration ("DEA"), which boasts over 10,000 employees in over 60 countries. Thanks to the "war on drugs," the USA has the infamous distinction of being the world's largest prison state, imprisoning more people than any other nation in the world (both in absolute numbers and proportionality). Roughly 1.5 million people are arrested each year for drug law violations, with 40% of them just for possessing marijuana. Heck, an American is arrested every 30 seconds for breaking one of the marijuana laws. Due to the "war on drugs," many people suffering from cancer (and other debilitating illnesses) are regularly denied access to their medicine or even arrested and prosecuted for using medical marijuana.

Let me explain the difference between the terms "hemp" and "marijuana" and "cannabis." The word "hemp" is English for a number of varieties of the cannabis plant, particularly the varieties like "industrial hemp" that were bred over time for industrial uses such as fuel, fiber, paper, seed, food, oil, etc. The term "marijuana" is of Spanish derivation, and was primarily used to describe varieties of cannabis that were more commonly bred over time for medicinal and recreational purposes (like *cannabis indica* and *cannabis sativa*).

Two cannabinoids are preeminent in cannabis – 1) THC, the psychoactive ingredient, and 2) CBD, which is an anti-psychoactive ingredient. "Marijuana" (which is actually a slang term to make it sound more "sinister") is high in the psychoactive cannabinoid, THC, and low in the anti-psychoactive cannabinoid, CBD. The reverse is true for industrial hemp, which has minimal THC and a much higher percentage of CBD. I prefer to use the terms "hemp" or "cannabis" for all varietals of the cannabis plant. Using the term "marijuana" is actually acquiescing to the pejorative intentions of the Medical Mafia that wants to ban this miracle plant ... not miracle "drug" ... miracle plant. You see, "marijuana" was one of the battle line words that marked the difference between "straights" and "stoners" ... between "Feds" and "heads."

Speaking of hemp, **did you know** that early laws in some American colonies actually required farmers to grow hemp, and they could go to jail for refusing to grow it? **Did you know** that, according to their diaries, many of our early presidents, including George Washington and Thomas Jefferson, grew hemp? **Did you know** that the American Declaration of Independence and the Constitution of the USA were both drafted on hemp paper? **Did you know** that Henry Ford built an experimental car body out of hemp fiber, which is 10 times stronger than steel? **Did you know** that the first Model-T was actually built to run on hemp gasoline?

I'll bet you didn't!

For millennia, hemp has been used in medicinal teas and tonics because of its healing properties. And, yes, it is an effective treatment for cancer. It not only relieves pain and helps with the appetite of cancer patients; it also has been shown to have curative properties. The chemicals in hemp (aka cannabis or marijuana) which are responsible for many of the medical benefits are called "cannabinoids." The most notable cannabinoid is "Delta-9-tetrahydrocannabinol" but most folks call it "THC."

As late as the 1930s in the USA, medicinal hemp tinctures with THC were available in most pharmacies. But in the 1940s, hemp was made illegal. But why would the US government outlaw a **plant** which has a plethora of useful applications? I'll tell you why. One main reason was that at that time, William Randolph Hearst and the Hearst Paper Manufacturing Division of Kimberly Clark owned millions of acres of timberland. The Hearst Company, which supplied most of the paper products in the USA and also owned most of the newspapers, stood to lose billions because of the hemp industry. In 1937, Dupont patented the processes to make plastics from oil and coal. Dupont's Annual Report urged stockholders to invest in its new petrochemical division. Synthetics such as plastics, nylon, and rayon could now be made from oil. Natural hemp industrialization would have ruined over 80% of Dupont's business.

Andrew Mellon became President Hoover's Secretary of the Treasury and Dupont's primary investor. He appointed his future nephew-in-law (Harry J. Anslinger) to head the Federal Bureau of Narcotics and Dangerous Drugs. Secret meetings were held by these financial tycoons. Hemp was declared "dangerous" and a threat to their billion dollar enterprises. For their dynasties to remain intact, hemp had to go. They took an obscure Mexican slang word ("marijuana") and pushed it into the consciousness of America.

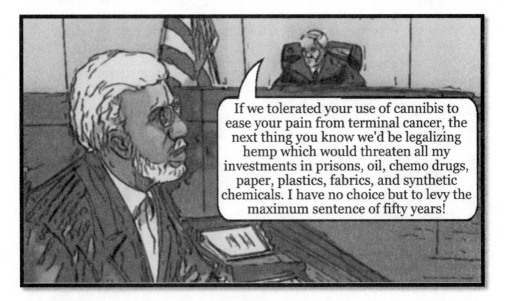

A media blitz of "yellow journalism" raged in the 1920s and 1930s; Hearst's newspapers ran stories emphasizing the horrors of "marijuana." Readers were led to believe that it was responsible for car accidents, loose morality, and countless acts of violence, incurable insanity, and brutal murders. Hollywood films like "Reefer Madness" and "Marijuana: The Devil's Weed" were nothing more than blatant propaganda designed by these industrialists to create an enemy. Their purpose was to gain public support so that anti-marijuana laws could be passed. Coupled with the fact that Big Pharma didn't like the non-toxic and inexpensive medicinal applications, and you have two main reasons for "criminalizing" a glorious, medicinal plant with numerous therapeutic and industrial uses. Hemp was plentiful and inexpensive, and to make matters worse for the Medical Mafia, it didn't cause any additional medical conditions that required prescriptions for more poison. So, it was **outlawed**.

The medical evidence for the effectiveness of THC at treating cancer and also reducing pain is overwhelming. We have known this since 1974 when the first experiment documenting marijuana's anti-tumor effects took place at the Medical College of Virginia at the behest of the US government and the National Institute of Health (NIH).

The purpose of the study was to show that marijuana damages the immune system and causes cancer. However, the study found instead that THC slowed the growth of three kinds of cancer in mice (lung and breast cancer, and a virus-induced leukemia). **OOPS!** We can't have that information made public can we? So, the DEA quickly shut down the Virginia study and all further research on the anti-cancer effects of marijuana ... even though the researchers found that THC **cures** cancer!

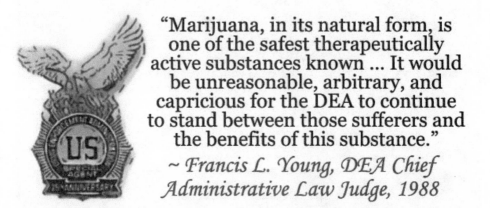

"Marijuana, in its natural form, is one of the safest therapeutically active substances known ... It would be unreasonable, arbitrary, and capricious for the DEA to continue to stand between those sufferers and the benefits of this substance."
~ *Francis L. Young, DEA Chief Administrative Law Judge, 1988*

In 2000, researchers in Madrid learned that the THC in hemp inhibits the spread of brain cancer through selectively inducing programmed cell death (apoptosis) in brain tumor cells without negatively impacting surrounding healthy cells. They were able to destroy **incurable** brain tumors in rats by injecting them with THC. But sadly, most Americans don't know anything about the Madrid discovery, since virtually no major US newspapers carried the story.

A 2007 Harvard Medical School study (published in *Science Daily*) showed that the THC in hemp decreased lung cancer tumors by 50% and significantly reduces the ability of the cancer to metastasize (spread). Other researchers have also shown that THC is an effective treatment for Hodgkin's disease and Kaposi's Sarcoma. A recent study out of Thailand demonstrated that THC can also fight bile duct cancer, which is rare and deadly. As a matter of fact, the International Medical Verities Association is including hemp oil on its cancer protocol.

On March 29, 2001, the *San Antonio Current* printed a story by Raymond Cushing titled, *"Pot Shrinks Tumors – Government Knew in '74"* which detailed government and media suppression of news about marijuana cancer benefits. Cushing noted in his article that it was hard to believe that the knowledge that cannabis can be used to fight cancer has been suppressed for almost thirty years and aptly concluded his article by saying: *"Millions of people have died horrible deaths and in many cases, families exhausted their savings on dangerous, toxic and expensive drugs. Now we are just beginning to realize that while marijuana has never killed anyone, marijuana prohibition has killed millions."*

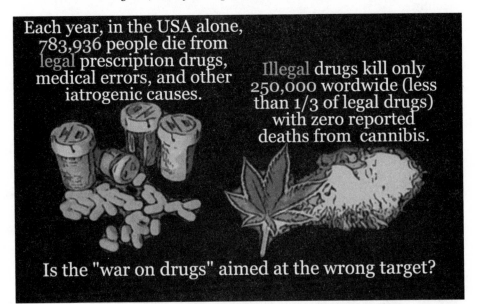

Each year, in the USA alone, 783,936 people die from legal prescription drugs, medical errors, and other iatrogenic causes.

Illegal drugs kill only 250,000 wordwide (less than 1/3 of legal drugs) with zero reported deaths from cannibis.

Is the "war on drugs" aimed at the wrong target?

Marijuana has also been proven to be effective in the treatment of alcohol abuse, ALS ("Lou Gehrig Disease"), arthritis, asthma, atherosclerosis, bipolar disorder, MRSA, depression, dystonia, epilepsy, hepatitis C, Parkinson's disease, psoriasis, sleep apnea, and anorexia nervosa. But the government has made it illegal to grow this amazing plant. Although you can't legally purchase this miracle plant (unless you live in one of the few states with legalized medical marijuana), you can still get all the booze you want. **Booze it up!** Alcohol, a legal and taxed drug in America, causes nearly 4% of deaths worldwide, more than AIDS, tuberculosis or violence, according to the World Health Organization. Approximately 2.5 million people in the world die from alcohol related causes each year.

It is impossible to overdose on marijuana; the "war on drugs" should actually be waged against legal prescription drugs and the drug-pushing doctors that prescribe them! Why? Because prescription drugs (the ones Americans get from their "omniscient" doctors to quell the symptoms of disease resulting from GMO food, fluoridated water, vaccines, heavy metal poisoning, MSG, and aspartame) are actually killing **more** people than the "illegal" drugs. According to the FDA's own website, legal prescription drugs kill over 100,000 people per year. According to a 2012 report from Brandeis University, prescription painkillers like methadone, oxycodone, and hydrocodone are responsible for more fatal overdoses (in the United States) than heroin and cocaine combined! According the CDC, enough prescription painkillers were prescribed in 2010 to medicate every adult American around-the-clock for an entire month.

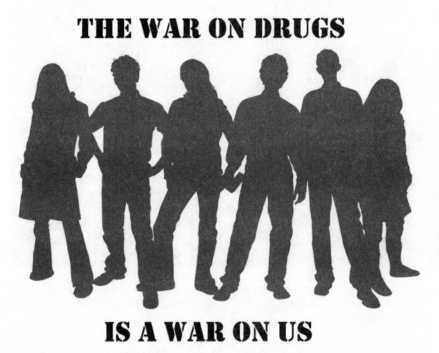

THE WAR ON DRUGS

IS A WAR ON US

While it should be more appropriately called a "war on people," drug prohibition is one of the biggest infringements on individual liberties in America today. To regulate what someone can or can't ingest or smoke is like regulating what they can or can't read, write, listen to, or speak. This is not an endorsement of drug use, but the realization that the "war on drugs" and unregulated government power are far more dangerous narcotics than drugs could ever be. Unconstitutional, warrantless "no-knock" SWAT raids (over 100 per day in America according to *Huffington Post*) are a direct consequence of the government's regulation of our blood content.

I'm sure that you're familiar with the Fast and Furious gun trafficking operation, in which the US government sold guns to known criminals and then the Department of Justice ("DoJ") repeatedly lied about it. It turns out that there was a policy in place at the highest levels in the ATF and the DoJ to transport weapons to Mexican drug cartels. In 2011, when Attorney General Eric Holder testified under oath before a Congressional committee that, *"I probably heard about Fast and Furious for the first time over the last few weeks."* He was lying, and was proved to be a liar in Fox News reports that ensued.

Remember Scooter Libby? He recalled the date of a meeting to the FBI differently than did others, and was convicted of a felony. However, unlike the case of Scooter Libby, Fast and Furious has resulted in the death of two US federal agents and at least 200 Mexicans killed by guns supplied to the drug cartels. The Watergate adage *"it's not the crime, it's the cover-up that matters"* comes to mind. The only difference is that the crime in Fast and Furious – supplying thousands of sophisticated firearms to a drug cartel resulting in the deaths of hundreds of people including two federal agents – dwarfs the magnitude of a third rate burglary. We'll revisit "Fast and Furious" later in the book.

But that's not all. According to a December 3, 2011 *New York Times* article, apparently, while the ATF was shipping weapons to the drug cartels, the DEA was helping them launder their cash. That's right! Many people know that Wachovia Bank had to admit to laundering $378.4 billion in drug money between 2004 and 2007 and that they paid a mere $160 million in fines to avoid prosecution. What they don't know is that the money was from a drug cartel in Mexico that the DEA and the DoJ supported as part of a program called "Divide and Conquer" which was designed to weed all the other drug gangs out and leave the one cartel (our cartel) in place. Of course, this was all done to "catch the bad guys" right?

So, I guess that in the District of Criminals, when you get caught doing something immoral (oh yeah, like morality factors into any equation in Washington DC anymore) and illegal, all you have to do is say you were doing it to "catch the bad guys." Providing weapons to murderous thugs in Mexico to destabilize the country? Just say you did it to "catch the bad guys." Laundering colossal amounts of drug money for off the books financing of your destabilization teams? Just say you were doing it to "catch the bad guys." Pretty simple, eh? And as long as you have overpaid bobble-head stenographers (posing as journalists) in the mindless mainstream media providing homogenized, pasteurized "news reports," the technique will work like a charm.

Want more examples of the phony "war on drugs"?

We can go back to the 1980s where the CIA was trading weapons with our enemy (Iran), even though they held 52 US students hostage for over a year. Why? Follow the money. The CIA was charging extravagant prices for the weapons in order to fund the Nicaraguan Contras, who were attempting to overthrow the democratically elected government in what equated to a fascist coup. Guess how else they funded the Nicaraguan Contras? With drug money. Yep. Crack cocaine. Traitor Oliver North can tell you all about this scandal. And so can "Freeway" Ricky Ross and Gary Webb who testified that the CIA created crack cocaine and sold it to the Crips and the Bloods in order to fund the Nicaraguan Contras. Gary Webb wrote "Dark Alliance" exposing this fact and when he turned up dead with two bullets in his head, they called it a "suicide." Hang tight. There's an entire chapter on Gary Webb later in the book.

We can go back to Mena, Arkansas (and the start of the Clinton rise to power) where it's known that the CIA was bringing in cocaine to fund its imperial ambitions. A bunch of people ended up dead in that area. People associated with Mena. Just do a search for "Kevin Ives" and "Don Henry" to get you started. On a personal note, I have a friend who used to have a nationally syndicated radio show in the 1990s. He had scheduled an interview with an ex-CIA agent and airline pilot who was lifelong friends with soon-to-be President of the USA, William Jefferson Clinton ("Bill"). The ex-CIA agent asked to remain anonymous, so let's just call him "Ed." My friend met Ed the day before the interview at a local restaurant, where Ed shared the following true story with him, giving him unambiguous instructions **never** to share his identity in relation to this story, or he would deny it, fearing for the life of his family. The only reason Ed is still alive today is that he was childhood friends with Clinton.

One day, while the lifelong friends were hanging out at the Governor's mansion in Little Rock, Bill asked Ed if he wanted to be in the CIA. Ed wasn't sure how this would be possible since he had never applied and had never submitted to a background check. "No problem" said Bill. Within 2 weeks, Bill called him and welcomed him to the CIA. Ed was not really all that surprised, since he knew that Bill had techniques of "getting things done." Ed's first assignment was flying a plane (full of unmarked boxes) from Central America to a small airport in Mena, Arkansas. Then another ... then another.

After a few trips, Ed got a little curious as to what "cargo" he was actually transporting, so he opened one of the boxes. To his surprise, it was cocaine. "Candy cane" ... "white horse." You get the picture, right? So, as soon as he landed the plane in Mena, Ed headed straight for the Governor's mansion in Little Rock. *"Bill, you have a serious problem,"* he told his friend. *"Those planes I've been flying for you are full of cocaine."*

At that moment, Ed said that Bill put his feet up on his desk, leaned back, and took a puff on his cigar, smiled, and said, *"Welcome to the big time."* Realizing that he was "in deep," Ed then asked Bill, *"What do you think (then President) Bush will do to us if he finds out?"* To which Bill replied, *"Who do you think is running the show?"* **True story.** Every word.

On August 23, 1987, in a rural community just south of Little Rock, police officers murdered two teenage boys (Kevin Ives and Don Henry) because they witnessed a police-protected drug drop. The drop was part of a drug smuggling operation based at a small airport in … yes … Mena, Arkansas. Of course, the official story is that they were run over by a train. The coroner, Dr. Fahmy Malak, ruled it an accidental death. Even though he had never tested their THC levels, he claimed they had smoked so much marijuana that they "fell asleep" on the railway tracks and did not wake up when the train approached. **Seriously.** That was the gist of his report, which was nothing more than a fairytale to cover up their murder. Malak's report makes about as much sense as saying that they were "hobbits" who were put under an evil spell by the Eye of Sauron.

The mistake with Malak's monumental myth is that the train conductor saw bodies on the track and applied the train whistle and emergency brakes. It would have been impossible for someone not to awaken from that! Later on, the bodies were exhumed and another autopsy was performed. The second autopsy found the cause of death to be blunt force trauma. In other words, the boys were murdered then dumped on the railway tracks. It was also determined that Malak had tampered with the evidence trying to hide that fact. Turns out there were several murder cases that Dr. Malak ruled as suicides – including one man who allegedly shot himself five times and one man that was beheaded – which forces us to question why Governor Bill Clinton was so supportive of such an incompetent buffoon. The fact is that Ives and Henry were *"Arkancided"* because they saw something they weren't supposed to see, and Clinton needed Malak to cover it up. Just do a search for "Clinton body count."

Did you hear about the CIA plane that crashed in Mexico on April 25, 2012, only seventeen months after an American-registered DC9 airliner was busted with **5.5 tons** of cocaine? This was the second drug trafficking incident in Mexico's Yucatan which involved an American-registered Gulfstream II business jet owned by a dummy CIA front company named "Donna Blue Aircraft Inc." of Coconut Beach, Florida. FAA records show that the jet with tail number N987SA crash-landed with **3.7 tons** of cocaine aboard. Coincidentally (or maybe not), the same jet with tail number N987SA has been involved in the transport of extraordinary rendition victims to Guantanamo Bay. Logs also show that the plane flew twice between Washington, D.C. and Guantanamo and once between Oxford, Connecticut and Guantanamo. The American flights would have been CIA and Pentagon interrogators being ferried to interrogations at Guantanamo.

Have you heard of Barry Seal? He was a CIA agent who is said to have smuggled between $3 billion and $5 billion worth of drugs into the USA. According to friends, he was about to "come clean" and "spill the beans." Before that could happen, he was brutally murdered in 1986 in Baton Rouge. Seal's murder would openly expose (for all the world to see) the sordid underbelly of America's duplicitous "war on drugs," and how drug smuggling was, in fact, sanctioned by powerful men in order to advance a hidden agenda. Seal's life (and death) was the subject of a "made-for-TV" movie, *Double Crossed*, which starred Dennis Hopper as Seal.

Let's play a game of "Logic 101" here, shall we? Since it's actually the **US government** providing the weapons, the protection from prosecution, the lethal hits on the competition, and the resources to launder the cash, then isn't it actually the **US government** who is the drug cartel? I mean, after all, we are guarding the heroin fields in Afghanistan. Guess someone wants a monopoly on all the illicit drugs in the world just like they want a monopoly on the oil fields, healthcare, cancer treatments, GMO corn, and the central banks.

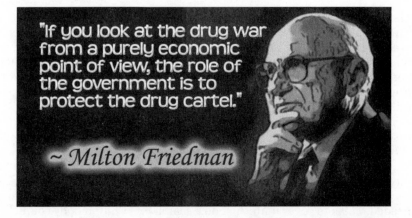

The "war on drugs" has become a war on families, a war on public health, and a war on our constitutional rights. Want to learn more about this phony war? I suggest you watch an excellent documentary entitled *American Drug War* (http://americandrugwar.com). Inspired by the death of four family members from "legal drugs," Texas filmmaker Kevin Booth set out to discover why the "war on drugs" has become such a big failure. Three and a half years in the making, the film follows gang members, former DEA and CIA agents, narcotics officers, judges, politicians, prisoners, and celebrities. Most notably the film befriends "Freeway" Ricky Ross (the man many accuse for starting the crack epidemic) who, after being arrested, discovered that his cocaine source had been working for the CIA ("Cocaine Import Agency").

The film shows unequivocally that the phony "war on drugs" has given rise to millions of Americans being incarcerated for low-level, nonviolent drug offenses. Archaic drug laws and mandatory minimums have driven an enormous spike in the prison population over the past few decades, leading many states to literally run out of jails, and have given rise to the "for-profit" prison industry.

RESOURCES

Websites
http://www.tpuc.org/content/marijuana-conspiracy
www.alternet.org/story/9257
http://americandrugwar.com/
http://americandrugwar2.com/

Videos & Movies
"Hemp For Victory"
http://www.youtube.com/watch?v=Y36Wjkt9iTk
"Run from the Cure" (Rick Simpson)
http://www.youtube.com/watch?v=aGjC4HReFL0
"American Drug War" (Kevin Booth)
http://www.youtube.com/watch?v=6CyuBuT_7I4

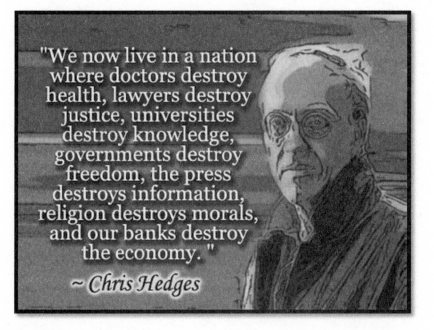

"We now live in a nation where doctors destroy health, lawyers destroy justice, universities destroy knowledge, governments destroy freedom, the press destroys information, religion destroys morals, and our banks destroy the economy."

~ Chris Hedges

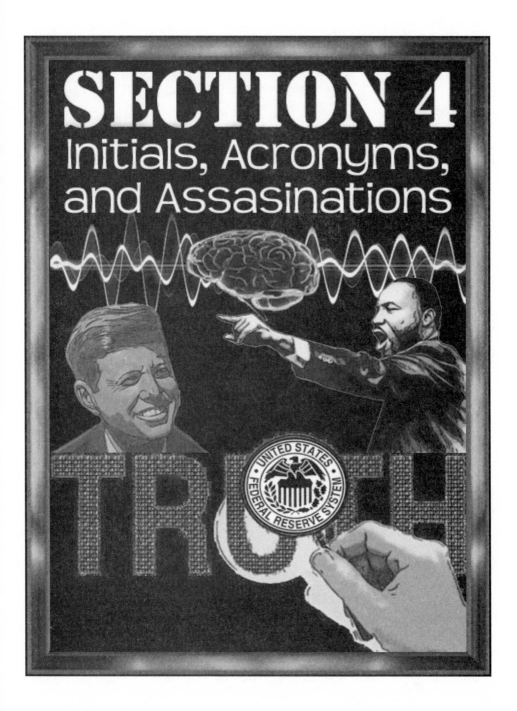

SECTION 4
Initials, Acronyms, and Assasinations

Chapter 15

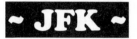

MONUMENTAL MYTH

President John F. Kennedy ("JFK"), the 35th President of the USA, was shot in Dallas by Lee Harvey Oswald, a Communist, anti-American, ex-military "lone nut." The "kill shot" was from over 260 feet as Oswald was located on the 6th floor of the Texas school book depository building. Oswald used a rifle he obtained via mail-order using a false name. While in the custody of Dallas police, Oswald was shot two days later by Jack Ruby. Ruby eventually died in prison. Case closed.

CAN YOU HANDLE THE TRUTH?

There are so many anomalies involved with the assassination of JFK that I can't possibly cover all of them. But I'll cover enough to convince you that something smells fishy in Norway, as the saying goes. My good buddy, Liam Scheff, wrote an incredible book, Official Stories, in which he covered the assassination of JFK. His book was an inspiration for this chapter, and I'll be quoting from it throughout. So, are you ready to take the red pill and stay in Wonderland? Ready to feel like a nut? Ready to go deep down the rabbit hole? I hope so, because we're heading south ... way south ... like Antarctica ... with the penguins!

Anomaly #1 – The Magic Bullet

To believe the monumental myth concerning JFK's assassination by "lone nut" Oswald, one must believe that the laws of physics were somehow "suspended" for a couple of seconds on the afternoon of November 22, 1963. As Liam wrote, for a single bullet to achieve *"what no piece of metal fired from a gun has ever achieved. Seven wounds in two people across shifting planes, through a back and neck, a ribcage, a wrist and into a thigh, at jumpy angles over most of 2 seconds, emerging unscathed – not smashed, bent or squashed due to impact, but only lightly scuffed and nearly pristine."*

Why does the government's mythical story require a magic bullet? Let's look at the facts. The Secret Service and the FBI reported that three cartridge cases were found at the scene. This information was given to the Warren Commission and it became their "ball and chain" because they were forced to work within those parameters (i.e. three bullets and three bullets **only**).

So let's account for all three bullets, shall we?

One bullet hit JFK in the back. The best evidence of this exists in the form of his suit coat and shirt. **One bullet** hit JFK in the head. This evidence is found in the Zapruder film, and attested to by numbers of witnesses. **One bullet** hit Governor Connally, and **one bullet** missed, injuring James Tague. The Warren Commission admitted this fact of the missed shot.

This forced them into the "magic bullet" scenario that combines the back shot and the Connally hit. According to Arlen Spector, who came up with what is now known as the "magic bullet" theory, Oswald fired his gun in a right-to-left trajectory, and the bullet went through the back of JFK's neck, exited the front of his neck, turned right to enter into Governor Connolly of Texas, who was sitting in the front seat. The bullet entered right behind his armpit, then changed angles, crushing a rib, exiting the front of his chest, then changed angles again, moved upward and then angled down, going through his wrist, changed angles again, and eventually lodged in his thigh. Seven wounds ... one bullet. Eventually, like most bullets do (sarcasm intended), it plopped out of his leg and deposited itself on a gurney next to the governor, where it was later found by an employee at Parkland Memorial Hospital. Oh yes, it was in pristine condition.

Seriously? They want us to believe that? Hey, I know what happened! A miniature leprechaun leapt out of the gurney and transformed the bullet back into perfect condition. Yeah, that's what happened! It was ... a leprechaun! That's the ticket! Oh, by the way, for his "magic bullet" balderdash theory, Arlen Spector was made Senator, practically for life. A non-zombie, thinking person knows that there were **at least** four bullets fired. We all know the precise timing of the shots by means of the Zapruder film. We all know that the indisputable "fourth" bullet means at least one more gunman. Two (or more) gunmen mean a conspiracy. This is the pin that bursts the balloon of the mainstream media's monumental myth that Oswald was a "lone wolf nut." From here on out the discussion is purely academic, relatively trivial, and mostly contrived. The official story is all done with *"Four bullets, Two gunmen."* **Game Over!** But I'll continue just to humor you...

Anomaly #2 – Secret Service Behavior

JFK's motorcade was scheduled to head straight down Main Street. It wasn't supposed to turn right on Houston and then left on Elm, slowing down to around 10 miles per hour, with the bullet-proof bubble top removed, under open windows. Isn't it the sole responsibility of the Secret Service to protect the President, to evaluate the landscape and identify potential risks, and to keep the motorcade away from dead-ends and potential areas of triangulated fire?

Where were the Secret Service agents? Do a web search for "*secret service stand down*" and you'll find dozens of videos in which you can watch Secret Service agents Clint Hill and John Ready (who were jogging alongside JFK's limo) being waved off by Special Agent In Charge Emory Roberts. You can see them argue with him as they appear flabbergasted at the order to leave JFK with no bodyguard while riding in an open car. Their body language screams, "*What? You want us to do WHAT?*" They shrug their shoulders then follow orders.

Is this the kind of conduct you would expect from an agency that routinely sends an advance team to a city a month (or more) prior to the President's arrival in order to make preparations? The assassination of JFK would have been very difficult if those agents had been flanking the limo, which they always did. This is stunning in itself, but is only one of more than fifteen indications that the Secret Service set up JFK for the hit, which include that two agents were left behind at Love Field, that the vehicles were in the wrong order, that the 112th Military Intelligence Unit was ordered to "stand down" rather than provide protection throughout the city, and that the motorcycle escort was reduced to four, who were instructed not to ride forward the rear wheels. Open windows were not covered and the crowd was allowed to spill out into the street – totally violating protocol. Surprised? I'm not. I mean, didn't the Praetorian Guard pull away from Caesar and allow the mob to remove him from his throne?

And after all, the purpose was to get rid of JFK. And they did. Less than a minute later, JFK's brains were splattered all over the limo. After the assassination, Secret Service Agent Roy Kellerman essentially had to steal JFK's body from Parkland Memorial Hospital to prevent the coroner, Dr. Earl Rose, from performing an autopsy (an honest autopsy) as required under Texas law. There was a loud, ugly altercation between Dr. Rose and Kellerman at Parkland, and the Secret Service agents eventually had to show their weapons in order to snatch JFK's body away from the hospital. Why would they not want an autopsy by the Dallas medical examiner? Let's examine that question in the next section.

If you get the chance, read the work of Vincent Palamara. He has interviewed many of the JFK Secret Service men and reveals many details unknown before.

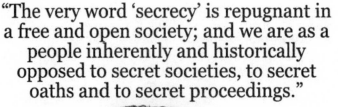

"The very word 'secrecy' is repugnant in a free and open society; and we are as a people inherently and historically opposed to secret societies, to secret oaths and to secret proceedings."

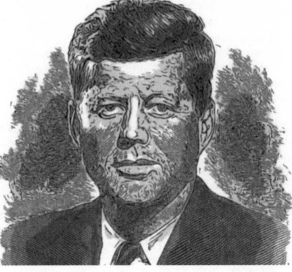

Anomaly #3 – The Post Mortem

From where did the fatal shot come? What exactly happened on that historic Friday in 1963? What did the autopsy conclude? Let's examine a few quotes from people who were at Parkland Memorial Hospital and who saw JFK's body up close and personal.

According to Dr. Charles Crenshaw, surgeon at Parkland Hospital: "*The head wound was difficult to see when he was laying on the back of his head. However, afterwards when they moved his face towards the left, one could see the large, right rear parietal, occipital, blasted out hole, the size of my fist, which is 2½ inches in diameter. The brain, cerebral portion had been blurred out and also there was the cerebellum hanging out from that wound. It was clearly an exit wound from the right rear, behind the ear. A right occipital area hole, the size of my fist.*"

Doris Nelson, emergency room nurse at Parkland Hospital, stated: "*We wrapped him up .... and I saw his whole head ... There was no hair back there ... It was blown away. Some of his head was blown away and his brains were fallen down on the stretcher.*" Then we have Dr. Kemp Clark, neurosurgeon, who stated: "*I was called because the President had sustained a brain injury. It was apparent the President had sustained a lethal wound. A missile had gone in and out of the back of his head, causing extensive lacerations and loss of brain tissue. Shortly after I arrived, the President's heart stopped. We attempted resuscitation, initiating closed chest heart massage, but to no avail. We were able to obtain a palpable pulse by this method but again to no avail. President Kennedy died on the emergency table after 20 minutes.*"

There are more. Dozens more. People that have two things in common. 1) They all saw JFK after he was shot, and 2) they all testified that there was a huge wound at the **back** of JFK's head. Not the front. At the **back**.

So where did the fatal shot come from? While one straightforward official investigation (like the 1963 Warren Commission) should have settled this matter, but in this case it didn't. On a side note, in the words of Liam Scheff, "*Who did the Warren Commission appoint to investigate all intelligence leads and witnesses for the official story? Our friend from the Central American Banana Wars, the United Fruit Company, lawyer for Bush family interests in Germany, kingpin of coup d'états, former head of the CIA and proud member of the don't-worry-about-that-swastika-school-of-international-banking – the man you know as: Allen Welsh Dulles. Go figure. Fired from the CIA to investigate the murder of the guy who fired him. I guess they really wanted to get away with it.*"

There were three additional, publicized probes: those of the so-called "Clark Panel" in 1968, the Rockefeller Commission in 1975, and the House Select Committee on Assassinations (HSCA) in 1978. And there was also another one conducted without public disclosure in 1966 and 1967 by the US Justice Department. Yet despite repeated investigations, there still remain glaring gaps in the "evidence." For example, all five groups of investigators failed to question at least one key medical witness, the President's personal physician, Admiral George Burkley. The admiral was the only physician who was intimately involved with both JFK's emergency care in Dallas and with his autopsy at the Naval Hospital in Bethesda, Maryland. Yet he was not asked to testify by any of the investigators. The ironic tragedy of this omission is that Burkley had repeatedly said he believed there had been a conspiracy. But they didn't want anyone even insinuating the "C" word. No, a lone nut did it. That's what they told us. That's what we were supposed to believe. "*Don't think about it. Don't investigate it. Just shut up and repeat the official story. Don't worry about the anomalies and glaring inconsistencies.*"

Among the glaring issues that cry out for explanation is the multiple delivery of JFK's body to the Bethesda morgue on the evening of the assassination. After JFK was declared dead at Parkland Hospital in Dallas, his body was wrapped in sheets and placed into an extremely expensive, heavy, ornate casket. The casket was taken from Parkland and delivered to Dallas Love Field, where it was placed into the back of Air Force One, the plane in which the new president, Lyndon Johnson, was traveling. A few hours later, the plane landed at Andrews Air Force Base outside Washington, D.C. The casket was removed from the plane and placed into an automobile (carrying Jackie Kennedy) which slowly made its way to Bethesda Naval Hospital where JFK's casket was officially carried into the morgue at 8:00 PM

There was one big problem. Something Jackie didn't know. The casket did **not** contain JFK's body. Unbeknownst to her, his body had secretly been removed from the Parkland casket and placed into a body bag and a cheap shipping casket which (with JFK's body inside it) was secretly placed into a black hearse containing a team of men in suits. They transported the casket to the back of the Bethesda Naval Hospital, where the morgue was located. A waiting team of soldiers carried the cheap shipping casket into the morgue at 6:35 PM, even while Jackie was still slowly traveling from Andrews Air Force Base to the Bethesda facilities under the erroneous assumption that JFK's body was inside the casket that was in the back of her car.

How do we know this happened? Because it was witnessed by several Navy and Marine enlisted men who were there and saw it happen. Moreover, their eyewitness accounts are supported by two documents that were discovered in the 1990s by the Assassination Records Review Board, the agency that had been created in the wake of the storm over government secrecy in the JFK assassination produced by Oliver Stone's 1991 movie *JFK*.

According to his incredibly documented article *"The Ongoing Kennedy Casket Mystery,"* Jacob G. Hornberger explains, *"The first document was a written report of the funeral home that handled the embalming of the president's body. It contained the following notation: 'Body removed from metal shipping casket at NSHN at Bethesda.' The second document was an official military report filed four days after the assassination by Marine Sgt. Roger Boyajian, which stated in part: 'The detail arrived at the hospital at approximately 1800 [6:00 PM] and after reporting as ordered several members of the detail were posted at entrances to prevent unauthorized persons from entering the prescribed area…. At approximately 18:35 [6:35 PM] the casket was received at the morgue entrance and taken inside.' "*

What about the photos? Here's where the rabbit hole gets deep. The **autopsy** photos show that the back of JFK's head was virtually without a blemish, except for a small red spot near the top of the back of the head, with a large wound at the front. However, the autopsy photos were inconsistent to photos taken at Parkland Memorial Hospital, where doctors had testified that JFK's gaping skull wound was not in front, but in the back. So what happened?

The preponderance of the evidence renders a nearly unavoidable conclusion: that sometime between Dallas and Andrews Air Force Base, unidentified US government agents secretly removed JFK's body from the expensive, elaborate casket into which it had been placed at Parkland and then secretly delivered it in a cheap shipping casket to the Bethesda morgue at 6:35 PM How did the "wound to back of the head" disappear and morph into a "wound to the front"? Did someone altar the corpse of JFK prior to the autopsy?

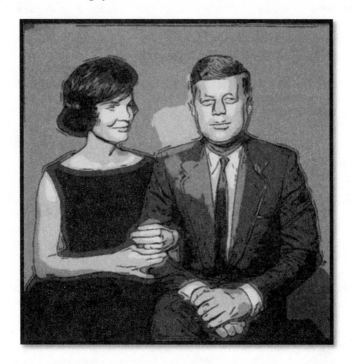

In the previous section, I posed the question, *"Why would they not want an autopsy by the Dallas medical examiner?"* Are you getting the picture? What was the purpose of the secret, early delivery of JFK's body to the Bethesda morgue? Why was the entire episode kept secret?

Think. Be **logical** – not emotional. There is only one conclusion. They needed to change JFK's wounds prior to the start of the official autopsy to hide evidence of shots having been fired from the front. They needed to cover up the huge hole in the back of JFK's head and clean up all the brains. Because a large hole at the back of the head indicates a shot from the front, which then would have ruined the official "lone nut" Oswald story.

Don't forget, after all, that the team of doctors that treated JFK at Parkland held a press conference immediately after the president had been declared dead, at which they announced that the hole in the front of Kennedy's neck was an entry wound. Don't forget also that several witnesses verified that there was a big hole in the back of JKF's head that denoted an exit wound, indicating that he was shot from the front. It is undisputed that Oswald was situated behind JFK and, therefore, could not have fired any shots from the front.

You see, now it starts to make sense that the team of Secret Service agents at Parkland Hospital (led by Roy Kellerman) brandished guns and threatened to use force to prevent Dr. Earl Rose (the Parkland coroner) from conducting the autopsy, as Texas law required.

It would also explain the need to place the autopsy under the control of the military, which could be relied upon to follow orders, do their duty, and keep the entire episode top secret.

Anomaly #4 – The *Christchurch STAR*

I used to live in New Zealand. I never could get used to the fact that the time in the USA was approximately 18 hours **behind** the time in New Zealand (depending upon the particular time zone). I frequently had problems converting the time, especially when I was trying to watch the Super Bowl (in the middle of the night).

Apparently, the "powers that be" also have problems with time zone conversions. You see, JFK was hit at 12:30 PM on Nov 22nd, Dallas time, which was 6:30 AM November 23rd in Christchurch, New Zealand. The *Christchurch STAR* reported JFK's assassination in the Saturday edition. It is evident that much of the "news" items about the assassination that appeared in that issue of the *STAR*, had to have been written **before** the shooting took place. The paper had to have been printed **before** Oswald had been arraigned for the crime of killing JFK.

Keep in mind that Oswald, although picked up by the police on suspicion for the murder of a Dallas Patrolman (J.D. Tippet) only 35 minutes after Kennedy was shot, was not arraigned for the assassination of JFK until 11:26 PM on November 22nd, which was 6:26 PM on November 23rd in Christchurch. It was typical for the *STAR* to be "on the streets" between 1 PM and 2 PM each afternoon, which was between 7 PM and 8 PM on

November 22nd in Dallas. Here's the kicker. The *Christchurch STAR* printed an article stating that Oswald was arrested under suspicion of shooting JFK ... **before** he was charged! On the following page is the actual photo from the 11/23/1963 *Christchurch STAR*. I have enlarged the caption to make it easier to read.

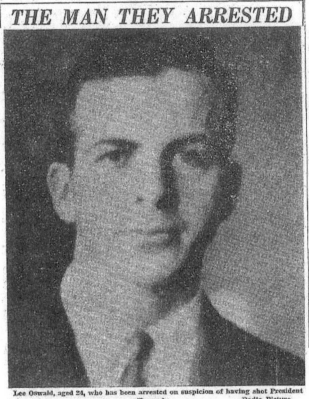

THE MAN THEY ARRESTED

Lee Oswald, aged 24, who has been arrested on suspicion of having shot President Kennedy. —Radio Picture

Lee Oswald, aged 24, who has been arrested on suspicion of having shot President Kennedy.

Are you getting the picture? Do the math. A newspaper on the streets between 1 and 2 PM on the 23rd, in Christchurch, had to have been printed and on the streets at least 4 to 5 hours **before** Oswald had been arraigned for JFK's murder.

Amazingly, this early afternoon newspaper, published in New Zealand, contained many columns of Lee Harvey Oswald's biography that must have been assembled, written, and transmitted around the world many hours before Oswald had been arraigned. Other papers were given the same material about Oswald. They printed it too. Keep in mind that

Oswald was picked up by the police as a suspect in the crime of killing a Dallas policeman and **not** for killing JFK! As a matter of fact, Oswald didn't even know what he had been charged with, and once he found out he was charged with murdering JFK, he uttered his infamous words: "*I'm just a patsy.*" He claimed that he hadn't even been at the window when the President was shot. He was sitting floors below, eating his lunch. And, for the record, his supervisor agreed with him.

Back to the *Christchurch STAR* story. In the lower left-hand corner of the front page there is a story under the heading, "*Arrested Man Lived in Russia.*" At that time the STAR, and other papers around the world, also published a fine studio photo of Oswald. There is no way that the newspapers could have run that select photo unless it had been provided to them before the murder and his arraignment. There were not picture quality scanning machines in 1963! There was no email, thus images could not be transmitted electronically. Plus, Oswald, who had yet to be charged, was wearing street clothes that day, not a suit coat and tie. There can be no question but what this "Oswald biography" that was flashed around the world even before he was charged with the crime was a preplanned part of the monumental myth.

Anomaly #5 – The Weapon

Early reports from newsmen and authorities on November 22, 1963 indicated that the weapon allegedly used to assassinate JFK was a 7.65 German Mauser bolt action rifle. The rifle had been found by Dallas police on the sixth floor of the Texas School Book Depository, a building which overlooked the Presidential motorcade at the time of the assassination. The man who found the gun, Deputy Eugene Boone, signed a sworn affidavit claiming the weapon in question had been identified as a Mauser. So did Deputy Constable Seymour Weitzman. Deputy Sheriff Roger Craig, who was present when the rifle was found, even claims to have seen "*7.65 Mauser*" written stamped on the murder weapon. Dallas District Attorney Henry Wade passed on this bit of information to the press with a moderate degree of certainty, and various news anchors such as Walter Cronkite presented the Mauser claim as fact to the American public. Why not a 7.63 Mauser? Why not a 7.90 Mauser? Why? Because they found a **7.65 Mauser**. That's what they saw. The truth is the truth.

Not widely reported in the annuals of the Mauser controversy is the Warren Commission testimony of Malcolm Price. On October 26, 1963 Price was at the Sports Drome Rifle Range in the next booth over from Lee Oswald and took note of the rifle he was using. He reportedly talked to Oswald about the rifle and was allowed to handle it. He identified the weapon as a German Mauser with a Tascosa brand scope. Anyway, back to November 22, 1963. Within a matter of hours, these initial reports about the 7.65 Mauser were "corrected" and news-hungry Americans were informed that the alleged murder weapon was actually a 6.5 Italian Mannlicher Carcano bolt action rifle with a leather strap and telescopic sight. So when did the switcheroo take place? Your guess is as good as mine. In the end, the rifle was traced to the post office box of A.J. Hidell, an alias used by Oswald.

How could three police officers, all experienced with firearms and the identification of weapons, miss pinpointing this important piece of evidence? And why would Oswald use a Mannlicher Carcano, since in Texas he could have bought a superior rifle for cash without a paper trail? Can you grasp the sheer stupidity of it all? In the Texas of 1963 Oswald could have bought a rifle across the counter with few if any questions asked. He could have done so and risked only a future debatable identification by some gun shop worker. Instead, we are told, Oswald ordered the murder weapon by using the alias "A. Hidell," gave his own post office box number, committed his handwriting to paper, and then went out to assassinate the President of the United States with this same "Hidell"-purchased rifle and while carrying a "Hidell" ID card in his wallet! Oh yes, I almost forgot, the Dallas police said nothing about the fake ID card until the FBI later announced that the alleged murder weapon had been ordered by an "A. Hidell." Can anybody say, *Patsy*"?

Seriously folks. The Mannlicher Carcano is not exactly the gun that an ex-Marine would use if he were planning to kill the President from almost the length of a football field. It's a lousy gun because it's so inaccurate. It's a carbine, for Pete's sake! A carbine is a short barreled rifle that originated many years ago for use with cavalry. Very inaccurate. So, if he did it, he must have been the first sniper to use a carbine, because no real sniper uses that type of rifle. And the actual gun supposedly used to kill JFK had a misaligned scope, which would have made it even more difficult to make the kill shot, especially for Oswald, who was not a very good shot, according to his military peers. Add the fact that it is nigh impossible to take 3 shots in 5.6 seconds with a manual bolt-action rifle like the Mannlicher Carcano. Since the shooting, which was over 40 years ago, numerous attempts have been made to duplicate this amazing feat, to no avail. Not one FBI sharpshooter, military or private citizen, or marksman has been able to reproduce the alleged shots by Oswald. Not even with a superior rifle and immobile object, much less with a bad scope and a moving target.

Interestingly, there was no gun powder residue on Oswald's hands when he was arrested. Odd, in light of the fact that he allegedly took several shots from that infamous 6th floor window. In addition, after his arrest, according to Dallas police testimony, there we no fingerprints on the rifle. None. Miraculously, after Oswald was shot and killed, the rifle somehow developed his palm print on the gun barrel. **Very odd.**

Strange. Almost sounds like something that would be accomplished by placing someone's hand on it in the morgue. Incidentally, Paul Groody (director of the funeral home that buried Oswald) told investigative reporter Jim Marrs that the FBI showed up with the gun and pressed Oswald's dead palm to the rifle. In his own words, "*I had a heck of a time getting the black fingerprint ink off of Oswald's hands.*"

Back to the law enforcement officers that found the rifle. Eventually, officers Boone and Wetizman recanted their stories of finding a Mauser. How could this be? Here are men that had given numerous reports and testimony under oath, that the rifle they had discovered was a Mauser carbine. A weapon that Craig said Weitzman had examined up close. Did somebody get to these men? Sounds like it to me. Importantly, it should be pointed out that no signed or sworn affidavit by any police officer (involved in the finding of the rifle) listed it as a Mannlicher Carcano. All sworn affidavits listed a **Mauser**.

However, Deputy Sheriff Roger Craig never would recant. Some people insist he was a liar, others claim he was an American hero. Either way, he went to his grave insisting that the gun found that day on the sixth floor of the Texas School Book Depository was unquestionably a 7.65 German Mauser. And the sad series of occurrences which led Mr. Craig to that grave is perhaps one of the most heartbreaking footnotes to the Kennedy Assassination tragedy. Craig's refusal to change his story about the Mauser, like all the other officers had done, caused him to be ostracized by his peers. He was fired from the Dallas Police Department in 1967, apparently for discussing sensitive information with a journalist. Roger Craig never found steady work again, he lost his wife, and then began suffering a series of bizarre accidents. He was shot at, driven off the side of the road, and at one point his car engine mysteriously exploded. The injuries induced by these incidents left Mr. Craig in almost constant physical pain. In 1975, Roger Craig took his own life.

Anomaly #6 – The Body Count

The problem with a crime as big as the assassination of JFK in broad daylight in downtown Dallas was that there were countless witnesses, investigators, reporters, Secret Service agents, etc. Hundreds. So they should all corroborate the government's story, if that's actually what went down, right?

Oddly enough, since that auspicious day in 1963, there have been over one thousand murders, suicides, and mysterious deaths of the people who were either eyewitnesses or otherwise involved with the investigation of the JFK assassination. Quite honestly, investigations were thwarted by the number of material witnesses who died in the first few years after the assassination and in periods of renewed interest in the case during the 1970s. Many key people died at strategically significant moments.

Here are a few of the more "attention-grabbing" cases, many of them gleaned from Carl Oglesby's paper entitled "Who Killed JFK":

- **Jack Ruby** died of cancer. He was taken into the hospital with Pneumonia. Twenty eight days later, he was dead from cancer.
- **David Ferrie**, a militant anti-Castroite and associate of Oswald, died of an apparent brain embolism in February 1967. He was just about to be arraigned for conspiracy in the JFK assassination by New Orleans District Attorney Jim Garrison, whose investigation convinced him that the CIA was involved. He supposedly left two suicide notes.
- **Eladio Del Valle**, a friend and political comrade of David Ferrie's, was shot at close range the day after Ferrie's death. Jim Garrison had been trying to find Del Valle for questioning.
- **Dr. Mary Stults Sherman** was found stabbed and burned in her apartment in New Orleans. Dr. Sherman had been working on a cancer experiment with David Ferrie.
- **Albert Guy Bogard**, an automobile salesman who worked for Downtown (Dallas) Lincoln Mercury, showed a new Mercury to a man using the name "Lee Oswald." Shortly after Bogard gave his testimony to a Commission attorney in Dallas, he was badly beaten and had to be hospitalized. Upon his release, he was fearful for his safety. He was found dead in his car at the Hallsville (Louisiana) Cemetery on St. Valentine's Day in 1966. A rubber hose was attached to the exhaust and the other end extending into the car. The ruling was suicide. He was just 41 years old.
- **Gary Underhill**, a CIA agent who claimed the CIA was involved in the JFK assassination, died of a gunshot to the head in May 1964. His death was ruled a "suicide."
- **Guy Banister**, a former FBI agent and acquaintance of Oswald, died of an apparent heart attack in June 1964. Files containing information on his anti-Castro activities were missing by the time authorities reached his office.
- **Mary Meyer**, a mistress of JFK during the White House years and the estranged wife of CIA veteran Cord Meyer, was murdered in October 1964 in a park in Washington, DC. Cord Meyer was a fishing companion of CIA counter-intelligence chief, James Jesus Angleton, who seized Meyer's diary after her death.
- **C.D. Jackson**, senior vice president of *Life* magazine, died of unknown causes in September 1964. Jackson arranged for *Life* to buy the Zapruder film soon after the Dealey Plaza shooting and then locked it away. (The film was not widely seen by the public until it was shown on ABC's Goodnight America in 1975.)

- **Rose Cheramie**, a prostitute and strip dancer in Jack Ruby's Dallas nightclub, died in a Texas hit-and-run accident in September 1965. Two days before the assassination, she told police in Louisiana she overheard two men plotting to kill JFK.

- **Delilah Walle** was a worker at Jack Ruby's strip club. She was married only 24 days when her new husband shot her. She had been working on a book of what she supposedly knew about the assassination.

- **Jack Zangetty**, the manager of a modular motel complex near Lake Lugert, Oklahoma, remarked to some friends (on the day after JFK was killed) that *"three other men – not Oswald – killed the President."* He also stated that *"A man named Ruby will kill Oswald tomorrow and in a few days a member of the Frank Sinatra family will be kidnapped just to take some of the attention away from the assassination."* Two weeks later, Jack Zangetty was found floating in Lake Lugert with bullet holes in his chest.

- **Dorothy Kilgallen**, a prominent columnist and TV personality, was ruled a suicide by drug overdose in November 1965. She had just completed a lengthy interview of Ruby in prison and told friends privately that she was about to "break" the JFK case.

- **Hale Boggs**, House majority leader and a member of the Warren Commission, was killed in a plane crash in Alaska in 1972. He had begun to express public doubts about the Warren Commission's findings.

- **J.A. Milteer**, the far-right Miami activist, died when his heater exploded in February 1974. He predicted an attempt on JFK's life and the capture of a scapegoat shortly before events in Dealey Plaza – and a man looking a lot like him was picked up by the police that November afternoon.

- **George de Mohrenschildt**, who befriended Oswald in Dallas, was found dead of a gunshot wound, deemed self-inflicted, in March 1977. Two hours before his death, an investigator for the House Assassinations Committee came to interview him about the JFK case, but de Mohrenschildt was not at home. In a manuscript found afterwards, de Mohrenschildt supported Oswald's view of himself as "a patsy."

- **Charles Nicoletti**, also on the House Committee's witness list, was shot three times in the back of the neck in the parking lot of a suburban Chicago shopping center in March 1977, less than 48 hours after de Mohrenschildt's death. Nicoletti was said to have been a "handler" (that is, supervisor) of Mafia assassins in the ClA-Mafia plots.

- **Carlos Prio Socarras**, a president of pre-revolutionary Cuba, was found dying of a pistol shot in April 1977, just six days after Nicoletti was gunned down. His death was ruled a suicide. He, too, was on the House Committee's witness list because of his alleged links to Jack Ruby and anti-Castro Cuban militants.

- **Lieutenant Commander William Bruce Pitzer** was the technician who filmed the JFK autopsy. He died in October 1966. It was ruled a "suicide" despite the fact that he was shot in the right temple and was left-handed.
- **Lou Staples**, a radio announcer who was doing a good many of his radio shows on the JFK assassination, lost his life May 13, 1977 near Yukon, Oklahoma. He had been having radio shows on the assassination since 1973 and the response to his programs was overwhelming. Lou's death was termed "suicide," but the bullet ending his life entered behind his right temple and Lou was left handed.
- **Roger Dean Craig** died of a massive gunshot wound to the chest. Supposedly, it was his second try at suicide and a success. Craig was a witness to the slaughter of JFK and testified at the Jim Garrison trial. Only Craig's story was different from the one the police told. Dallas Police Department's "1961 Man of the Year," Craig lost his job because he would not change his story of the assassination. Craig wrote two manuscripts of what he witnessed: "When They Kill A President" and "The Patient Is Dying." Craig's father was out mowing the lawn when Craig supposedly shot himself.
- **Sam Giancana**, mafia boss of Chicago, was shot to death in the basement of his home while in the Federal Witness Protection Program in June 1975. At the time of his murder, Giancana was scheduled to testify to the Senate Intelligence Committee on the CIA's alliance with the mafia in an attempt to kill Castro.

Anomaly #7 – Oswald's Associates

Lee Harvey Oswald was undoubtedly an ex-Marine, possibly a "nut," but he was definitely not "alone." Oswald worked in Guy Banister's office at the heart of the "intelligence community" (CIA, FBI, Secret Service, Navy) in New Orleans. Banister was a former FBI agent who "ran guns" to Cuba and hated Castro. He also hated JFK. Also working at Banister's office were David Ferrie and Clay Shaw. Ferrie was a bizarre, nervous, nasty, anti-Castro mercenary and gunrunner, skilled pilot and known deviant pedophile. Clay Shaw was a wealthy, powerful homosexual businessman who ran the International Trade Mart. Shaw also had CIA connections and was a known CIA "handler."

Oswald was one of Shaw and Ferrie's operatives. In 1963, prior to the assassination of JFK, Oswald was seen handing out **pro**-communist literature. However, the address on the pamphlet was 544 Camp Street, which was one of two doors on intersecting streets that led to the same corner office. The address of the other door that led to the same office was 531 Lafayette Street. Interestingly, the office to which both doors (with different addresses) led was the office of **anti**-communist, Guy Banister. David Ferrie, that peculiar pervert pedophile, initially met Oswald when he was only fifteen. Ferrie also knew Barry Seal, whom I talked about in the "war on drugs" chapter. Both Seal and Oswald trained under Ferrie in a civilian branch of the military, called the Civil Air Patrol.

Another interesting associate of Oswald was Jack Ruby, the man who killed him. That's right, Jack Ruby knew Oswald, Ferrie, Shaw, and Bannister. As a matter of fact, Oswald and Ruby were quite frequently seen in New Orleans night clubs. But that's not the only place Ruby and Oswald were seen together. You see, Ruby owned the Carousel Club, which was a strip bar in Dallas, and was also a well-known figure in the Dallas underworld. Jada Conforto, a stripper at the Carousel Club, told friends about the Ruby-Oswald connection on the night JFK was killed. She was killed in a motorcycle accident before she could testify for the Warren Commission. According to an article in the *Dallas Times Herald* (May 22, 1975), Kathy Kay, also a stripper at the Carousel Club, danced with Oswald a few nights before the assassination at the club. Sharri Angel confirmed Kathy Kay's account, adding that Ruby told Kay to do the "bump and grind" while dancing with Oswald to embarrass him.

Sharri Angel's husband was Wally Weston, the master of ceremonies at the Carousel Club until five days before the assassination. Weston recalled hitting Oswald at the Carousel for saying he thought Weston was a communist. According to Jim Marrs' excellent book, <u>Crossfire: The Plot That Killed Kennedy</u>, Weston mentioned this incident to Ruby when Ruby was in jail. Weston also related an incident that occurred on his last night at the Carousel Club, November 17, 1963. Ruby introduced him (but not by name) to "some friends from Chicago." Weston left the club and tried to get back in, but he was told to stay outside. Inside, according to one of the attendees, Myron Thomas Billet (aka Paul Bucilli), were Jack Ruby, Lee Harvey Oswald, Sam Giancana, John Roselli, an FBI agent, and Billet. The discussion was about a hit on JFK. Giancana and Billet left, not wishing to take part.

Well, as you know, JFK **was** killed five days later on November 22, 1963. Then, on November 24th, Ruby managed to stroll into Dallas police headquarters with a loaded gun. Amidst dozens of cops and reporters, he fatally shot Oswald in the stomach. According to Liam Scheff, in <u>Official Stories</u>, "*All of this was filmed and broadcast live on national television. Which is an effective way to send a message to the American public. 'The man who shot the President is dead – and you all saw it.'* "

Before his death in prison, Jack Ruby went on record. He said (and I quote): "*Everything pertaining to what's happening has never come to the surface. The world will never know the true facts of what occurred – my motives. The people that had so much to gain and had such an ulterior motive for putting me in the position I'm in, will never let the true facts come above board to the world."*

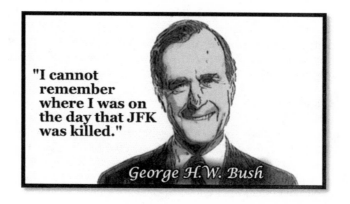

"I cannot remember where I was on the day that JFK was killed."

George H.W. Bush

Anomaly #8 – Bush?

Despite his protestations to the contrary, a Freedom of Information Act (FOIA) lawsuit memo unearthed in 1977-78 proves that former President George H. W. Bush was a member of the CIA and the recipient of a full briefing on the day after the assassination of JFK. According to CIA agent Frank Sturgis (victim of a covered-up poisoning death in October 1992 prior to the Bush-Clinton November election), FBI Director J. Edgar Hoover wrote the memo referring to the Bush briefing and on the night before JFK arrived in Dallas, Hoover met with Bush, Richard Nixon, and others at the Dallas ranch of Texas oil baron and Dallas Cowboys owner Colin J. "Clint" Murchison, Jr.

I'm sure you've seen the movie "Mission Impossible" with Tom Cruise. His character, Ethan Hunt, was based upon the real life Bay of Pigs-Watergate-Nixon administration CIA agent named E. Howard Hunt, a major lieutenant in the CIA's "anti-Castro Cuban" program. According to his deathbed confession to his son, Saint John Hunt, he was in Dallas and involved in the assassination. Seriously. Just do a search for "*E Howard Hunt deathbed confession*" and you will be able to listen to Hunt's voice as he tells his son how they "dunnit." As a matter of fact, the April 5, 2007 issue of *Rolling Stone* featured Hunt's deathbed confession as recorded by Saint John.

In his book, <u>Bond of Secrecy</u>, Saint John states, "*According to my father, LBJ and it seems just about everyone else in the military industrial complex viewed Kennedy as a threat and wanted him out of the way. LBJ, knowing that if Kennedy served another term would place him completely out of the presidential throne, was open to suggestions and agreed to control the investigation and cover up in return for his chance at the oval office. J. Edgar Hoover and the Kennedys had been virtually at war, with Hoover having the edge and aligning himself with Johnson. It is known that just prior to the assassination, LBJ and Hoover held a secret meeting witnessed by LBJ's mistress, Madeline Brown. Brown also has gone on record as being present when LBJ said in a moment of anger, that he was 'taking care' of Kennedy. Billy Sol Estes, close friend of LBJ, confided in his attorney Douglas Caddy that LBJ had told him he was part of the move to kill Kennedy."*

So ... Hunt admitted that he was directly involved in the murder of JFK, and Bush supervised Hunt. But Bush probably supervised a lot of CIA agents, not all of whom were directly involved in the assassination. A high-ranking officer may be connected to all of the acts of all of his troops, by reason of his being their commander. But it's not a direct connection. It doesn't establish that the officer knew about, or approved of, or was involved in, all the actions of those troops.

Let's continue. Until recently, Bush still claimed that he "can't remember" where he was the day JFK was shot. **Really?** The mere claim itself is extraordinarily incriminating. Everyone who was alive can remember where they were on 9/11. And everyone who was alive in 1963 can tell you exactly where they were when they heard about JFK. Except Bush. Until recently. More on that in a moment. For now, check out the following page, where I have included the US government memo dated 11/22/63 with the subject line *"Assassination of President John F. Kennedy."* You'll notice that it records Bush's phone call to the FBI at 1:45 PM from Tyler, Texas. This seems odd, doesn't it? Bush couldn't remember where he was when he made this phone call? Seriously? Walter Cronkite made the announcement that JFK was dead at 1:38 PM and then Bush makes a phone call only seven minutes later, but he doesn't remember where he was? Even though the memo says Tyler, Texas. Huh?

James Fetzer wrote an article entitled, "Was George H.W. Bush Involved in the Assassination of JFK?" In the article, Fetzer asserts, *"It only makes sense that Bush was staying at the Dallas Sheraton because his duty assignment was in Dallas. His phone call to the FBI cannot have been random. This James Parrott worked for Bush as a sign-painter; he was not an assassin; this phone call is not what it purports to be; Bush was fulfilling some obscure under-cover function in making this call. So the phone call has to be seen as part of his CIA assignment; which was clearly connected to the assassination. This memo then establishes that Bush was in the Dallas area, and on duty; and that his duty assignment was connected to the assassination. And if his men were in Dallas shooting the President, as they were, he was certainly on duty supervising them. If he were not supposed to be supervising them, his bosses would have assigned him to be at his home office in Houston, Texas; or on his oil rigs in the Caribbean."*

UNITED STATES GOVERNMENT

Memorandum

TO : SAC, HOUSTON   DATE: 11-22-63

FROM : SA GRAHAM W. KITCHEL

SUBJECT: UNKNOWN SUBJECT;
ASSASSINATION OF PRESIDENT
JOHN F. KENNEDY

At 1:45 p.m. Mr. GEORGE H. W. BUSH, President
of the Zapata Off-shore Drilling Company, Houston, Texas,
residence 5525 Briar, Houston, telephonically furnished
the following information to writer by long distance
telephone call from Tyler, Texas.

BUSH stated that he wanted to be kept confidential
but wanted to furnish hearsay that he recalled hearing in
recent weeks, the day and source unknown. He stated that
one JAMES PARROTT has been talking of killing the President
when he comes to Houston.

BUSH stated that PARROTT is possibly a student
at the University of Houston and is active in political
matters in this area. He stated that he felt Mrs. FAWLEY,
telephone number SU 2-5239, or ARLINE SMITH, telephone
number JA 9-9194 of the Harris County Republican Party
Headquarters would be able to furnish additional information regarding the identity of PARROTT.

BUSH stated that he was proceeding to Dallas, Texas,
would remain in the Sheraton-Dallas Hotel and return to his
residence on 11-23-63. His office telephone number is
CA 2-0395.

ALL INFORMATION CONTAINED
HEREIN IS UNCLASSIFIED
DATE 10-15-93 BY 9803 ADO/KSR
(JFK)

GWK:djw
(2)

Schmidt -
of
Jackson

62-2115-6

SEARCHED____ INDEXED____
SERIALIZED 2214 FILED 2214
NOV 16 1963
FBI - HOUSTON

Fetzer continues, "*But, even in context, this memo and the phone call it describes is still weird, no? I mean, how could Bush have been so stupid as to make this insanely incriminating phone call? Without this FBI memo, recording this phone call, we don't know, or even have a good clue as to where Bush was, or what he was doing the day of the assassination. Do we? Bush has, until recently, simply said that he did not remember what he was doing the day of the assassination. But with this memo, Bush tells us where he was and what he was doing — he hands us his head on a silver platter. What could possibly have motivated him to make such a stupid error as making this phone call to the FBI? It's a valid question. It's not an essential question. We can still value this memo, and extract a great deal of important content from it without answering the question of why, but the question remains. And we can make a stab at answering it. Russ Baker in his fine book, Family of Secrets, suggests that Bush was attempting to establish an alibi. Now, by making this phone call, he, in fact, establishes that he was in the Dallas area, and that he was on duty, related to the assassination. So if he's trying to establish an alibi to cover-up where he actually was and what he was actually doing, what he is trying to cover up must be some pretty bad stuff, some pretty incriminating stuff, if it's worse than what he gives us with this alibi. And what could be worse than what he gives us? Well, obviously, he must have actually been in Dallas. In fact, I think, this situation suggests he must have actually been in Dealey Plaza. I mean seriously. Think about it. He's so panicked about the truth coming out, that he puts his head in a noose and hands it to us. It makes me think he must have been in Dealey Plaza, he must have been in the company of the shooters, and he must have felt that there would be evidence to prove that.*"

Looks like an alibi to me. But, hey, I'm not a rocket scientist. Of course, this is just speculation, but it makes sense, doesn't it? If a guilty party is in a panic, trying to cover evidence connecting them to a crime, they may invent an explanation (alibi) that seems like a good idea at the time, but in reality creates a very damaging admission.

Then we have the bizarre Bush behavior at the funeral of President Gerald Ford, where Bush looks gleeful and laughs when he mentions the murder of JFK. **Seriously**. Do a search for "*Bush Laughs at JFK Shooting*" and you can watch it for yourself. In the YouTube video, you see Bush state, "*... after a deluded gunman assassinated President Kennedy,*" and then he chuckles. I'm not sure what's funny about JFK's brains splattering all over the car. But apparently Bush thinks something is funny about the "deluded gunman" theory. Does he know something?

Back to the "*I can't remember where I was.*" Until recently, Bush had nothing more to say about his whereabouts the day of the assassination than that he didn't remember where he was. However, now Bush has apparently concocted the story that he was speaking at the Tyler Rotary

Club. I guess it took Bush almost 40 years to remember where he was on that day. **Do you believe that?** I don't. He didn't even include this in his autobiography. Sure sounds made up to me. Hey, maybe he was hanging out with the Easter Bunny and Santa Claus at the North Pole. Yeah, that's it. That's the ticket!

Bush was eventually made head of the CIA. According to John Hankey, who produced the documentary, *JFK 2 – The Bush Connection*: *"George Herbert Walker Bush helped to supervise the assassination of President Kennedy, and from that point on, his political future was made – he was a 'made man.' He lost the race for Senate; they gave him a seat in Congress. He lost again for Senate; they have him a job in the White House. He lost the primaries to Reagan; they made him Vice President and he ruled while Reagan napped for 8 years."*

Who says the wicked never prosper?

Anomaly #9 – The Lady in Red

Jean Hill, a Dallas schoolteacher, was an eyewitness to history. To JFK assassination buffs, she is known as "the lady in red" because of the red raincoat she was wearing on November 22, 1963. She was not the anomaly, but what she said she saw was definitely incongruous to the official story of the assassination.

Standing less than 10 feet from JFK's passing limousine, Jean Hill and her friend, Mary Moorman, were taking Polaroid pictures of the motorcade, when Hill saw the shadowy figure of a man fire at President Kennedy from behind the picket fence, atop what is now commonly referred to as the "grassy knoll." She watched the President have his brains blown out, backward, onto the trunk of the car. Only seconds later, she also saw a man running from the direction of the School Book Depository, towards the Grassy Knoll. Jean Hill later identified that man as Jack Ruby.

As she ran up to the grassy knoll area to find out what was going on, two men in trench coats grabbed her, confiscated the picture of the assassination, took her to the Dallas County Records Building, and proceeded to interrogate her. When she told them what she had seen and heard (four to six shots fired), the agents told her that she didn't see what she saw, that there was nobody on the grassy knoll, and the shots all came from the window.

In her own words, *"They (Secret Service agents) took me to the Records Building and we went up to a room on the fourth floor. There were two guys sitting there on the other side of a table looking out a window that overlooked the killing zone, where you could see all of the goings on. You got the impression that they had been sitting there for a long time. They asked me what I had seen, and it became clear that they knew what I had seen. They asked me how many shots I had heard and I told them four to six. And they said, 'No, you didn't. There were three shots. We have three bullets and that's all we're going to commit to now.' I said, 'Well, I know what I heard,' and they told me, 'What you heard were echoes. You would be very wise to keep your mouth shut.' Well, I guess I've never been that wise. I know the difference between firecrackers, echoes, and gunshots. I'm the daughter of a game ranger, and my father took me shooting all my life."*

Hill later testified before the Warren Commission that she heard between four and six shots, and she was certain that some of the shots came from the grassy knoll. In interviews on television after the assassination, Hill said she saw "a little white dog" in the rear seat of the limo. As there was no dog in the car, the reliability of Hill's witness statement was undermined. However, 25 years later, it was revealed that a small white stuffed animal **was** on the back seat of the car. A child had presented it to Jackie Kennedy at the beginning of the tour of Dallas. This information was suppressed in order to discredit Hill as a reliable witness.

For many years, Hill refused to give interviews about the assassination of JFK. However, in 1990, Hill agreed to work as a technical adviser on Oliver Stone's motion picture, *JFK*. In 1992, Hill published her book on the case, <u>JFK: The Last Dissenting Witness</u>. Jean Hill, who worked as a schoolteacher in Dallas for over twenty years, died on November 7, 2000.

But it wasn't just Jean Hill. The first people to say there was a shot from the grassy knoll were Secret Service agents and police officers on the scene. At least 34 witnesses would come forward to say they thought a gunshot had been fired from the grassy knoll area. However, the FBI studiously avoided interviewing eyewitnesses, like Bill and Gayle Newman, who were approximately 15 feet from JFK's car, and both of whom said JFK was killed by a shot fired from the front. The Warren Commission never took the Newman's testimony. Reporters of the *New York Times*, the *Washington Post* and other national newspapers never sought to interview the witnesses who said a shot had come from the front.

The Big Question – "WHY?"

Good question. Why would "they" want JFK dead? Since November 22, 1963, there have been over 2,000 books, dozens of television programs and countless movies filled with theory, conjecture and myth as to why

JFK was gunned down in broad daylight on a downtown street in Dallas. I have my suspicions that he was murdered for three main reasons involving the CIA, Vietnam, and FRNs. And my friend, Liam Scheff, covers this topic quite nicely in <u>Official Stories</u>, so I'll paraphrase some of his arguments while I elaborate and summarize.

The three men that ran the CIA in the early 1960s were General Charles Cabell, Allan Dulles, and Richard Bissell. They all hated JFK ... thought he was a weak, mama's boy, pill-popping, traitor, especially after the Bay of Pigs, where he refused to bomb and invade Cuba. In 1961, the Joint Chiefs presented JFK with Single Integrated Operational Plan for Fiscal Year 1962, or "SIOP-62." It was a plan to preemptively attack any country in the world that had a nuclear bomb and was not our ally. Oh yes, with nuclear arms, by the way! An ELE ("extinction level event") perhaps. It's reported that JFK was so irritated after the meeting that he said in disgust to Secretary of State Dean Rusk at the conclusion of the meeting, "*And we call ourselves the human race.*" He nixed the plan. The Joint Chiefs were miffed. No unilateral destruction. Back to the drawing board.

The CIA presented plan B – perhaps you've heard of it – called "Operation Northwoods." Wait'll you get a load of this. The plan, which had the written approval of the Chairman and every member of the Joint Chiefs of Staff, called for innocent people to be shot on American streets; for boats carrying refugees fleeing Cuba to be sunk on the high seas; for a wave of violent terrorism to be launched in Washington, D.C., Miami, and elsewhere. People would be framed for bombings they did not commit; planes would be hijacked. Using phony evidence, all of it would be blamed on Castro, thus giving Lemnitzer (Joint Chief) and his cabal the excuse, as well as the public and international backing, they needed to launch their war.

As Liam said, they wanted to "*whip America into a war-frenzy against that terror of a banana-growing republic*" of Cuba – a country that had **not** attacked the USA, but that Americans **thought** had attacked us. This is what is typically called a "false flag." We'll learn more about false flags in a few chapters. When presented the plan, JFK said, "*Have you lost your freaking marbles?*" Well, maybe not in those exact words, but he also nixed this plan. Then he proceeded to fire Cabell, Dulles, and Bissell. He told his advisors, "*I want to splinter the CIA into a thousand pieces and scatter it to the winds.*"

And that leads us to Vietnam. Adding insult to injury, on October 11, 1963, JFK signed a National Security Action Memo ("NSAM") #263, which did something unimaginable – it began a total pullout of CIA "advisors" from Vietnam. JFK was going to end the war before it started. That can't be good for the imperialistic "war machine" we call the USA. Liam Scheff puts it in perspective in his book, <u>Official Stories</u>: "*General Cabell had called Kennedy a traitor. He said it loud enough for people to hear. Cabell gave a talk in New Orleans. He was introduced by none other than Clay Shaw, Lee Oswald's rabid anti-Castro, anti-Kennedy CIA handler. I'll bet Cabell also told his brother, Earle. Earle Cabell was mayor of the big town of Dallas, Texas. I'll bet it was Mayor Cabell, brother of General Cabell, who gave the orders to change the parade route, to leave the sniper windows open and to get the deeply corrupt and dirty police force their story before any of it even happened."*

On November 22, 1963, just hours after JFK was assassinated at Dealey Plaza, Lyndon B. Johnson (LBJ) became President of the United States. Just four days later, on November 26, 1963, LBJ signed a NSAM #273 as guidance for future Vietnam plans and policy. This brief directive most significantly initiated changes reversing JFK's Vietnam policy of NSAM #263, in which JFK had decreed then that *"the bulk of US personnel would be out of Vietnam by the end of 1965."* Despite NSAM #263, there has been much speculation and debate on what JFK would or would not have done in Vietnam had he not been killed. If I were to engage in speculation, I would tend to believe that the man who twice refused to submit to the Joint Chiefs and the CIA on bombing and invading Cuba (a mere ninety miles from our shore) would not have consented to sending hundreds of thousands of US troops half way around the world to slaughter Vietnamese peasants.

Then, on August 4, 1964, multiple US warships were attacked by North Vietnamese PT Boats in the Gulf of Tonkin – an incident that kicked off US involvement and initiated full-scale conflict in Vietnam. LBJ wanted war with Vietnam and he got it, without even declaring it. Except, ummm, well, it never happened. What? The August 1964 Gulf of Tonkin incident was actually a "false flag." It's an American tradition. Big lies launch wars. Manufactured pretexts initiate them. Mass killing and destruction follow.
It would take over thirty years for the truth to emerge that the Gulf of Tonkin incident was a staged event that **never** actually took place. LBJ later admitted that he lied and that the Gulf of Tonkin attack never happened. He also said, showing his discomfort, that he believed there was a conspiracy to murder JFK.

Lastly, JFK was killed because of FRNs. What's an FRN? A "Federal Reserve Note" printed by the Federal Reserve Bank ("the FED"). In a nutshell, the FED is a consortium of private banksters that own the US government via their ability to "print money" out of thin air and loan it to the government. We will talk more about the FED later in the book. On June 4, 1963, a virtually unknown Presidential decree, Executive Order 11110, was signed with the authority to basically strip the FED of its power to loan money to the US government at interest. With the stroke of a pen, JFK declared that the privately owned FED would soon be out of business. "United States Notes" were issued as an interest-free and debt-free currency backed by silver reserves in the US Treasury.

Let's compare a "Federal Reserve Note" (issued from the FED) with a "United States Note" from the US Treasury issued by JFK's Executive Order. They almost look alike, except one says "Federal Reserve Note" on the top while the other says "United States Note."

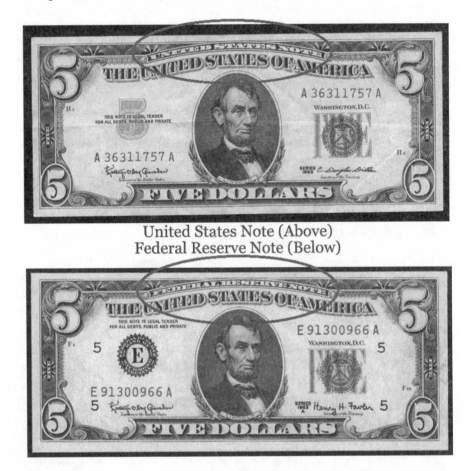

United States Note (Above)
Federal Reserve Note (Below)

JFK knew that if the silver-backed United States Notes were widely circulated, they would have eliminated the demand for Federal Reserve Notes. This is a very simple matter of economics. JFK was assassinated on November 22, 1963 and the United States Notes he had issued were immediately taken out of circulation.

Because of his quest for world peace, his struggle to preserve the human race from a devastating thermonuclear war, and his desire to restore America to a real monetary system, our last "real" President, John Fitzgerald Kennedy, was slaughtered by those who were tasked with protecting him.

Perhaps the assassination of JFK was a warning to all future presidents not to interfere with the Fed's control over the creation of money. It seems very apparent that JFK starkly challenged the ominous "shadow government" that exists behind the USA. With true patriotic courage, JFK boldly faced the two most successful vehicles that have ever been used to drive up debt: 1) the Vietnam War and 2) the creation of money by a privately owned central bank. Here is an interesting quote by JFK which shows that he knew about the shadow government: *"The very word 'secrecy' is repugnant in a free and open society; and we are as a people inherently and historically opposed to secret societies, to secret oaths and to secret proceedings."*

Interestingly, in contrast to the conclusions of the Warren Commission, the United States House Select Committee on Assassinations (HSCA) concluded in 1978 that Kennedy was probably assassinated as a result of a conspiracy. The HSCA found the original FBI investigation and the Warren Commission Report to be seriously flawed. The HSCA stated that there were at least four shots fired (only three of which could be linked to Oswald) and that there was *"...a high probability that two gunmen fired at (the) President."*

Oh yes, I almost forgot about Jackie Kennedy. Right after the assassination, they wanted her to change her dress since it was stained with JFK's blood. She said, *"No, I want the American people to see what **they** did to my husband."* What "**THEY**" did. She didn't believe the "lone nut" crap either.

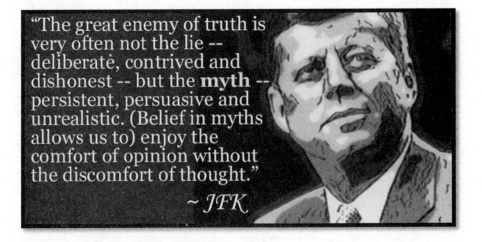

"The great enemy of truth is very often not the lie -- deliberate, contrived and dishonest -- but the **myth** -- persistent, persuasive and unrealistic. (Belief in myths allows us to) enjoy the comfort of opinion without the discomfort of thought."

~ JFK

RESOURCES

Websites
http://www.thirdworldtraveler.com/CIA/Who_Killed_JFK.html
http://www.veteranstoday.com/2011/11/16/was-george-h-w-bush-involved-in-the-assassination-of-jfk/

Movies
"JFK II – The Bush Connection"
http://www.youtube.com/watch?v=gsMKMMlleOE
"The Killing of a President"
http://www.youtube.com/watch?v=ocZAiIgQ9jI

Videos
"Secret Service Standdown"
http://www.youtube.com/watch?v=XYo2Qkuc_f8
"Conspiracy Theory: JFK Assassination" (Jesse Ventura)
http://www.youtube.com/watch?v=sfDASCapA9Q
"Deathbed Confession of E. Howard Hunt"
http://www.youtube.com/watch?v=bknUDgKdEJQ

Books
Official Stories (Liam Scheff)
Crossfire: The Plot That Killed Kennedy (Jim Marrs)
They Killed Our President: 63 Reasons to Believe There Was a
Conspiracy to Assassinate JFK (Jesse Ventura)

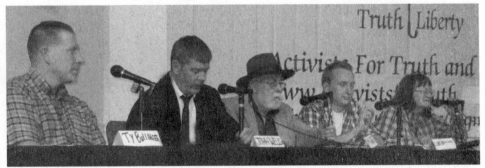

I was honored to participate in a roundtable discussion in Dallas on November 21, 2013 (the day before the 50 year anniversary of JFK's assassination). Other participants were John B. Wells (host of "Coast to Coast AM"), Jim Marrs (author of Crossfire: The Plot That Killed Kennedy, Luke Rudkowski (founder of "We are Change"), and Judyth Vary Baker (Lee Harvey Oswald's girlfriend and author of Me and Lee).

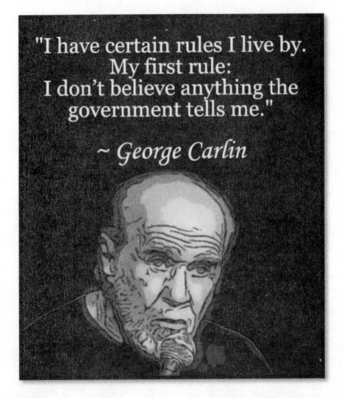

Chapter 16

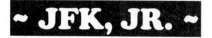

MONUMENTAL MYTH

On Friday, July 16, 1999, John F. Kennedy, Jr. ("John-John") was piloting a Piper Saratoga airplane en route to Hyannis Port, Massachusetts, traveling with his wife, Caroline, and her sister, Lauren Bessette. The weather was bad and there was almost no visibility. John-John was not IFR ("instrument flight rules") certified, so he was unable to fly a plane using instruments. Due to the inclement weather, poor visibility, and his inexperience, he lost his bearings and was unable to control the plane.

At 9:40 PM, approximately 13 miles shy of the local airport off the coast of Martha's Vineyard; the plane went into a steep vertical "death spiral" and crashed headlong into the sea, killing all aboard. According to the NTSB and FAA, radar records indicate that John-John was changing altitude and direction somewhat erratically and rapidly in the minutes preceding the crash.

The mainstream media's much-ballyhooed official story was that John-John was a reckless pilot who died because of his own carelessness.

CAN YOU HANDLE THE TRUTH?

Christopher Condon wrote an incredible article entitled *"What Actually Happened to John F. Kennedy, Jr.?"* which was very enlightening to me, so I'll be quoting from it and also paraphrasing some of his arguments. Actually, his article was a summary of an illuminating DVD documentary entitled *The Assassination of John F. Kennedy, Jr.* by John Hankey, so many of the information, quotes, and thought processes were his.

Before we dive into the actual details of the crash, let's highlight a couple of interesting facts about Kennedy. First of all, John-John was not your average "spoiled rich kid." He was a thinker. He may have been handsome, wealthy, and a "Kennedy," but he was not one of the globalist scumbags. He was a man with a strong social conscience and anti-fascist roots who had his own magazine, *George*, as a forum.

Strap on your seat-belts. We're going to take a fast roller-coaster ride through the enigmatic facts that surround the 1999 crash which took the lives of John-John, Caroline, Lauren, and possibly another person ...

The Weather

Let's take a look at the mainstream media's myth that the visibility at Martha's Vineyard was poor. In the words of John A. Quinn with NewsHawk® Inc., *"FAA Flight Specialist Edward Meyer of LaGuardia Airport in Queens N.Y., tapped by FAA administrator Jane Garvey to prepare the FAA's official report of weather conditions when Kennedy's plane was destroyed, stated in the report that visibility in the region was at least very good on the evening of July 16th. Meyer himself became so distressed by endless spewing of erroneous disinformation about these weather conditions by government agencies and mass media, he took the unprecedented step of issuing a public statement on his own – which thoroughly slammed this onslaught of 'dis-informational noise' as complete, total nonsense, utterly unsupported by the facts."*

To quote from Meyer's personal statement as released to mass media: *"The weather along his flight was just fine. A little haze over eastern Connecticut. I don't know why the airplane crashed, but what I heard on the media was nothing but garbage."*

The Crash and "Disappearing" Evidence

John-John checked in with the FAA Tower at Martha's Vineyard at 9:39 PM, just **one minute** prior to the crash. He mentioned that he was 13 miles from the airport and making his final approach. He was in control of the plane at that time. No issues with weather. No issues with visibility. Then, one minute later – **BOOM!** – the plane began to nosedive and crashed into the Atlantic Ocean. FAA radar showed the plane went into a dive and dropped 1,200 feet in just 12 seconds. Of course, there is a miniscule possibility that immediately after the radio call, there was some sort of catastrophic mechanical failure or John-John somehow suddenly lost total control of the plane. Or both.

At approximately 12:30 PM the next day, Petty Officer Todd Burgun (with the Public Information Office of the Coast Guard) made a routine press announcement. At least, he thought it was routine. He indicated that he had been advised by FAA that at 9:39 PM (on the night of the crash), John-John's plane was holding steady and contacted air traffic control at Martha's Vineyard to clear for final descent.

But then something strange happened: Burgun's announcement was "disappeared" from the media, the FAA and Coast Guard were silenced, and all press communication was taken over by the Pentagon. Why the Pentagon? Kennedy was not a member of the military. He was not flying a military aircraft. His flight had no military purpose. Perhaps Pentagon officials were complicit in the plane crash and were ready to cover it up.

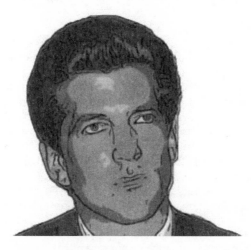

What do I mean that Burgun's announcement was "disappeared"? According to John A. Quinn with NewsHawk® Inc., *"our associate obtained irrefutable proof that the reported fact of this radio contact was deliberately removed from archived tape transcripts of WCVB-TV Channel 5's broadcast of July 17, 1999, during which – at approximately 12:35 PM – US Coast Guard Petty Officer Todd Burgun reported to WCVB the fact of JFK Jr.'s radio contact the night before. By later in the evening on July 17th, this vital information was being actively covered up by WCVB and some other mass media outlets, as it has been in all subsequent government and mass media reports."*

Even more damning, when the tape of WCVB's broadcast of July 17, 1999 was obtained from Corporate Media Services (which archives tapes of TV broadcasts), it was inexplicably cut just as Burgun began his report on the 9:39 PM radio call from John-John! I'm not kidding! Then it resumes with WCVB's broadcast from 6 PM that evening – approximately 5½ hours later! How do you like that? The tape is "mysteriously" cut right as the 9:39 PM radio communication is being mentioned, and then the tape picks up over five hours later! I'm sure it was just "coincidence" ... an unfortunate "accident." Sure it was ...

Why was Burgun's announcement "disappeared" down the memory hole? It's simple: When a plane contacts the FAA, its radar blip is logged into the FAA system by its tail-number, and if that plane descends below 100 feet outside its normal landing area, an automatic alert is sounded and a search is launched at the point where the transponder-generated radar signal disappeared. Furthermore, once a plane has contacted FAA and has been cleared for landing, if that plane does not land within five minutes, a search is automatically launched.

So, we're back to the same question that I've been asking throughout the book: "*If you have nothing to hide, then why are you hiding something?*"

Oh yes, I almost forgot. Also reported by WCVB news anchors during that 5½ hour portion of the broadcast which was "accidentally" cut, is the fact that a reporter for the (Martha's) *Vineyard Gazette* who was on the beach on the night of the crash reported an airborne explosion ("*a big white flash in the sky*") in the vicinity where John-John's plane went down. Several local news reports initially reported that dozens of people saw and heard an explosion in the air over the same area at the same time John-John's plane went down. It was probably just an alien spacecraft shooting off fireworks – nothing to worry about. In addition, during that 5½ hour portion of the broadcast, the 9:39 PM radio contact is referred to numerous times as a rock-solid fact. Oh yes, you can actually see it in Hankey's documentary. He obtained the "uncut" video.

The Mainstream Media Begins to Lie

So, what do you think were the first words out of the mouth of the mainstream media bobble-heads when the WCVB tape resumed at 6 o'clock on the evening of July 17th? Any guesses?

The teleprompter reading "press-titute" for the evening, stuttering, hands fidgeting, twitching, and scrabbling for words; looking anxious, troubled, and flustered, made the following muddled and highly unpersuasive statement: "*Something that we had **thought** earlier may not be true: that there was actually no radio communication with JFK Jr.'s plane after it left New Jersey. We had hoped that there was some radio communication of course, most recently at Martha's Vineyard. This this (uncomfortable pause) last night at about **nine o'clock, nine-thirty**, when perhaps things started to go wrong. We had hoped we could learn from that, but it seems that there (another uncomfortable pause) **may be no evidence** because there **may be no recording** to listen to to get these details from.*"

Wow! Where do I start with this mangled mess of a "confession" (I mean "newscast")? I have bolded the words in the quote that I want to address. First of all, the 9:39 PM call wasn't something that they had previously "thought." It was the unambiguous report from the Coast Guard. No thinking involved. Secondly, she mentions *"nine o'clock, nine-thirty."* Why would she do this? Could it be that she was obviously aware of the fact that there actually **had** been radio contact and inadvertently gave the general time of the actual radio contact? It's almost like your mom walking in the kitchen right after you took a cookie from the cookie jar, and you say *"Hey Mom, I didn't just eat a cookie from the cookie jar because I know I'm not supposed to eat the cookies without your permission."*

Next, the news anchor states, *"there may be no evidence because there may be no recording to listen to to get these details from."* Almost reminiscent of the infamous *"the dog ate my homework"* line, isn't it? I mean, **seriously**? And then, after regurgitating the "official story" and beginning to spin the web of lies, the reporter has an immediate look of relief. Why didn't she just say, *"The Coast Guard was mistaken – there was no radio contact between John-John and the airport prior to the crash."*?

John-John's Qualifications & The Search

The "disinfo" machine was in full gear after the crash, claiming that John-John only had a couple hundred hours of experience and was a reckless pilot. I even heard some of the spooks spewing nonsense about him possessing some sort of "reckless" gene (never before heard of in the history of science, by the way) that made him take unwise risks.

So, what's the truth? Every personal flight instructor that John-John ever had indicated that he was an exceedingly careful, cautious, and proficient pilot; definitely not given to recklessness or risk-taking. Most pointedly, John McColgan (Kennedy's federal licensing instructor) stated that John-John had seventeen years of experience as a pilot and had accumulated over 700 hours of flight time. And, guess what? He had completed the IFR written test just a few months before the crash and had completed his hands-on tests for the IFR certification. All he needed to obtain his IFR certification was a few more hours with a Certified Flight Instructor (CFI).

Kennedy had flown the same route from Caldwell, New Jersey to Martha's Vineyard 8 times that summer, and all 8 times he took a CFI. And he had a good reason for this – on 5 of the flights, visibility was too poor to fly VFR (visual flight rules") without instruments. Of course, based on the testimony of FAA Flight Specialist Edward Meyer, we have already learned that John-John could have easily flown VFR on the night of the crash, since the weather was good. OK, so the weather was good and John-John was an excellent pilot. Back to the events which occurred right after the crash.

After the crash, no focused search was conducted for over 15 hours. That's right. John-John's contact with the FAA tower in Martha's Vineyard meant that there could be no viable explanation for the delay in the focused search. Therefore, the inconvenient radio communication was made to disappear. Why didn't they want to search immediately? I'll tell you why. They needed time to find the plane and remove the battery from the cockpit voice recorder, remove the Flight Log that listed all passengers, and remove the body of anyone else that was on the plane but wasn't supposed to be on the plane. More on that in a minute.

John-John was flying a Piper Saratoga, which is equipped with a flight voice recorder. But when that voice recorder was recovered, the battery necessary to preserve its content was missing. That's strange. And John-John always kept his Flight Log in an aquamarine duffle bag. But when the bag was recovered from the wreckage, there was no Flight Log. That's also strange, isn't it?

"Why would the Flight Log matter anyway?"

I'll tell you why. It contains a list of the passengers on that flight.

"But we already know who was on the flight, don't we?"

Not exactly. When Carol Ratowell, a Kennedy family friend, phoned the Coast Guard at 2:15 AM, she told them that there was a Certified Flight Instructor (CFI) on board. Are you ready for more strangeness? His body was never found. But not only that, one of the seats of the aircraft was missing.

"Why does it matter whether a CFI was on board?" Because the NTSB would eventually determine that there had been no mechanical failure of the airplane. In other words, they said that the plane crashed due to "pilot error." But if there were a CFI on board, then this is a far-fetched determination.

You see, removing the Flight Log would require being on the scene before the plane was "officially" found. Guess what? There is strong evidence to support this assertion. The official focused search didn't begin until the next afternoon, but Lt. Colonel Richard Stanley of the Civil Air Patrol had initiated a search for the missing plane on dry land off Martha's Vineyard by 7:30 AM and advised the news media that at that time (hours before the official focused search and discovery) he had seen Coast Guard helicopters circling the area. The only problem was that the Coast Guard said that the helicopters weren't theirs. So whose were they? Perhaps the helicopters belonged to whoever caused the plane to crash?

The fact of the matter is that John-John was still getting used to his new plane and had never flown it without a flight instructor. **Not once. Never.** And as I just mentioned, he had passed the written and hands-on tests for IFR certification that would permit him to fly it in any weather, and all he needed for the certification was to log additional hours with a CFI.

But that's not all ...

The airplane was equipped with an Emergency Locator Transmitter (ELT) – a beacon that goes off after a crash and signals via satellite the location of the crash site within feet to the FAA. I guess the beacon must have failed, eh? Nope. ABC news coverage had visuals of the precise location of the crash site as determined by the ELT, that the newscasters attributed to the ELT, with a little ELT logo to let you know the source of the data. The ELT was working just fine. So, again, I ask you. Why did it take them 15 hours before they began the focused search, in light of the fact that they most definitely knew where the plane had crashed? Think about it.

What About the Quote from John-John?

In a January 27, 2000 investigative report, NTSB interviewer David Muzio interviewed Robert Merena, a CFI who had previously flown with John-John many times. During the interview, Merena told Muzio that he had spoken to John-John on the day before he died, but when he offered to fly with him to Hyannis Port, Kennedy declined and said, "*I want to do it alone.*" I remember the quote making national headlines, as talk-radio hosts across the USA told their audiences that the rash, careless, reckless, hedonistic sybarite, John-John Kennedy, got what he deserved.

My question for the NTSB: Why did it take you six months to get around to interviewing a man who had this crucial information? One more question for the NTSB: Why didn't Merena mention this in his July 21, 1999 interview with Muzio (just 5 days after the crash)? According to the transcript of that interview, "*The instructor (Merena) was not aware of the pilot (Kennedy) conducting any flights in the accident airplane without an instructor aboard.*" So, in a nutshell, they want us to believe that 5 days after the crash, Muzio and Merena had an interview and John-John's final words ("I want to do it alone") were never discussed and Merena "remembered" these words six months later? **Seriously?** Are they smoking crack? Tripping on LSD, perhaps? Hey, maybe pigs really **can** fly!

One thing that Hankey brought up in the documentary was very telling. The Muzio report dated January 27, 2000 violates the cardinal rule of an NTSB interview – it fails to give the time, date, and place of the supposed interview. And it fails to have the interviewee sign the interview summary, as procedure requires.

Which leads us to the question: *"Did Muzio make up the quote?"*

On February 25, 2000, Merena's attorney, Peter V. Van Deventer, Jr., wrote a letter to the NTSB and answered this very question. The letter states that Merena and Kennedy had a conversation between 10 AM and 11 AM on the day in question. However, John-John **never** indicated that he intended to depart on the day or evening in question. There it is. Hidden in plain sight! Van Deventer, on behalf of Merena, is telling the NTSB that Muzio is lying through his teeth! He made it up. He fabricated the entire quote. Wow!

In the words of Michael B. Green, Ph.D., former Assistant Professor of Philosophy at the University of Texas, *"Hankey has given us a full-court satisfying proof that John Kennedy Jr. was murdered by a fascist ruling class in direct control of the Pentagon, FAA and subordinate governmental bureaucracies such as the NTSB, and with the media fully intimidated and controlled at its core by the owners and managers who belong to the ruling class, and who keep at bay, largely by suasion, bluff and distraction the relevant and penetrating inquiries of the front-line reporters."*

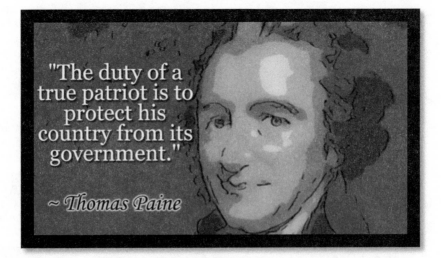

"The duty of a true patriot is to protect his country from its government."

~ Thomas Paine

Why?

It's very important to understand that John-John refused to believe the findings of the Warren Commission – that his father, JFK, was killed by a "lone nut." He also supported Oliver Stone's work on the movie, *JFK*. But what might have been the equivalent of "crossing the line," John-John published an article (in *George*) by Oliver Stone about how the rich and powerful had always assassinated their opponents, including his father, JFK. He also published another article entitled *"A Mother's Defense"* by Guela Amir, the mother of Yigal Amir, who was convicted of assassinating Yitzhak Rabin, the peace-loving Israeli Prime Minister. In the article, Amir said her son was a tool of the Mossad (the equivalent of the Israeli CIA) and he could never have penetrated Rabin's security if it weren't an "inside job." This exposé on the Rabin assassination alone was enough to have gotten him killed. John-John had also been vocal in his criticism of the US government's handling of Waco and Ruby Ridge.

Question: If you were part of the Project for a New American Century (PNAC) powers that were already hard at work in Florida to fix the 2000 Presidential Election and eliminate any "potential future resistance," would you want *George* and John-John around?

John-John was going to run for political office and he was going to expose his father's killers. He was a natural politician, with charisma and charm. He would have won **whatever** position he ran for. Period.

John F. Kennedy, Jr. was a political threat. Could it be that the plotters of 9/11 murdered him in anticipation of their future evil deed to assure his silence? Just asking a question, that's all. Think about it …

RESOURCES

Websites
http://archive.lewrockwell.com/orig11/condon-c1.1.1.html
http://rense.com/politics5/coverup.htm
http://911research.wtc7.net/essays/green/TheAssassinationOfJFKJr.html

Movies
"The Assassination of JFK, Jr."
http://www.youtube.com/watch?v=6EK2swspKgw
"John Kennedy Jr. Was Murdered?"
http://www.youtube.com/watch?v=dSziV-ajYz4
"The Assassination of JFK Jr. - Murder By Manchurian Candidate"
http://www.amazon.com/

"WHEN THE PEOPLE FEAR THE GOVERNMENT THERE IS TYRANNY. WHEN THE GOVERNMENT FEARS THE PEOPLE THERE IS LIBERTY."

Thomas Jefferson

Chapter 17

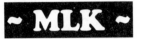

MONUMENTAL MYTH

I was about 2½ months old when it happened. On April 4, 1968, while standing on the balcony of the Lorraine Motel in Memphis, Dr. Martin Luther King, Jr. (MLK) was assassinated. The official story is that a single "lone nut" bumbling petty crook, James Earl Ray, was staying at a rooming house located at 422 South Main Street. In the back of this rooming house was a shared bathroom with a window that looked out onto the swimming pool of the Lorraine Motel.

Since the window in the bathroom was over his head, Ray stood on a bathtub and fired the shot that killed MLK. He then ran from the bathroom into the bedroom, bundled up the rifle and a bizarre collection of personal belongings into a blanket (ensuring that the rifle and belongings but not the bathroom door or the bedroom door had his fingerprints on them), ran the length of the rooming house (down a flight of stairs), dumped the bundle in the street, walked calmly to his waiting Mustang and drove away within the 90 seconds it took uniformed officers to reach the same location.

He drove off in his white Mustang and singlehandedly evaded a police dragnet in Memphis, drove a conspicuous white Mustang all the way to Atlanta, then left the country and journeyed as far as Portugal before finally being apprehended in London's Heathrow Airport on June 8, 1968 and charged with the assassination of MLK. Or so the myth goes...

CAN YOU HANDLE THE TRUTH?

In 1968, there were already a large number of people who didn't believe the official story that Lee Harvey Oswald had been the "lone nut assassin" of JFK. The previous chapter should have provided you with lots of "food" to chew on concerning the anomalies with the assassination of JFK. Not surprisingly, in light of the inquisitive atmosphere of the 1960s coupled with the incredulity concerning the official JFK story, public suspicions over the investigation of MLK's death surfaced almost immediately.

Truth be told, there is **no physical evidence** to prove that James Earl Ray shot MLK, and Ray spent his life in prison based solely on a coerced confession which he immediately retracted. None of the ballistics tests, which were performed on the rifle Ray allegedly used, were able to link that rifle to the actual bullet that killed MLK. In addition to these facts, there is a long list of "odd" events surrounding the shooting.

As you read through the chapter, here are several questions to ponder.

- How had so many police arrived so quickly on the scene (within moments of the shot being fired) yet failed to spot the assassin either arriving or departing?
- If, as the police claimed, the shot had come from the bathroom window, why did several people claim to have seen a gunman in the bushes across the street?
- Why were the bushes cut down the next morning?
- What about the role of Lloyd Jowers (owner of Jim's Grill)?
- Did you know that there were army photographers on the roof of the fire station that photographed the entire assassination?
- Did you know that the photographs are currently buried in the archives at the Department of Defense?

And you know **why** you did not know? Because there was **never** a police investigation of the MLK assassination. No house-to-house investigation. Neighbors as late as two weeks later stated *"they never knocked on my door."* In thirty years, they never talked to the Captain who ran the fire station across the street. He put the photographers up there. He took the stand and stated, *"yeah I put them up there. They showed me credentials saying they wanted to take pictures."* Where are those pictures? That proof has existed for all of these years. It's there. It has been buried. Right next to the 86 FBI videos of what really hit the Pentagon on 9/11. Right next to Jimmy Hoffa.

Should the US government be allowed to assassinate its own citizens? April 4, 1968 is an excellent day to examine, since on that day, the US government was part of a successful conspiracy to assassinate MLK. That's not just some kooky, wing-nut-job conspiracy theory. It's not a theory at all. It is a **fact**, according to our legal system.

I bet you didn't know that, did you?

That's right. In 1999, in Shelby County, Tennessee, Lloyd Jowers was tried before a jury of his peers (made up equally of white and black citizens, if it matters) on the charge of conspiring to kill MLK. The jury heard testimony for a full month. On the last day of the trial, the attorney for the MLK family (which brought suit against Lloyd Jowers) concluded by saying: *"We're dealing in conspiracy with agents of the City of Memphis and the governments of the State of Tennessee and the United*

States of America. We ask you to find that conspiracy existed." It took the jury only 2½ hours to reach the verdict: Jowers and *"others, including governmental agencies, were parties to this conspiracy."*

So let's backtrack and take a few minutes to explore several facets of the assassination and see if we can determine why the 1999 jury ruled that Ray was not guilty and that the government (amongst others) was responsible for the murder of MLK.

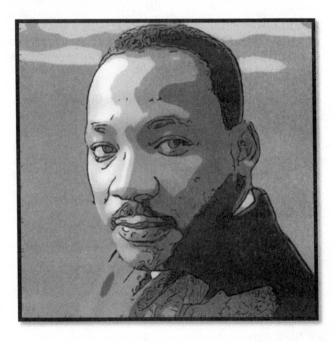

The Bullet & Rifle

Within minutes after the shooting of MLK, a local police officer discovered a Remington 30-06 rifle, several unused bullets, and other effects that belonged to James Earl Ray, wrapped inside a blanket, outside Canipe's Amusement store. The owner of the store recalled someone dropping the package at his door **before** the time of the assassination. Despite this evidence, it would be months before the FBI and police agencies began looking for escaped convict James Earl Ray as the alleged assassin of MLK.

The FBI told many dubious and inconsistent stories about their ballistics work in this case. They claimed that the rifle was not tested on retrieval to see if it had been fired that day, a simple and standard procedure, the omission of which strains credulity. I'd guess that it's more likely that the test **was** done and the rifle was found **not** to have been fired. But that's just my opinion.

Judge Joe Brown, who presided over two years of hearings on the rifle, testified that "...*67% of the bullets from my tests did not match the Ray rifle.*" He added that the unfired bullets found wrapped with it in a blanket were metallurgically different from the bullet taken from MLK's body, and therefore were from a different lot of ammunition. And because the rifle's scope had not been sited, Brown said, "*this weapon literally could not have hit the broadside of a barn.*" Holding up the Remington 30-06 rifle, Judge Brown told the jury, "*It is my opinion that this is **not** the murder weapon.*"

Perhaps the most telling evidence was the bullet fragment removed from the spine of MLK during an inadequate autopsy. The FBI tested this bullet fragment, along with the alleged murder weapon, in 1968, as did the House Select Committee on Assassinations (HSCA) in 1976, with the same result. The fatal bullet could **not** be conclusively linked to the Remington 30-06 rifle purchased by James Earl Ray. Yet the evidence presented at Ray's "trial" gave the impression that the bullet was proven to have been fired from the rifle.

The Eyewitnesses

There was much eyewitness evidence, at the time of the shooting, to suggest that the fatal shot that struck MLK did **not** come from the direction of a nearby rooming house bathroom window, thus James Earl Ray was **not** the killer.

Solomon Jones was MLK's chauffeur in Memphis. The FBI document, dated April 13, 1968, says that after MLK was shot, when Jones looked across Mulberry Street into the brushy area, "*he got a quick glimpse of a person with his back toward Mulberry Street. ... This person was moving rather fast, and he recalls that he believed he was wearing some sort of light-colored jacket with some sort of a hood or parka.*" When he was interviewed by the police at 11:30 PM on the day of the murder, Jones provided the same basic information concerning a person leaving the brushy area in a hurry.

Olivia Catling lived a block away from the Lorraine Motel on Mulberry Street. Catling had planned to walk down the street the evening of April 4th in the hope of catching a glimpse of MLK at the motel. She testified that when she heard the shot a little after six o'clock, she said, "*Oh, my God, Dr. King is at that hotel!*" She ran with her two children to the corner of Mulberry and Huling streets, just north of the Lorraine. She saw a man in a checkered shirt come running out of the alley beside a building across from the Lorraine. The man jumped into a green 1965 Chevrolet just as a police car drove up behind him. He gunned the Chevrolet around the corner and up Mulberry past Catling's house moving her to exclaim, *"It's going to take us six months to pay for the rubber he's burning up!!"*

The police, she said, ignored the man and blocked off a street, leaving his car free to go the opposite way. Catling later said that the man was definitely **not** James Earl Ray. She also testified that from her vantage point (the corner of Mulberry and Huling) she could see a fireman standing alone across from the motel when the police drove up. She heard him say to the police, *"The shot came from that clump of bushes,"* indicating the heavily overgrown brushy area facing the Lorraine and adjacent to the fire station.

Earl Caldwell was a *New York Times* reporter in his room at the Lorraine Motel the evening of April 4th. In videotaped testimony, Caldwell said he heard what he thought was a bomb blast at 6:00 PM. When he ran to the door and looked out, he saw a man crouched in the heavy part of the bushes across the street. The man was looking over at the Lorraine's balcony. Caldwell wrote an article about the figure in the bushes but was never questioned about what he had seen by any authorities.

And the only person to ever identify James Earl Ray as having been at the rooming house (never mind shooting) at the time of the murder was **Charlie Stephens**, a man so drunk a cab driver even refused to take him anywhere that day. Imagine how drunk you'd have to be for a cab driver to refuse service! Oh yes, did I mention that Stephens couldn't identify Ray when he was later shown a photograph? Did I mention that Stephens was the government's "star witness" in a trial that resulted in the conviction and imprisonment of Ray in March 1969? Oh yeah. Put the pieces together folks.

Didn't Ray Plead Guilty?

Yes, he did. The so-called trial took place suddenly on March 10, 1968 and, following a lengthy list of charges the state would have tried to prove, Ray pleaded guilty and was sentenced to 99 years. He immediately petitioned for a new trial, which was denied. He eventually died in jail in 1998.

Since he's dead, we can only speculate why James Earl Ray plead guilty, but certain anomalies stand out. Ray's lawyers were Percy Foreman and

Hugh Stanton (the Shelby County Public Defender). It is interesting to note that earlier Stanton had acted as lawyer to Charlie Stephens. Yep, the same Charlie Stephens that was the "star witness" for the prosecution. You know... the fellow who was too drunk to stand but then saw Ray running down the hallway, but then didn't recognize Ray in a photograph. Apparently no one thought that Stanton representing the prosecution's chief witness **and** the defendant was a "conflict of interest."

In December 1967, Foreman proposed to prosecutor Phil Canale that Ray could be convinced to plead guilty in exchange for a slightly reduced sentence and no death penalty. But Ray would have none of it. And it took more than two months for him to cave in, despite all manner of tactics employed to pressure him and his family into agreeing. Notwithstanding the fact that most of the evidence was in Ray's favor, Foreman told him there was a 100% chance he was going to be convicted and a 99% chance that he would get the death penalty.

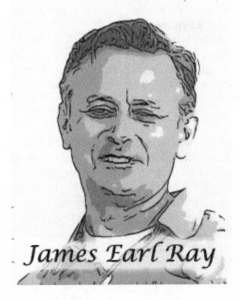

James Earl Ray

Memphis Police Department "Weirdness"

Remember the Secret Service stand down with JFK? Despite the presence of numerous people engaged in the surveillance of MLK, apparently not one of them spotted the assassin arriving, shooting him, or escaping the scene. Given that the Memphis Police Department had in the past provided extensive security for MLK on previous visits and was aware of the vulnerability of the Lorraine Motel, it seems incredible that a contingent of police bodyguards assigned to MLK on his arrival should have been removed the day of the shooting, apparently without the knowledge of the police chief, Frank Holloman.

Just two hours before the assassination the MPD's patrolling "TAC Units" (each comprising three cars) were pulled back five blocks from the vicinity of the Lorraine Motel. Police chief Holloman claimed that he did not know of that decision until afterwards. Furthermore, immediately after the shooting, no "All Points Bulletin" was issued. This would have ensured that the major escape routes out of Memphis were sealed. No satisfactory explanation has ever been provided for that failure.

In another bizarre incident, on the day of the assassination, an erroneous message was delivered by a Secret Service agent to the Memphis Police headquarters stating that there had been a death threat against a black police detective. The detective, Ed Redditt, was stationed at a surveillance post next to the Lorraine Motel. Shortly after the first message, a corrected message arrived saying that the threat was a hoax but the police intelligence officer who received it nevertheless, went to where Detective Redditt was stationed and ordered him to go home. This was two hours before the assassination. Why did the intelligence officer send Redditt home even though he knew the threat to be false?

The Pre-Crime, Crime Scene, and Clean Up

Leon Cohen, a retired New York City police officer, testified that in 1968 he had become friendly with the Lorraine Motel's owner and manager, Walter Bailey (now deceased). On the morning after MLK's murder, Cohen spoke with a visibly upset Bailey outside his office at the motel. Bailey told Cohen about a strange request that had forced him to change King's room to the location where he was shot. Bailey explained that the night before MLK's arrival he had received a call *"from a member of Dr. King's group in Atlanta."* The caller wanted the motel owner to change MLK's room. Bailey said he was adamantly opposed to moving MLK, as instructed, from an inner court room behind the motel office (which had better security) to an outside balcony room exposed to public view.

Within hours of MLK's assassination, the crime scene that witnesses were identifying to the Memphis police as a cover for the shooter had been "sanitized" by orders of the police. That's right, much like the thousands of tons of steel at the 9/11 crime scene were quickly exported to China, so the crime scene at MLK's murder was quickly cleaned up. In a 1993 affidavit from former SCLC official James Orange that was read into the record, Orange said that he *"... noticed, quite early the next morning around 8 or 9 o'clock, that all of the bushes and brush on the*

*hill were cut down and cleaned up. It was as though the entire area of
the bushes from behind the rooming house had been cleared."*

Maynard Stiles, who in 1968 was a senior official in the Memphis
Sanitation Department, confirmed that the bushes near the rooming
house were cut down. At about 7:00 AM on April 5th, Stiles told the jury
that he received a call from Memphis Police Department Inspector Sam
Evans *"requesting assistance in clearing brush and debris from a
vacant lot in the vicinity of the assassination. ... They went to that site,
and under the direction of the police department, whoever was in
charge there, proceeded with the clean-up in a slow, methodical,
meticulous manner."* Within hours of MLK's assassination, following
orders from the Memphis Police, the crime scene that eyewitnesses were
identifying as a cover for the shooter had been "sanitized."

What happened to the rifle? William Hamblin tells a story he was
told many times by his friend James McCraw, now deceased. McCraw
was the taxi driver who arrived at the motel to pick up Charlie Stephens
shortly before 6:00 PM on the day of the shooting. In a deposition read
earlier to the jury, McCraw said he found Stephens in his room lying on
his bed too drunk to get up, so he turned out the light and left without
him. Amazingly, only a few minutes later (according the official myth),
Stephens identified Ray as he was passing down the hall from the
bathroom. McCraw also said the bathroom door next to Stephen's room
was standing wide open, and there was no one in the bathroom. Why is
this important? Because that was the bathroom where James Earl Ray
was supposedly balancing on the tub as he was preparing to squeeze the
trigger and kill MLK.

At the trial, Hamblin told the jury that he and McCraw were close friends
for about 25 years. Hamblin said he probably heard McCraw tell the
same rifle story 50 times, but only when McCraw had been drinking and
had his defenses down. In that story, McCraw said that Loyd Jowers (the
owner of Jim's Grill in Memphis) had given him the rifle right after the
shooting. According to Hamblin, *"Jowers told him to get the [rifle] and
get it out of here now. (McCraw) said that he grabbed his beer and
snatched it out. He had the rifle rolled up in an oil cloth, and he leapt out
the door and did away with it."* McCraw told Hamblin that he threw the
rifle off a bridge into the Mississippi River.

Lloyd Jowers and the Mafia

In 1993, Lloyd Jowers told his story to Sam Donaldson on *Prime Time
Live.* He said he had been asked to help in the murder of MLK and was
told there would be a decoy (Ray) in the plot. He was also told that the
police *"wouldn't be there that night."* Jowers said the man who asked

him to help in the murder was a Mafia-connected produce dealer named Frank Liberto (now deceased) who had a courier deliver $100,000 for Jowers to hold at his restaurant (Jim's Grill), the back door of which opened onto the dense bushes across from the Lorraine Motel. Jowers said he was visited the day before the murder by a man named Raul, who brought a rifle in a box.

Other witnesses testified to their knowledge of Liberto's involvement in MLK's murder. Store-owner John McFerren said he arrived around 5:15 pm, April 4, 1968, for a produce pick-up at Frank Liberto's warehouse in Memphis. When he approached the warehouse office, McFerren overheard Liberto on the phone inside saying, "*Shoot the son-of-a-bitch on the balcony.*" Café-owner, Lavada Addison, a friend of Liberto's in the late 1970s, testified that Liberto had told her he "*had Martin Luther King killed.*"

Addison's son, Nathan Whitlock, when he learned of this conversation, asked Liberto point-blank if he had killed MLK. According to Whitlock, "*(Liberto) said, 'I didn't kill the n*gger but I had it done.' I said, 'What about that other son-of-a-bitch taking credit for it?' He says, 'Ahh, he wasn't nothing but a troublemaker from Missouri. He was a front man ... a setup man.'*"

Consider Myron Billett's story. If the name sounds familiar, yes, this is the same Myron Billett (aka Paul Bucilli) that was present at the meeting the night before the assassination of JFK at the Carousel Club in Dallas. And yes, his boss, Mafia chief Sam Giancana, was also at the meeting, along with Jack Ruby and Lee Harvey Oswald. According to a June 1989 interview with Myron Billett, in early 1968, Sam Giancana asked Billett (his chauffeur) to drive him, and fellow mobster Carlos Gambino, to a meeting at a motel in upstate New York.

Other major Mafia figures from New York were there as well as three men who were introduced as representatives from the CIA and FBI. There were a number of subjects on the agenda, including Castro's Cuba. According to Billett, one of the government agents offered the mobsters a million dollars for the assassination of MLK. Billett stated that Sam Giancana replied, "*Hell no, not after you screwed up the Kennedy deal like that.*" As far as Billett knows, no one took up the offer.

Billett relayed this information in an interview conducted just weeks before he died of emphysema. Given his condition, there appears to be no particular reason for him to lie. While his allegations are mentioned in the HSCA's final report, it makes no judgment as to their validity – the HSCA report simply states that is was unable to corroborate his story.

The 1999 Trial

According to a Memphis jury's verdict on December 8, 1999, in the wrongful death lawsuit of the King family versus Loyd Jowers *"and other unknown co-conspirators,"* MLK was assassinated by a conspiracy that included agencies of his own government. Almost 32 years after MLK's murder at the Lorraine Motel in Memphis on April 4, 1968, a court extended the circle of responsibility for the assassination beyond the late scapegoat James Earl Ray to the United States government.

The trial took 30 days with 70 witnesses and 4,000 pages of transcript. During the trial, the jurors heard a tape recording of a two-hour-long confession Lloyd Jowers made at a fall 1998 meeting with MLK's son (Dexter), former UN Ambassador Andrew Young, and Dr. William Pepper. Jowers said that meetings to plan the assassination occurred at Jim's Grill. He said planners included undercover Memphis Police Department officer Marrell McCollough (who now works for the CIA), Memphis Police Department Lieutentant Earl Clark (who died in 1987), a third police officer, and two men Jowers did not know but thought were federal agents. Jowers said that right after the shot was fired he received a smoking rifle at the rear door of Jim's Grill from Clark. He broke the rifle down into two pieces and wrapped it in a tablecloth. A man named Raul picked it up the next day. Jowers said he didn't actually see who fired the shot that killed MLK, but thought it was Clark, the MPD's best marksman.

Who was Raul? One of the most significant developments in the Memphis trial was the emergence of the mysterious "Raul" through the testimony of a series of witnesses. In a 1995 deposition by James Earl Ray that was read to the jury, Ray told of meeting Raul in Montreal in the summer of 1967, three months after Ray had escaped from a Missouri prison. According to Ray, Raul guided Ray's movements, gave him money for the Mustang car and the rifle, and used both to set him up in Memphis. In other words, Raul was Ray's "handler." Andrew Young and Dexter King described their 1998 meeting with Jowers at which Dr. William Pepper had shown Jowers a spread of photographs, and Jowers picked out one as the person named "Raul" who brought him the rifle to hold at Jim's Grill. Pepper displayed the same spread of photos in court, and Young and King pointed out the photo Jowers had identified as Raul. There were several other witnesses at the trial that identified Raul.

Testimony which juror David Morphy later described as "awesome" was that of former CIA operative Jack Terrell, a whistle-blower in the Iran-Contra scandal. Terrell, who was dying of liver cancer in Florida, testified by videotape that his close friend J.D. Hill had confessed to him that he had been a member of an Army sniper team in Memphis assigned to shoot "an unknown target" on April 4, 1968. After training for a triangular shooting, the snipers were on their way into Memphis to take up positions in a water tower and two buildings when their mission was suddenly cancelled. Hill said he realized, when he learned of MLK's assassination the next day, that the team must have been part of a contingency plan to kill King if another shooter failed.

Terrell said Hill was shot to death. His wife was charged with shooting Hill (in response to his drinking), but she was not indicted. From the details of Hill's death, Terrell thought the story about Hill's wife shooting him was a cover, and that his friend had been assassinated. In an interview, Terrell said the CIA's heavy censorship of his book <u>Disposable Patriot</u> included changing the paragraph on J.D. Hill's death, so that it read as if Terrell thought Hill's wife was responsible. Wow. That's pretty damning evidence, if you ask me!

Another witness was Walter Fauntroy, MLK's colleague and a 20-year member of Congress. In an April 4, 1997 article printed in the *Atlanta Constitution*, Fauntroy had said that he believed *"Ray did not fire the shot that killed King and was part of a larger conspiracy that possibly involved federal law enforcement agencies."* Later on, when Fauntroy talked about his decision to write a book about what he'd uncovered since the assassination committee closed down, he was promptly investigated and charged by the Department of Justice (DoJ) with having violated his financial reports as a member of Congress. His lawyer told him that he could not understand why the DoJ would bring up a charge on the technicality of one misdated check. Fauntroy said he interpreted the DoJ's action to mean: *"Look, we'll get you on something if you continue this way ... I just thought: I'll tell them I won't go and finish the book, because it's surely not worth it."*

At the conclusion of his testimony, Fauntroy also spoke about his fear of an FBI attempt to kill James Earl Ray when he escaped from Tennessee's Brushy Mountain State Penitentiary in June 1977. Congressman Fauntroy had heard reports about an FBI SWAT team having been sent into the area around the prison to shoot Ray and prevent his testifying at the HSCA hearings. Fauntroy asked HSCA chair Louis Stokes to alert Tennesssee Governor Ray Blanton to the danger to the HSCA's star witness and Blanton's most famous prisoner. When Stokes did, Blanton called off the FBI SWAT team, Ray was caught safely by local authorities, and in Fauntroy's words, *"we all breathed a sigh of relief."*

The 1999 trial (of course) was not covered, with very few exceptions. As a matter of fact, you've probably never even heard of it. But there was a narrow window of about 12 hours where there was some minor reporting. And then it just all went away and has never been heard of again. Except wherever it was raised, critics would start attacking, even though none of them had actually been there at the trial. In typical fashion, the critics attacked the judge. They attacked the defense counsel. They attacked the jury. They attacked the King family. They name-called. They mocked. They buried the story. Edwin Bernays would have been proud...

Drawing Some Conclusions

Perhaps the lesson of the MLK assassination is that our government understands the power of nonviolence better than we do, or better than we want to. In the spring of 1968, when MLK was marching, he was determined that massive, nonviolent civil disobedience would end the domination of democracy by corporate and military power. The "powers that be" took MLK seriously. **They dealt with him in Memphis.**

According to Dr. William Pepper who wrote the amazing book, <u>An Act of State: The Execution of Martin Luther King</u>: "*The assassination of Martin King was a part of what amounted to an on-going covert program in which they tried to suppress dissent and disruption in America.*" Much of the information in this chapter was gleaned from Pepper's book. I also obtained copious amounts of information from <u>The Murder of Martin Luther King Jr.</u> by John Edginton and John Sergeant.

A plethora of this chapter's contents came from an article by Jim Douglass in the Spring 2000 issue of *Probe Magazine*, entitled *"The Martin Luther King Conspiracy Exposed in Memphis."* Douglass was one of only two reporters who attended the 1999 trial in Memphis from start to finish. Writing in the spring of 2000, he stated, "*Thirty-two years after Memphis, we know that the government that now honors Dr. King with a national holiday **also killed him**.*"

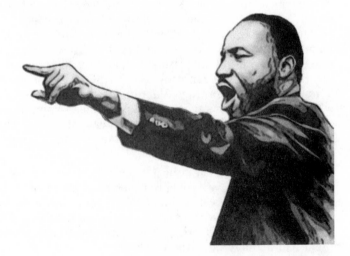

Let's summarize: Under US Civil Law, covert US government agencies were found guilty of the assassination of MLK, who was the leading figure of the Civil Rights Movement, a Nobel Peace Prize winner, and widely recognized as one of the world's greatest speakers for what it means to be human. The King family's conclusion as to motive was to prevent MLK from ending the Vietnam War because the government wanted to continue its ongoing covert and overt military operations to control foreign governments and their resources.

It is therefore a factual statement that under US Civil Law, the US government assassinated MLK.

RESOURCES

Websites
http://mcadams.posc.mu.edu/weberman/MLK.txt
http://www.ratical.org/ratville/JFK/Unspeakable/MLKconExp.html

Movie
"Media Mayhem: MLK Assassination Conspiracy"
http://www.youtube.com/watch?v=DF25N_549GE

Books
Orders to Kill: The Truth Behind the Murder of
Martin Luther King (Dr. William F. Pepper)

An Act of State: The Execution of Martin Luther King
(Dr. William F. Pepper)
The Murder of Martin Luther King Jr.
(John Edginton and John Sergeant)

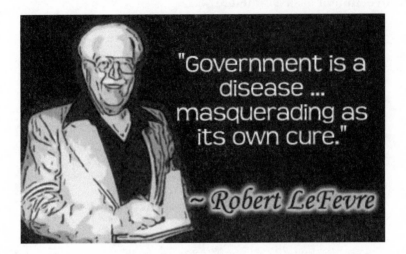

"Government is a disease ... masquerading as its own cure."

~ Robert LeFevre

Chapter 18

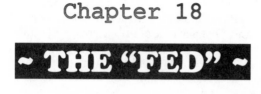

MONUMENTAL MYTH

The Federal Reserve, a branch of the US government and the nation's central bank, provides America with a safe, flexible, and stable monetary and financial system.

CAN YOU HANDLE THE TRUTH?

The Federal Reserve ("The Fed") is the biggest Ponzi scheme in the history of the world, and if the American people truly understood how it really works, they would be screaming for it to be abolished immediately. Henry Ford (founder of the Ford Motor Company in 1903) stated: *"It is well that the people of the nation do not understand our banking and monetary system, for if they did, I believe there would be a revolution before tomorrow morning."*

I remember in 2008 when Congress was attempting to pass the $700 billion "bailout," I was sitting in the San Antonio airport waiting for a flight to Nashville. I watched several "financial experts" express their opinions on the pros and cons of the bailout, and as I listened, it seemed that at least once per sentence someone would refer to "The Fed." I had to chuckle to myself as these mind-controlled bobble-heads were obviously oblivious to the truth about "The Fed."

You see, the simple truth is that The Federal Reserve System is **neither** "federal," **nor** does it have any "reserves." The Fed is a system of private banks, owned by rich foreign and American bankers. It is the biggest scam ever perpetrated upon the American people. But don't take my word for it. The Ninth Circuit Court put that issue to rest in 1982 when they adjudicated: *"Examining the organization and function of the Federal Reserve Banks, and applying the relevant factors, we conclude that the Reserve Banks are not federal instrumentalities for purposes of the FTCA, but are independent, privately-owned and locally controlled corporations."* [Lewis vs. US, 680 F. 2d 1239, 1241]

Still want more proof? Try taking a peek at a Washington, D.C. phone book. Here's what you'll find. The D.C. phone book is divided into four sections: a) general information b) residential numbers c) the Blue Pages - United States and District of Columbia governmental listings, and d) business listings. Now, where do you think the Federal Reserve should be included? If the Fed were part of the government, then it should be in section 3 – the Blue Pages. But no! Guess where it is. Yup – section 4, under **business** listings!

"But wait a minute! Doesn't the US government control The Fed? Doesn't the President appoint the Chairman of the Federal Reserve?" Well, yes, the President does appoint the Chairman, but **no**, the US government does **not** "control" The Fed.

Quite the opposite. The Fed actually controls the US government. Baron M. Rothschild once wrote, *"Give me control over a nation's currency and I care not who makes its laws."* Well, The Fed not only controls the US currency, but it also controls our politicians. The Fed is the reason we have inflation and an enormous national debt, which, by the way, will **never** be paid off, since The Fed would rather have the interest on the loan (the national debt) than the principal, because they make **trillions** of dollars from the US being in debt.

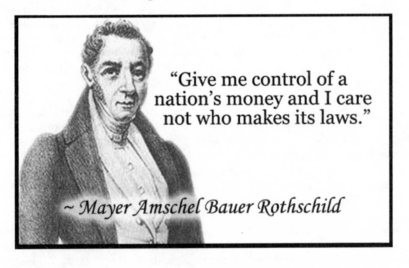

"Give me control of a nation's money and I care not who makes its laws."

~ Mayer Amschel Bauer Rothschild

The Meeting at Jekyll Island

Let's hop into our time machine (you know, the DeLorean with a flux capacitor) and travel back over a century to the year 1910. At that time, Jekyll Island (an island off the coast of Georgia) was privately owned by a small group of millionaires from New York, including William

Rockefeller and J.P. Morgan. Their families would travel to Je to spend the winter months. There was a brilliant structure clubhouse, which was the center of their social activities. The .... since been purchased by the state of Georgia, converted into a state park and the clubhouse has been restored. However, if you were to visit the clubhouse and walk downstairs, you would come to a door with a plaque stating: *"In this room the Federal Reserve System was created."*

In November of 1910, Senator Nelson Aldrich sent his private railroad car to the railroad station in New Jersey. From there, he and six other men traveled under the cloak of secrecy to Jekyll Island. They were told to arrive separately at the railroad station, not to eat together, not to speak to each other, and to act like they were strangers. They were told to avoid newspaper reporters since they were well-known people, and reporters would have wondered why these seven prominent men were all traveling together.

Once they got on board the train, the deception continued. They were told to use first names only, not to use their last names at all. A few of the men used pseudonyms. Once they arrived at Jekyll Island, they spent over a week hammering out the details of what eventually became the Federal Reserve System. When they were done they went back to New York. After the meeting at Jekyll Island, for several years, these men denied that there ever was a meeting. It wasn't until after the Federal Reserve System was established in 1913 that they then began to talk openly about their secretive trip and meeting at Jekyll Island. As a matter of fact, they wrote books, magazine articles, and gave interviews to reporters, so now it's possible to go into the public record and learn exactly what happened there off the coast of Georgia.

Who Were The Seven Men?

Senator Nelson Aldrich, whom I have already mentioned, was a Republican Senator and was the chairman of the National Monetary Commission. He was also the very important business associate of J. P. Morgan and was the father-in-law of John D. Rockefeller, Jr. and was the grandfather of Nelson Rockefeller.

Also in attendance at Jekyll Island was **Abraham Andrew**, who was Assistant Secretary of the Treasury. **Henry Davison**, senior partner of the J.P. Morgan Company, was in attendance, as was **Charles Norton**, the President of the First National Bank of New York. **Benjamin Strong**, the head of J. P. Morgan's Banker's Trust Company, was at Jekyll Island, and in 1913, when the Federal Reserve Act was passed, Strong became the first head of The Fed.

Frank Vanderlip, the President of the National City Bank (NCB) of New York, was an attendee at Jekyll Island. NCB just happened to be the largest of all of the banks in America representing the financial interests of William Rockefeller and the international investment firm of Kuhn, Loeb & Company.

Finally, there was **Paul Warburg** who was almost certainly the most important at the meeting because of his familiarity with banking as it was practiced in Europe. Paul was one of the wealthiest men in the entire world. He was a partner in Kuhn, Loeb & Company and was a representative of the Rothschild banking dynasty in France and England. He maintained very close working relationships with his brother, Max Warburg, who was the head of the Warburg banking consortium in Germany and the Netherlands.

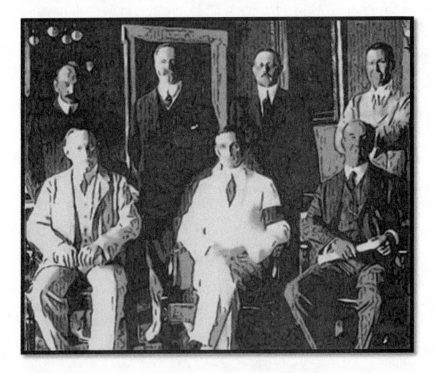

These were the seven men aboard that railroad car who were at Jekyll Island. According to G. Edward Griffin, author of The Creature from Jekyll Island, as amazing as it may seem, they represented approximately **1/4 of the wealth of the entire world**! These are the men that sat around the table and created the Federal Reserve System.

Why Was Secrecy Important?

You might ask, *"What is the big deal about a group of bankers getting together in private and talking about banking?"* According to Vanderlip, *"If it were to be exposed publicly that our particular group had gotten together and written a banking bill, that bill would have no chance whatever of passage by Congress."* You see, the purpose of the bill was to break the grip of what was referred to as the *"money trust,"* which was the concentration of wealth in the hands of a few large banks in New York on Wall Street ... and it was written by the money trust! Had that fact been known from the beginning, the US would never have had a Federal Reserve System because as Vanderlip said, Congress would never have passed it. It would have been like hiring the fox to install the security system at the henhouse. This was why secrecy was so important. The goal was to create a "central bank" much like those in existence in Europe for centuries.

How could they conceal that from the American people? Congress was already on record as saying they did not want a central bank in America. Their challenge was to create a central bank that nobody would know was a central bank. This was their strategy: first, they would give it a name and including the word "Federal" so that it appears to be an official government entity. Then they would add the word "Reserve" so that it would appear there were reserves somewhere. Then, they would add the word "System" so that it would appear that there was a system of regional banks which would spread power over the entire country and remove the concentration of financial power from New York City. When you analyze it, you will realize that what they created there was **not** federal, there are **no** reserves, and it's **not** a system at all in the sense of diffusion of power. It was brilliant strategy.

Convincing the Public

The next thing was to "sell" The Fed to the public. The first draft of the Federal Reserve Act as it was presented to Congress was called the Aldrich Bill (*named after the sponsor, Senator Nelson Aldrich*). However, since Aldrich was so identified with big business interests, the people were outraged and Congress voted it down. But, just like Congress does today, they took the bill, rearranged the paragraphs, took Aldrich's name off the bill and found a couple of Democrats (Carter Glass and Robert Owen) to sponsor the new bill. Since everybody "knew" that the Republicans represented big business and that Democrats represented the "common man," this was a brilliant move. The Aldrich Bill had morphed into the Glass-Owen bill, and the new bill was perceived as being totally different from the Aldrich Bill.

The next step was for Aldrich and Vanderlip to give speeches and interviews to newspaper reporters **condemning** the Glass-Owen Bill. They would frequently state that the new bill would be *"ruinous to banking and terrible for the country."* By the time the American public would read that comment in the local newspaper, he would gullibly say, *"Gee whiz, I reckon if the big bankers don't like the bill very much then it must be pretty good."* With this kind of expert tactics and deception, the public didn't stand a chance. It is no surprise that popular support was finally gained for the bill and on December 22, 1913 the bill was passed by Congress and the following day was signed into law by President Wilson.

As author G. Edward Griffin states, *"...the creature from Jekyll Island finally moved into Washington, DC."* After the passage of the Federal Reserve Act, Congressman Charles Lindbergh stated: *"This Act establishes the most gigantic trust on earth....When the President signs this Act, the invisible government by the money power, proven to exist by the Money Trust Investigation, will be legalized....The new law will create inflation whenever the trust wants inflation....From now on, depression will be scientifically created."* That's right! Lindbergh stated that future depressions would be "created" by the bankers.

Louis McFadden, Chairman of the House Banking Committee during the 1930s, said about the stock market crash of 1929: *"It was not accidental; it was a carefully contrived occurrence. The international bankers sought to bring about a condition of despair so that they might emerge as ruler of us all ... This evil institution has impoverished and ruined the people of these United States, has bankrupted itself, and has practically bankrupted our Government. It has done this through the defects of the law under which it operates, through the maladministration of that law by the Fed and through the corrupt practices of the moneyed vultures who control it."* Since 1913, the Federal Reserve Act has been amended over 100 times, with each amendment expanding the power and reach of the Federal Reserve System to *"create money out of nothing."*

The "Mandrake Mechanism" – Money Out Of Nothing

The passage of the Federal Reserve Act in 1913 was the creation of the partnership between a cartel of international private bankers and the US government. This is **very** important. Cartels often go into partnership with governments because they need the force of law to enforce their cartel agreement. I have heard many economists refer to The Fed's process of creating money from nothing as the *"Mandrake Mechanism"* named after the comic-book character of the 1940s, Mandrake the Magician, who could create something out of nothing. Perhaps in the current day vernacular, we would call it the *"Gandalf the Grey Gadget,"* but let's stick with "Mandrake Mechanism" because that's how it's more commonly known.

Let's take a simplified look and see how the banksters create money through the Mandrake Mechanism. Here's how it works. It starts with the government side of the partnership (Congress) which only knows how to **spend, spend,** and **spend**.

Suppose Congress needs an extra billion dollars today so it goes to the treasury and says *"we need a billion dollars"* and the Secretary of the Treasury says *"you're crazy, we're plum out of money, we ran out of the tax money back in May."*

Congress then gets together and strolls down Constitution Avenue and stops at the local Kinko's and prints off some "official" US Government bonds, which are really nothing more than fancy IOU's. After printing a billion dollars' worth of these bonds, they offer them to the private sector (i.e. the American "sheeple").

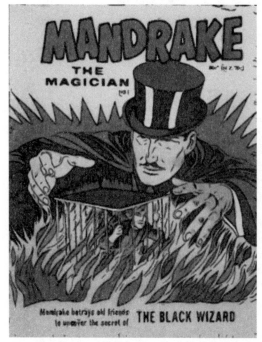

Well, tens of thousands of Americans are anxious to lend their money to the government, since they've been told by their trusted investment advisors that this is the soundest investment that you can make, since these bonds are backed by the *"full faith and credit of the US government."* They're not quite sure what that means but it sure sounds good.

Now, after selling half a billion of US bonds, Congress still needs more money...after all, they've got a spending addiction. They've already milked the American public with the issuance of the bonds, so the next day they stroll down to the Federal Reserve building. The Fed has been waiting for them – that's one of the reasons it was created. By the time they get inside the Federal Reserve building, the Fed officer is already opening up his checkbook, and he writes a check to the US Treasury for half a billion bucks.

Where Does The Money Come From?

You might be asking, *"Where did The Fed get half a billion dollars to give to the US Treasury?"* Did they have $500,000,000 in their account? The startling answer is there is **no money** in the account at the Federal Reserve. **None.** In fact, technically, there isn't even an account, there is only a checkbook. That billion dollars "springs into being" at precisely the instant the officer signs that check and, if you remember in Economics 101, that is what the professor called *"monetizing the debt."* I still remember Dr. Capone – the scrawny, peculiar, insolent, yet shrewd economics professor at Baylor University. I took two of his classes, but I never did understand exactly what *"monetizing the debt"* was while I was in college. Honestly, as bright as he was, I'm not sure that Dr. Capone did either.

Anyway, this is how the government gets its instant access to any amount of money at any time without having to go to the taxpayer directly and justify it or ask for it. Otherwise, they would have to come to the taxpayer and say we're going to raise your taxes another $7,500 this year. Of course, if they did that, then the American taxpayer would vote them out of office quick, fast, and in a hurry. No, Congress really likes the Mandrake Mechanism because it's a "no questions asked" source of instant cash.

Now, this is where it really gets interesting. Let's go back to that half billion dollar check that the Fed official just wrote. The Treasury official deposits the check into the government's checking account and all of a sudden the computers indicate that the government has a billion dollar deposit. So now the government can write a billion dollars in checks against that deposit, which Congress does very quickly, as they are going through withdrawals from not having enough money for their "spending sprees." For the sake of our simplistic analysis, let's just follow $1000 out of that half a billion.

Let's say Congress writes a $1000 check to Johnny, who cuts the lawn at the White House. He gets a check for $1000, completely clueless that only a day before, this money didn't even exist, but he doesn't care, so he deposits it into his bank account. Now, the bank manager sees that a $1000 deposit has been made he runs over to the loan window and opens it up and says *"Attention, attention, we now money to loan."* Everyone is thrilled since that's one of the chief reasons that people go to banks, right? They want to borrow money.

Well, it just so happens that Freddie (Johnny's neighbor) needs to borrow $900 for a home renovation. The Federal Reserve System requires that the banks hold no less than 10% of their deposits in reserve, so the bank holds 10% of that $1000 in reserve ($100) and it loans

Freddie the $900 he needs for his home renovation. What do you think Freddie does with the $900? He wants to spend it so he puts it into his checking account.

When he puts this $900 into his checking account, it's considered a deposit, then the bank is only required to keep $90 in deposits and can turn around and loan out $810. The next fellow also needs a loan, so he borrows the $810, deposits it into his checking account, and then the bank has more deposits which can, in turn, create more loans. At the end of the day, the bank can eventually loan out $9000 based on the initial $1000 deposit, as a result of the 10% fractional reserve requirement.

Where did the $9000 come from? The answer is the same as when the Fed officer wrote the check... **there was no money**. The money is "created" precisely at the point at which the loans are made. Think about this for a minute. This money was created out of nothing and yet the banks collect interest on it which means that they collect interest on **nothing**. What a racket, huh? Gandalf and Mandrake have nothing on the banksters that control the Fed, do they?

"Money Soup"

But the story doesn't stop there. This newly created money goes out into the economy and it **dilutes** down the value of the dollars that were already out there. My lovely wife Charlene cooks an amazing homemade chicken tortilla soup. The broth is amazing. Now, if I were to add a gallon of water to the cauldron, it would ruin the broth. But this is analogous to what's happening with the money supply. Injecting this "money created from nothing" into the economy is like pouring water into a wonderful pot of soup.

So by throwing more and more money into the US "economic soup," the money gets weaker and weaker and weaker and we have the phenomenon called inflation which is the appearance of rising prices. But inflation is just the "appearance" of rising prices. In reality, prices are not really rising. Inflation is a result of our money falling in value, more commonly referred to as the "devaluation of the dollar." If this dollar devaluation continues, our money will be more useful as toilet paper than as a medium of exchange.

And with the recent housing crisis, I'm sure that you are all familiar with the fact that, when you get that bank loan of money created out of nothing, the bank wants something from you. It wants you to sign on the dotted line and pledge your house, your car, your inventory, your assets so that in case for any reason you cannot continue to make your payments they get your assets. The banks are **not** going to lose anything on this. Whether its expansion or contraction, inflation or deflation, the banks are covered and we like sheep go right along with it because we haven't figured it out, we don't know that this is a **scam**.

Want some statistics? OK, I'm a CPA. I can do that. According to a *Yahoo Finance* article dated 9/13/2013, the Federal Reserve has "created" approximately $2.75 trillion (out of thin air) and injected it into the financial system over the past five years. This has artificially inflated the stock market (currently soaring to unprecedented heights), but it has also caused our financial system to become precariously unstable. According to the limited GAO audit of the Fed that was mandated by the Dodd-Frank Wall Street Reform and Consumer Protection Act, the Federal Reserve made a whopping $16.1 trillion (that's right ... **trillion**) in "secret loans" to the big banks during the last financial crisis (from 2007 to 2010).

The following is a list of loan recipients that was taken directly from page 131 of the report...

Citigroup	$	2.513	trillion
Morgan Stanley	$	2.041	trillion
Merrill Lynch	$	1.949	trillion
Bank of America	$	1.344	trillion
Barclays PLC	$	868	billion
Bear Sterns	$	853	billion
Goldman Sachs	$	814	billion
Royal Bank of Scotland	$	541	billion
JP Morgan Chase	$	391	billion
Deutsche Bank	$	354	billion
"All Other Borrowers"	$	4.446	trillion

How's that? Looks to me like the only **real** financial crisis was with "*we the people*." Apparently, the big banksters never had any worries. Also, did you notice the foreign banks? Barclays, RBS, Deutsche Bank? Why were our dollars being used to bail out foreign banks while tens of millions of American families were genuinely suffering?

I've spoken to many people about the issue of the Fed and the fractional reserve system. And I've heard all the remarks and retorts and criticisms. "*Your paranoid ... Your nuts ... You're a conspiracy theorist ... You're a worry wart .... What? Buy gold and silver? Why? You're crazy ... You fear monger.*" I understand. Honestly, I do. I know that it's easier just to go back to sleep and crawl back into the "matrix."

Remember Cypher? The character in movie, "The Matrix," who decided to take the blue pill and continue in the dream? His quote rings true for many people: *"You know, I know this steak doesn't exist. I know that when I put it in my mouth, the Matrix is telling my brain that it is juicy and delicious. After nine years, you know what I realize? Ignorance is bliss."*

The only difference between Cypher and your average American is that one day, in the near future, it's going to be made crystal clear that the Federal Reserve issued "steak" (i.e. the dollar) isn't juicy and delicious, but is, in fact, rotten and full of gravel. And not only that, but the steak is poison and will kill you. And it will kill the country. It's already killing the country.

In Summation

Let's hear from one of the most influential Founding Fathers of the USA:

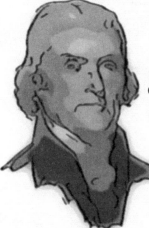

"If the American people ever allow private banks to control the issue of their money, first by inflation and then by deflation, the banks and corporations that will grow up around them, will deprive the people of their property until their children will wake up homeless on the continent their fathers conquered ... I sincerely believe the banking institutions having the power of money, are more dangerous to liberty than standing armies."

~ Thomas Jefferson

Our fundamental document (the US Constitution) states in Article 1, Section 8: *"The Congress shall have the power to coin money and regulate the value thereof."* Nowhere is there the slightest hint of authorization to delegate that power even to another governmental institution — much less to a private banking system.

Well, I guess you now have taken a "crash course" on the Federal Reserve System. I can assure you that you now know more about The Fed than you probably would if you enrolled in a four year college course in economics because they don't teach this stuff in school.

If you want to learn more about the Federal Reserve System, I strongly recommend The Creature from Jekyll Island by G. Edward Griffin. It is the "magnum opus" of books on this topic.

I leave you with this thought: In the Bible, we learn that the debtor is a slave to the lender. That is the relationship of the USA to The Federal Reserve System. In essence, we are all **slaves** to the international private bankers who own The Fed.

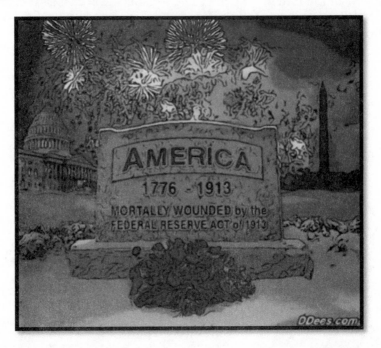

RESOURCES

Websites
http://www.healthfreedom.info/Federal_Reserve_Fraud.htm
http://alittletruth.hubpages.com/hub/Federal-Reserve-System-Biggest-Scam-in-History

Movie
"History of the Federal Reserve (The Money Masters)"
http://www.youtube.com/watch?v=EeIM-4hJO44

Book
The Creature from Jekyll Island (G. Edward Griffin)

Chapter 19

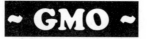

MONUMENTAL MYTH

Genetically modified organisms ("GMO") have been thoroughly tested and have been proven to be safe. They are needed to feed the world since they result in higher yield crops. Nobody ever got sick or died after eating GMO food.

CAN YOU HANDLE THE TRUTH?

Before we get rolling on this issue, I want to clarify the difference between GMO and hybrid plants. Farmers and gardeners have been cultivating new plant varieties for thousands of years through selective breeding. They did this by cross-pollinating two different (but related) plants over multiple generations, eventually creating a new plant variety. Hybrid seeds are just as natural as their historic counterparts, since they are merely cross-pollinated from two different (but related) plants.

Genetic modification, on the other hand, involves the laboratory process of artificially inserting genes into the DNA of food crops or animals. The result is called a genetically modified organism ("GMO"). GMO can be engineered with genes from bacteria, viruses, insects, animals, or even humans. The primary reason the plants are engineered is to allow them to basically *drink poison*. They're inserted with foreign genes that allow them to survive otherwise deadly doses of poisonous herbicides, fungicides, and insecticides. Genetic engineering creates combinations of plant, animal, bacteria, and viral genes that do not occur in nature. Scientists are putting fish genes into tomatoes and strawberries, human genes into corn and rice and sugarcane, jellyfish genes into corn, and even spider genes into goats!

Except for the "spider-goat" mentioned above, these techniques create different characteristics in the "franken plant," such as resistance to chemicals like Roundup® (glyphosate). When glyphosate is sprayed on GMO crops, they resist the herbicide. It kills the weeds, but not the crops. Farmers love it because they may get a higher yield from their farms. But how to these crops affect the people that eat them? This is the $64,000 question.

Imagine that you spray an insecticide on a plant, but you are unable to wash it off prior to eating it, because it has become part of the plant! Guess what happens when you eat the plant. You ingest that insecticide. **Case in point**: Monsanto has crossed genetic material from bacteria known as *Baccilus thuringiensis* ("Bt") with corn. This is one of the most common GMO traits, and crops that contain the Bt toxin are designed to kill insects and pests by breaking open their stomachs.

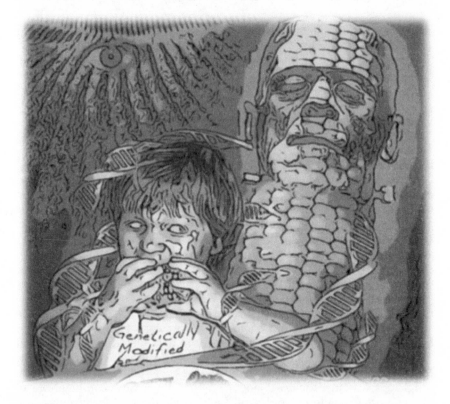

The resultant GMO plant (known as *"Bt Corn"*), is itself registered as a pesticide with the EPA, since the Bt toxin actually becomes part of every cell of the plant. In other words, if you feed this corn to your cattle, your chickens, or yourself, you'll be feeding them an actual pesticide, not just a smidgeon of pesticide residue. Bt corn has been implicated in the deaths of cows in Germany, and horses, water buffaloes, and chickens in the Philippines.

Speaking of intestines, the proliferation of GMO has corresponded with upticks in bowel diseases such as diverticulitis, colitis, and irritable bowel syndrome (IBS), Crohn's disease, leaky gut, and, especially in children, allergies. Coincidence? I don't think so. It's a massive human experiment, and we **all** are the guinea pigs.

Leaky gut syndrome takes place when fissures open between cells lining the gastrointestinal tract. Partially digested food particles ooze through those fissures into the body and appear to be foreign invaders. The immune system activated to do what it does best: seek and destroy. This is one of the main problems with GMO – they introduce gene sequences that the body has never seen before. Our immune systems then attack the GMO as if it were a harmful pathogen (which it actually is).

A 2009 study by Italian researchers (Benachour and Seralini) published in *Chemical Research in Toxicology* examined the toxicity of four popular glyphosate based herbicide formulations on human placental cells, kidney cells, embryonic cells, and neonate umbilical cord cells. What they found was shocking: **Total cell death** of each of these cells within 24 hours. In an interview at the European Parliament, Professor Andrés Carrasco (Argentine government scientist) reported that childhood cancer increased by 300% and babies with birth defects by 400% during the past decade in parts of Argentina, where GMO soy is grown to supply European farmers with cheap GM animal feed. He also noted that Argentinian children were consuming so much GMO soy that they began developing breasts from the estrogenic effects. His studies show glyphosate exposure can cause defects in the brain, intestines, and hearts of fetuses. Moreover, the amount of Roundup® used on GMO soy fields was as much as 1,500 times greater than that which created the defects!

In the past two decades, GMO have completely infiltrated our farm fields, grocery stores, and kitchens to such an extent that most folks have no idea how many GMO they actually consume daily. If you ingest processed foods, bread, pasta, crackers, cake mixes, canola oil, mayonnaise, soymilk, veggie burgers, corn tortillas, corn chips, corn oil, corn syrup, or anything else made from corn, soy, or cotton, you are usually consuming GMO. The first GMO food hit the market in 1994 (the "Flavr Savr" tomato). Since then, sugar beets, potatoes, corn, squash, rice, soybeans, vegetable oils and animal feed have all been manipulated. Each year, American farmers plant over 200 million acres of GMO crops. It is estimated that each person in the USA eats about 200 pounds of GMO foods per year!

But, hey, at least the GMO crops produce higher yields so we can "feed the world" right? **Think again.** In a 2013 study funded by the USDA, University of Wisconsin researchers refuted the "higher yield" argument for GMO. The researchers looked at data from that compared crop yields from various varieties of GMO corn between 1990 and 2010. While some GMO varieties delivered small yield gains, others did not. With the exception of one commonly used trait, the authors concluded, *"we were surprised **not** to find strongly positive transgenic yield effects."* Please allow me to translate: Both the glyphosate-tolerant (Roundup® Ready) and the Bt toxin (for corn rootworm) caused yields to drop. That's right. They found that GMO crops produce **less** rather than more food!

In an article from the Cornucopia website, Maria Rodale cites a number of independent studies that point to the dangers of GMO. One study she cites, taken from a journal entitled *Nature Biotechnology*, states *"after we eat GMO soy, some of the GMO genes are transferred to the microflora of our intestines and those GMO genes are still active."* She goes on to state that a study found in the journal *Reproductive Toxicology*, *"found Bt-toxin (used in genetically modified Bt corn) in the blood of 93% of the pregnant women studied and their babies."*

"But my doctor told me that GMO are safe."

Is that the same doctor that used to recommend smoking cigarettes for healthy lungs? OK, sorry, I couldn't pass it up. Anyway, if your doctor thinks GMO are safe, perhaps he/she hasn't been listening to the American Academy of Environmental Medicine (AAEM), because they certainly don't think so. As a matter of fact, AAEM reported that *"several animal studies indicate serious health risks associated with GM food,"* including infertility, immune problems, accelerated aging, faulty insulin regulation, and changes in major organs and the gastrointestinal system. The AAEM asked physicians to advise patients to avoid GMO foods, and due to the serious health risks, in 2009, they called for a moratorium on GMO foods, safety testing, and labeling. In their own words, *"There is more than a casual association between GM foods and adverse health effects. There is causation."*

Most people don't realize that before the FDA decided to allow GMO into food without labeling, FDA scientists had repeatedly warned that GMO foods can create unpredictable, hard-to-detect side effects, including allergies, toxins, new diseases, and nutritional problems. They urged long-term safety studies, but were ignored.

Am I being fair? Only giving one side of the story? God forbid! So let's check out Monsanto's own website and see what they say about GMO. After all, they are one of the largest producers of GMO. On their website (www.Monsanto.com), they refer to *"a large body of documented scientific testing showing currently authorized GM crops safe"* through a body called the Center for Environmental Risk Assessment (CERA). They were even kind enough to give a link to CERA's website.

Thanks Monsanto!

So, when I visited the CERA website (www.CERA-gmc.org), I found a list of people who make up the Advisory Council for CERA, which their website says *"is to act in an advisory and consultative capacity for CERA's Director and staff."* One of the members of this advisory council is Dr. Jerry Hjelle, Ph.D. Take a guess as to whom he works for. Can you guess? C'mon. Take a guess. Yep. **Monsanto!** Dr. Hjelle is Monsanto's VP for Science Policy. So, let me get this straight. One of the advisors for the organization that "researches" the safety of GMO also works for one of the largest companies that manufacture GMO. Are you kidding me? This takes *"the fox is guarding the henhouse"* to another level!

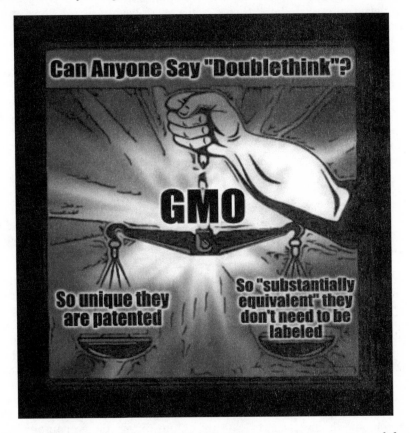

Of course, this is pretty typical with Monsanto. As a matter of fact, because of Monsanto, the only "testing" for safety that is required is for the GMO producer to submit a self-authored report on the safety of the new GMO. This scam was devised by Michael Taylor, a former FDA lawyer who established the "no testing" policy by reasoning that GMO's are "substantially equivalent" to food, and food has already been determined to be safe. Taylor (second cousin to Tipper Gore) is notorious for his "revolving door" employment within the US government and Monsanto and was chosen by Obama as the FDA Deputy

Commissioner for foods (aka the "food safety czar") in July 2009. While at Monsanto, Taylor's main responsibility was gaining regulatory approval of the GMO cancer-causing bovine growth hormone (rBGH).

And then we have Margaret Miller, a former Monsanto researcher who wrote a report on whether rBGH was safe. Soon after the report was completed, the FDA came knocking on her door. *"Maggie, how would you like a job?"* they asked. Miller was hired by the FDA as the Deputy Director of the Office of New Animal Drugs. Can you take a guess at what her first "job" at the FDA was? Yes indeed, her first job was to "approve" the very report that she authored while at Monsanto. Effectively, in the area of American food safety, we now have the "fox" guarding the "henhouse."

I'm shocked! (Not really.) Especially in light of the fact that Monsanto is the same company that manufactured DDT, Agent Orange, PCB, and dioxin. Cancer is being linked to PCB exposure. Thousands of US soldiers as well as Vietnamese civilians have cancer because of being exposed to Agent Orange during Vietnam. These people are suffering the horrible consequences of this chemical being sprayed in the jungles, leaching toxic and deadly chemicals into the water, soil and the air. Children are being born with birth defects, and thousands are dying of cancer caused by the exposure. The controlled mainstream media and Medical Mafia have both participated in many cover-ups and lies about the toxic effects of these chemicals. But hey, what do you expect? Many of them are criminals! And the mainstream media has long since been "bought and paid for" by the banksters that own the Fed.

Even though 93% of Americans believe that GMO should be labeled, proponents of GMO labeling are facing a bruising "food fight," given that the Big Agra and the biotech industry have spent massive amounts of money to combat prior GMO-labeling proposals. For example, California's "Proposition 37" was narrowly defeated in 2012 after companies such as Monsanto, Pepsico, and Kraft poured $46 million into lobbying against it. Then, in 2013, the same companies spent over $27 million into lobbying against Washington's "Initiative 522," which was also defeated. So this begs the question: If GMO are so "good for you," then why is Big Agra spending tens of millions of dollars to keep us in the dark about whether or not GMO are on our dinner plate or in our kids' lunchboxes?

And as I previously mentioned, they have not been adequately tested. One of the most glaring faults in the current regulatory GMO "testing" regime is the short duration of animals feeding studies. The industry limits trials to 90 days at most, with some less than a month. Short studies could easily miss many serious effects of GMO. It is well established that some pesticides and drugs, for example, can create effects that are passed on through generations, only showing up decades later. Nearly all GMO crops are described as "pesticide plants" because they either tolerate doses of weed killer (such as Roundup®), or produce an insecticide like Bt toxin. When regulators evaluate the toxic effects of pesticides, they typically require studies using three types of animals, with at least one feeding trial lasting 2 years or more. Typically, at least 1/3 (or more) of the side effects produced by these toxins will show up **only** in the longer study and **not** the shorter ones.

Case in point: Scientists in France, led by Gilles-Eric Seralini of the University of Caen, recently conducted feeding tests in rats over a period of two years. They fed the animals GMO corn sprayed with Roundup®. In the late summer of 2012, I remember when the results of the study (along with the photos of the rats with grotesque tumors) were published in the journal *Food and Chemical Toxicology*. Some of the tumors were so large the rats even had difficulty breathing. The authors stated: *"Scientists found that rats exposed to even the smallest amounts, developed mammary tumors and severe liver and kidney damage as early as four months in males, and seven months for females ... the animals on the GM diet suffered mammary tumors, as well as severe liver and kidney damage."* According to Dr. Michael Antoniou (molecular biologist), *"This research shows an extraordinary number of tumors developing earlier and more aggressively - particularly in female animals. I am shocked by the extreme negative health impacts."*

No, the Seralini study has not been debunked. Remember, any time you challenge mainstream dogma, you will be attacked. And so was Seralini. So let's debunk the debunkers, shall we? According to my friend Mike Adams ("the Health Ranger"), *"Not long after being published, Seralini's study was maliciously ripped apart by 'skeptics,' the media and many industry-backed institutions that claimed it was a badly-designed cancer study. But the truth is that Seralini's study was actually a chronic toxicity study, and one that met or exceeded all accepted scientific standards. ... The chorus of whining that ensued about how Seralini's study allegedly contradicted all other similar studies is also invalid, as no other similar studies have ever been conducted – Seralini's study is the only long-term study involving Monsanto's NK603 GM corn that has ever been conducted. Another popular criticism involves the Sprague-Dawley (SD) variety of rat used by Seralini in his study. This same variety has been used by Monsanto on many occasions in its 90-day 'safety' studies on GMO."*

Simply put, Seralini used the **same** type of rats and the **same** type of GMO corn that had been used in the previous Monsanto tests. The only difference was that, rather than pulling the plug at 90 days like Monsanto had done, Seralini continued the study for one year. And guess what. At between 120 and 150 days, the rats started developing tumors. Hmmm ... do you think Monsanto knew this might happen? Do you think this is why they always pulled the plug at 90 days?

Unbelievably, many people still don't want to know the truth about GMO. I suppose they'd rather live in their dreamland in the sand than believe the studies. So, if you're one of those folks who still want your GMO, please ... Don't listen to me. Don't listen to Seralini. Don't listen to Mike Adams or Liam Scheff or Robert Scott Bell or Dr. Joseph Mercola or Jeffrey Smith.

Keep eating your GMO. Feed them to your kids. They're "good for you." Stay asleep. Take the blue pill. Remain in the matrix. Avoid the "conspiracy nuts." Nothing to see here. Move along...

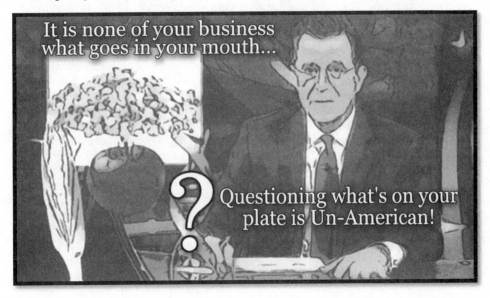

RESOURCES

Websites
http://www.responsibletechnology.org/
http://tahomaclinicblog.com/wp-content/uploads/2013/09/Seralini-2012.pdf
http://www.naturalnews.com/037249_gmo_study_cancer_tumors_organ_damage.html

Movies
"GMO Explained by the Health Ranger"
http://www.youtube.com/watch?v=b8qvskYvnH8
"Genetic Roulette – The Gamble of Our Lives"
http://geneticroulettemovie.com/

Chapter 20

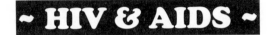

MONUMENTAL MYTH

A chimpanzee or a monkey somewhere in Africa transmitted simian immunodeficiency virus (SIV) to a human, and the virus "trans mutated" into human immunodeficiency virus (HIV). HIV, which is either a virus or retrovirus, somehow damages or stimulates or does something else to the immune system, eventually (mystifyingly) causing acquired immune deficiency syndrome (AIDS). HIV or AIDS (or both) are spread sexually, through intravenous drug use, and/or blood transfusions. AIDS is a fatal, incurable disease.

CAN YOU HANDLE THE TRUTH?

Ask your physician where AIDS came from and he/she will probably tell you the epidemic started when monkeys or chimps in the African bush transferred the AIDS virus (aka HIV) to a person while butchering primate meat for food or through an animal bite. Others will tell you that a homosexual and a monkey fell in love and ... well ... the rest is history. Regardless of the hypothetical origin, the fact of the matter is that there is no relationship between AIDS and HIV. The relationship is a **myth ... a fairytale ... a fable ... a legend.**

No, AIDS is not a monkey-gay-pervert disease. The multi-billion dollar HIV/AIDS industry is based on the monumental myth that AIDS is a disease caused by the "HIV" virus. The truth of the matter, which I will attempt to prove in this section of the book, is that the diagnosis of "HIV positive" means nothing of any relevance to health. It can be triggered by vaccines, malnutrition, the flu, leprosy, hepatitis, MS, measles, papilloma virus wart, pneumonia, antibiotic damage, Epstein Barr virus, glandular fever, malaria, syphilis, and over fifty other conditions. In the words of Liam Scheff, *"A diagnosis of 'HIV positive' is like a diagnosis of 'Yes, he's breathing.' "* The diagnosis of "HIV positive" has created the "AIDS" epidemic and the multi-billion dollar "AIDS research and treatment" racket ... err ... ummm ... I mean "industry."

There is no scientific evidence that exists today that proves the existence of HIV. No, I'm not saying that AIDS is fake. No, I'm not saying that people aren't suffering from very real immune suppression disorders. They are. What I am saying is that **HIV** is entirely fake. There is no such thing as a virus (or retrovirus) that causes AIDS. You see, the modern Medical Mafia's explanations of HIV and AIDS are a monumental medical myth (at best) and outright quackery (at worst).

In his book, Official Stories, Liam Scheff covers the official story about HIV and AIDS. His book was an inspiration for this chapter, so I'll be quoting from it throughout. So kick back, pull up a chair, prop your feet up on a pillow, grab some whisky (I mean orange juice), and get ready to learn some information that you've likely never heard before. Don't dismiss it. Just read it, chew on it, and then decide if it makes sense.

Dr. Robert Gallo

The tale of Dr. Robert Gallo's role in the discovery of the "virus" that causes AIDS is one of those stories that wouldn't be believable as fiction. While the phony "war on cancer" was looking for a virus which caused cancer, failed National Cancer Institute (NCI) "virus hunter," Robert Gallo, went from claiming that the same class of virus that caused massive cellular proliferation (cancer) now causes cellular death (AIDS).

You see, in 1976, Gallo (a young, belligerent, arrogant researcher at the NCI) claimed to have discovered a "cancer retrovirus" he called "HTLV-1" – a retrovirus that caused T-cells (a type of white blood cell) to go nuts and become cancerous. Sounds dangerous, doesn't it? Better watch out for that retrovirus! However, one of Gallo's contemporaries, Peter Duesberg, pointed out that in a group of over 600,000 people who tested positive for "HTLV-I," only 339 people had leukemia. That's only .06%. Six-hundredths of a percentage point. Six people out of a thousand. You get the point. HTLV-I causes leukemia ... except 99.9435% of the time.

Gallo had stimulated lab cultures of leukemia cells to produce an enzyme called Reverse Transcriptase (RT). It was assumed that when RT was found, retroviruses were at work. However, it turns out that RT is not unique to retroviruses at all and is not even a meaningful indicator, because the cells normally produce this enzyme. Tricky tricky tricky, Mr. Gallo! Shame on you. Pure junk science. A load of crap.

Gallo then discovered "HTLV-II" which causes ... well ... it doesn't cause anything. But hey, it was another notch in his belt, and Gallo wanted to be famous. So, a few years later, Gallo claimed that RT was a specific marker for another retrovirus, "HTLV-III," which he later called "HIV." Gallo claimed to find "virus like particles" (which he labeled HIV), but what he failed to mention (*"oops, my bad"*) was that his actual finding was regenerative proteins created by the cells when put under stress with hydrocortisone, which inhibits the production of nitric oxide and promotes the formation of regenerative proteins, which he called HIV.

Translation: he created a normal by-product in the lab and then labeled it HIV! Scientific fraud. Quackery.

Liam Scheff covers Gallo quite nicely in <u>Official Stories</u>, so I'll paraphrase some of his arguments while I elaborate. Even though Gallo had already tried to pull the same scam twice before (with HTLV-I and HTLV-II), apparently the third time was a charm, because a swarm of researchers had contracted "virus fever." Well, not literally. Maybe "money fever" would better describe the condition, because they **really really** wanted to find a new "bug" to do what polio had done for their forerunners. Polio had turned penurious researchers into multi-millionaires. So, in the end, the "RT" enzyme became synonymous with "retrovirus" ... even though everybody knew it really wasn't. Think about it! A "retrovirus" blamed for cellular proliferation (cancer) was now being blamed for cell death (AIDS)!

In 1984, Gallo's original papers proclaiming a new retrovirus was the cause of AIDS were published in *Science* magazine on May 4th. And this became the basis of the entire AIDS industry! Gallo actually "borrowed" most of his information (without asking) from Luc Montagnier, who was awarded the Nobel Prize in 2008 for discovering AIDS. Interestingly, in the 2009 film "House of Numbers," Montagnier stated to filmmaker Brent Leung: *"We can be exposed to HIV many times without being chronically infected. Our immune system will get rid of the virus in a few weeks, if you have a good immune system."*

According to Jad Adams in <u>AIDS: The HIV Myth</u>, *"It's not even probable, let alone scientifically proven, that HIV causes AIDS. If there is evidence... there should be scientific documents which... demonstrate that fact... There are no such documents."*

Coincidentally, Robert Gallo announced that HIV was the cause of AIDS the same day he patented a test for HIV. Since then, Gallo has obtained approximately 80 HIV/AIDS related patents which have earned him over **$1 billion** in the private sector. All of this fame, all of this money, for a virus that doesn't even exist. In light of these facts, it sure appears to me that Gallo was a "huckster," right up there in the ranks of Louis Pasteur. Heck, getting paid billions of dollars to treat a non-existent disease almost makes him a "magician."

I wonder if he took lessons from Merlin? Or Mandrake? Or Gandalf the Grey?

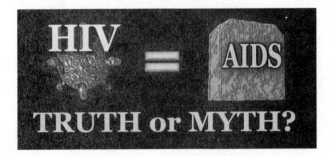

The HIV Test

HIV tests are protein tests. They look for reactions between proteins in the test kits and proteins in your blood. The only problem (well, actually one of many problems) with the HIV test is that it was constructed out of entirely normal proteins which occur in sick people **and** healthy people. According to the official HIV/AIDS myth, these proteins supposedly originated from some monkey (or chimp) virus.

According to Liam Scheff: *"HIV infection is inferred from a test that, in fact, has no standards for determining the presence or absence of HIV infection and comes up positive for an unknown number of conditions. These include: Pregnancy, flus, colds, vaccination, drinking, drugging and sex. Or just being alive. Or being around animals. Or being an animal. A mouse, dog, or cow, for example. HIV is believed to be a retroviral particle, which is considered 'fragile, wily, never the same,' and which cannot be purified or isolated. Various photos of putative 'HIV' tend to resemble every other kind of normal budding particle coming out of both healthy and sick cells."*

He continues, *"Furthermore, HIV has never been observed in any way, shape, or form, eating, humping, squeezing, biting, being angry at, stimulating, flattering with false praise, or in any other way, molesting or infecting T-cells. How HIV causes AIDS remains a rather profound mystery. And, besides a bit of colorful language, that's still official. It's just not what they put on billboards."*

Manufacturers of the HIV tests do not even claim that they work! Here are some disclaimers from the manufacturers themselves:

+ *"At present there is no recognized standard for establishing the presence or absence of HIV-1 antibody in human blood."* ~ Abbott Laboratories

- *"Do not use this kit [Western blot] as the sole basis of diagnosing HIV-1 infection."*

- *"...in the general population, which the CDC estimates to have a prevalence of HIV infection of 0.006%, using a test with a specificity of 99%, the result is that 94% of all positives will be false positives."* ~ The Western blot

- *"The Amplicore HIV-1 Monitor test is not intended to be used as a screening test for HIV or as a diagnostic test to confirm the presence of HIV infection."*

Huh? What did they say? Why would the manufacturers say such things? Let me paraphrase Liam Scheff in Official Stories, without some of his "colorful language." Why the disclaimer? I'll tell you why. Because when someone tells them, *"You lied to me; this test doesn't test for HIV. It's worthless. You ruined my life. I'm going to sue you!"* The manufacturers will pull out the paper, flip them off, and say, *"Get lost. We never said it tested for HIV."* Imagine that ... HIV tests that are **not** intended to be used to screen for HIV! The fact is that the AIDS industry and medical "experts" have stated, in no uncertain terms, that HIV tests are a complete and utter fraud that have given rise to the monumental myth that AIDS is a transmissible sexual disease.

The fraudulent HIV test is biased to give more false positives (actually all the test does is give false positives) for targeted groups – namely blacks. Africans are being wiped out because of a false test. In Africa, they diagnose multiple distinct diseases as "AIDS," oftentimes without even administering a test! By claiming that almost thirty separate diseases are actually the untreatable, incurable, terrifying AIDS, Africans are given a death sentence, rather than treatment. If you get a chance, check out Dr. Robert E. Willner, who inoculated himself with the blood of Pedro Tocino (a HIV-positive hemophiliac) on live Spanish television. You can still watch the video on YouTube.

Of course, from a monetary perspective, the HIV test was a huge success. I mean, who doesn't know what "HIV-positive" means? And when you hear those words, much like the "big C" word, you are stricken with fear and panic. You see, when you combine the diagnosis of "HIV-positive" and the prediction (stated or implied) that "You will die of AIDS," you have one of the most impressive pieces of medical "black magic voodoo" in history. Heck, people have committed suicide on the basis of the ludicrous diagnosis of "HIV positive" alone! So, what do they want? *"Give me the treatment!"* And what was (and is) the treatment?

Azidothymidine ...

AZT

Azidothymidine (AZT) began as a "cancer drug" but was withdrawn for being too toxic. Sort of like being thrown out of the Gestapo for being too cruel, I suppose. Even though it had failed at cancer, AZT was resurrected and put through a sham trial. Despite the fact that 169 out of 172 people taking AZT died in the trial, it was released for use in people that were "HIV-positive." Like most chemotherapy drugs, AZT works by stopping cell reproduction. It devastates the bone marrow, which, by the way, produces blood and also is a key component of the lymphatic system, producing lymphocytes which support the immune system. AZT is also a super-antibiotic. It destroys intestines, bowels, and livers. **It is toxic.** As a matter of fact, the actual label features a skull and crossbones.

The effects of AZT include cancer, hepatitis, dementia, seizures, anxiety, impotence, leukopenia, severe nausea, ataxia, etc. and the termination of DNA synthesis. Nevertheless, AZT was distributed like candy to tens of thousands of healthy folks who were "HIV-positive," and the AIDS death rate, which had been declining, mysteriously began to rise. Not too surprisingly, AZT eventually kills almost everyone who takes it. Like my friend Michael...

Back in the late 1980s and early 1990s, I was a competitive bodybuilder. One of my buddies was a man named Michael. We trained at World Gym together in Austin, Texas. Michael was healthy. He was also gay. I still remember the day that Michael was told by his doctor that he was "HIV-positive." He dropped by my apartment, and I noticed that his normally tan face was white as a sheet. I knew something must be wrong. And he told me. The doctors were going to start him on AZT immediately.

Let's backtrack for a moment. Michael was healthy and strong. He was not sick. He didn't have any symptoms that I can remember. Until the day he went to the doctor for a checkup, we would train together in the gym, and he was as strong as an ox. His heart was healthy and his muscles were strong. Seriously. He probably was 180 pounds and in great physical condition... until they started him on AZT. Once he began the "treatment," he seemed to, all of a sudden, look sick. His complexion changed from tan to pale. His face became emaciated and his body began to shrivel up. I can still remember this very vividly. In my heart, I knew that something was wrong, but I was still too naïve to understand (or wouldn't let myself believe) that they were killing him. And he died within three months of beginning treatment. A healthy thirty year old man was gone. He died alone in a hospital room, less than 100 pounds, with his liver destroyed. I still recall the night he died. I cried. That's all I have to say about that.

According to Dr. Peter Duesberg, *"The most toxic drug that has ever been licensed for long term consumption in the free world. ... AZT is a prescription drug and according to the manufacturer itself it causes symptoms that are indistinguishable from AIDS. So I would say it is not arrogant for me to say that AZT is AIDS by prescription."*

Celia Farber, a rare journalist who tried to be honest about the AIDS epidemic, was at an AIDS conference in 2008, where she was talking to a representative of Glaxo, the company that manufactures AZT. She wrote up the following story for Liam Scheff, which he included in <u>Official Stories</u>, and she also posted to her website. She stated, *"So speaking of reality, I wanted to ask you to tell me something honestly. And it's not an accusation, I just want to know your perspective. If I were to say to you, that it seemed clear to us all in the late 80s, that people were dying very rapidly from high dose AZT–not from 'AIDS' but from high dose AZT, I mean 1200 mg, 1000, mg, and so forth, the early years ... if I were to say that as a statement of fact, that high dose AZT was killing gay men outright in those years, would you think I was wrong?"* The drug rep then answered resolutely, *"Of course not, you'd be right."* And then came the hammer. Looking right into my eyes, not even blinking, she said: *"Why do you think we lowered the dose?"*

Yep, the rep admitted that they were killing AIDS patients with mega-doses of AZT. According to Liam, *"by the mid-90s, AIDS doctors finally understood that they'd killed a hundred thousand young gay men and stopped giving AZT as a primary treatment and radically lowered its dose (down to 100 or 200 milligrams). The death rate followed suit and dropped down close to pre-megadose-AZT levels. It's a really, really funny story, isn't it? If you're amused by mass murder. Now AZT is pumped into pregnant women. That's the primary market for the drug. Pregnant women who test positive."*

He continues, *"On the drug they have more miscarriages, birth defects and deaths than those not poisoned to death. Not surprising, is it? Today the AIDS drug business rolls on, still making AZT and its many clones. In the mid-90s, they added protease drugs, which alter physiology, melt the fat in the arms and face, leaving skin and bones, whittling muscle to nothing, redistributing fat into humps on the neck and back, bloating the stomach beyond proportion and making legs into toothpicks. This is what these drugs do. It even says so on the warning labels. Guys go blind, lose part of their colon, have plastic surgeries to stuff silicon into their calves and under their cheekbones - it's a whole industry that rides codicil to the AIDS drug business."*

AZT is yet another instance of Big Pharma and the Medical Mafia keeping us deaf, dumb, and blind to ourselves. We enthusiastically pay them to experiment on us, poison us, and kill us, with a smile on our face.

The Gay Community

The homosexual community hasn't changed much over the past 30 years. It's still like the Eagles' song, "Life in the Fast Lane." At the gay clubs, on any given night, you'll see a plethora of "uppers" (like cocaine, crack, and ecstasy) and "downers" (like valium, Xanax, and Quaaludes). You'll see LSD and heroin, too. Oh yeah, I almost forgot the alcohol and cigarettes. And crystal meth ... and PCP ... and "poppers."

Liam describes why poppers are so dangerous: *"Poppers weren't even considered a drug, but a party favor, like a beer at a game or glass of wine with dinner. These inhalant drugs came in bottles that said, 'flammable; fatal if swallowed' on the label, but were snorted and huffed from bottles and rags all night. Why? Because they gave a great rush, extended libido and erections far beyond the boundaries of normal human fatigue. More than that, because they rendered the user insensible to pain, the muscles in the sphincter would relax. Taken with methamphetamines, a lot of sex was (and is) had that was more intense, invasive and penetrating of the body than anything anyone had seen or done before. It was done in groups, with multiple partners and night after night – after night."*

He continues, *"And, no, condoms are not de rigueur, not that they'd do much against the kind of intestinal tearing that you get while fisting. This practice, of getting an arm up someone's colon, was attractive to the meth and popper set. No, it's not good for you. You stretch and rip the colon, you're spilling poop and bacteria into the blood. You now have sepsis, systemic fungal infections and internal wounds. If you have sex with two or five or eight guys in a night; or 10, 20, 30 or 50 in a week - and this was happening - you're going to have such a collection of STDs, that you could open a microbial zoo and charge admission to see the strange creatures you're carrying around. To deal with this, these guys popped antibiotics - they were in dishes and bowls in the bath houses, where so much of this sexual activity took place. Drugs like tetracycline and other broad-spectrum, gut-stripping chemicals. Antibiotics are gut bombs. They wipe out all of the essential bacteria in your intestine, so you can't really digest. You have diarrhea, no appetite and you begin to starve. Add to it your pile-up of STDs and what happens is you lose your functional immune system."*

So, what happened next? Well, in light of the fact that 70% to 80% of the immune system resides in the intestines, which were being decimated (in gay men) by the drugs, antibiotics, and rectal probing, it's not surprising. Liam states, *"Gay men started showing up in emergency rooms, pale, skinny, weak, used up, destroyed; unable to cope with the mildest bacteria and fungi that live on our bodies. The doctors plied* *them with antibiotics – but they were already on antibiotics. And they died. A lot of them. Quickly, painfully."*

What Causes AIDS? Ask The Experts...

From the inception of the AIDS paradigm in 1984 to the present, the answer is the same: *"We don't know, but please keep sending us your money."* Below are a few telling quotes from the AIDS "experts":

- *"We are **still very confused** about the mechanisms that lead to CD4 T-cell depletion, but at least now we are confused at a higher level of understanding."* ~ Dr. Paul Johnson, Harvard Medical School

- *"We still **do not know how,** in vivo, the virus destroys CD4+ T cells.... Several hypotheses have been proposed to explain the loss of CD4+ T cells, some of which seem to be **diametrically opposed**."* ~ Joseph McCune, immunologist

- *"Despite considerable advances in HIV science in the past 20 years, the reason why HIV-1 infection is pathogenic is still debated... There is **a general misconception** that more is known about HIV-1 than about any other virus and that all of the important issues regarding HIV-1 biology and pathogenesis have been resolved. On the contrary, what we know represents only a **thin veneer on the surface** of what needs to be known."* ~ Mario Stevenson, virologist

- *"Twenty-five years into the HIV epidemic, a complete understanding of what drives the decay of CD4 cells – the essential event of HIV disease – **is still lacking**...."* ~ W. Keith Henry, Pablo Tebas, and H. Clifford Lane

- *"Although twelve years have passed since the identification of HIV as the cause of AIDS, **we do not yet know how HIV kills its target, the CD4+ T cell,** nor how this killing cripples the immune system."* ~ T.H. Finkel, National Jewish Center for Immunology and Respiratory Medicine

Earlier in this chapter, I mentioned "House of Numbers." In this film were a series of telling quotes by Dr. Jay A. Levy, MD, director of the Laboratory for Tumor and AIDS Virus Research at UCSF. Levy initially states, *"HIV does **not** necessarily kill the cells it infects."* But then, one minute later, he contradicts that statement as he says, *"Some T-cells **are directly killed** by HIV and other T-cells keep the virus in check."* Then, just three minutes later, Adams states, *"How HIV depletes the T-cells so an individual advances to AIDS is probably due to multi-factorial elements. One is that **it will kill the cell** ... that it infects."* Huh? Levy contradicted himself twice in the span of four minutes! Wow! Does he have a clue?

What you're reading in these incredible quotes is billions of wasted tax-payer dollars. And hundreds of thousands of patients killed by extremely toxic drugs like AZT, used to "kill the virus" that "kills T-cells" – except they aren't sure how (or if) HIV actually kills the T-cells. Yep, it's still a "puzzle" to the so-called "experts." Do T-cells die when in the presence of "HIV" DNA? No. Yes? What is it? The official answer is, *"We're confused at a much higher level of understanding."* Gosh, these experts do seem to be having trouble, don't they?

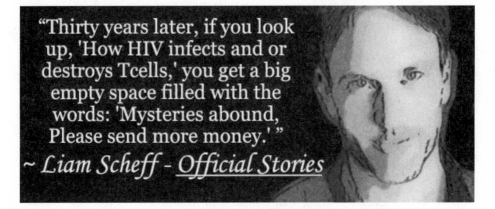

"Thirty years later, if you look up, 'How HIV infects and or destroys Tcells,' you get a big empty space filled with the words: 'Mysteries abound, Please send more money.' "

~ *Liam Scheff - Official Stories*

The Immune System and "GRID"

The gut doesn't just digest food. It kills pathogens and gives rise to the immune function that is so vital to maintain health. As I mentioned above, 70% to 80% of the immune system resides in the intestines. The bacteria in the gut are responsible for the formation, signaling, and distribution of our immune system cells (including T- and B-cells). Remember Gallo's "HTLV-1"? You know, the retrovirus that caused T-cells to go nuts and become cancerous? Well, Gallo was full of crap on this issue, but T-cells do have much to do with our health. The AIDS research from 30 years ago was largely focused on T-cells as well, and the health and functionality of your T-cells is directly dependent on the integrity of your intestines and all the happy critters that live down there. The friendly fauna. The good bacteria. Whatever you want to call them. I personally like "colon critters."

But, in the words of Liam Scheff, the gay men were (and still are) *"destroying their intestines at both ends, giving themselves sepsis and putting nuclear bombs into their guts. As a result, they got very sick and went to the hospital, where western medicine finished the job. Because western medicine does not know how to care for the human body. It is good at sewing parts back together after an explosion, because that's what it was developed for: war. Our emergency room medicine is just a progression of WW1 battlefield surgery. We have no 'official cures' for cancer, 'AIDS,' obesity, diabetes, chronic fatigue, M.S., fibromyalgia and a dozen other conditions that sprout up daily. Because all of western medicine emerges from one single idea: There is a pathogen, we must kill it. That's Pasteur's model. Put a gun down the throat and shoot the patient until the 'virus' or 'bacteria' is dead. If the patient survives, so much the better. If not, we'll have to shoot bigger bullets next time."*

What is "GRID"? According to a researcher named Tony Lance, who also happens to be gay, GRID stands for "gay related intestinal dysbiosis." His theory, which makes very good sense, is that the immune failure known as "AIDS" in the gay male community may actually be caused by damage to the intestinal flora due to common sexual and hygiene practices, such as rectal douching and the use of some sexual lubricants, as well as the high rate of antibiotic abuse in some subsets of gay men. According to Lance, the activities most associated with AIDS (in the 1980s)were drug use and also being the receptive partner. In other words, most of the men who got sick were on the receiving end and were using poppers and other drugs. Incidentally, AIDS was initially called "GRID" by a California physician. In this case, GRID stood for "gay related immune deficiency." But this was too offensive to gay activists, so they called it AIDS.

Summing It Up

In the words of Mike Adams, *"I've finally put the pieces together on this. It turns out that AIDS propagandists are just like some of the global warming scientists: They've already decided what's true and they viciously attack anyone who even dares to ask an intelligent question about the validity of their so-called science ... It doesn't even matter whether they're right or wrong – their unwillingness to even tolerate sensible questions obliterates any credibility they might have previously had. A credible scientist, you see, is happy to answer questions or even critics. Credible scientific study stands up to scrutiny. It can withstand scientific challenges and weather the storm. But none of the conventional AIDS theories are allowed to be questioned at all. And why not? Because if an intelligent, evidence-based inquiry into conventional AIDS propaganda were to ever be conducted, the whole fraudulent system would collapse like, well, a house of cards. (Hence the* name 'House of Numbers' for the documentary.) But that can't be allowed to take place. Much like we see with vaccines and cancer, too much money is riding on conventional AIDS mythology, and it's too late to change their story."

Over two thousand (and rising) of the world's scientists are now disputing the HIV/AIDS hoax. Either scientists do not see evidence for a lethal virus called HIV (saying that it has never really been isolated) or they assert that the virus is harmless. In any case, it is helpful to remember that, in science, correlation is not causation. Needless to say, their efforts are being continually suppressed by the AIDS establishment, Big Pharma, the mainstream media, and political and media lackeys. Of course, the mere mention of any intent to question conventional HIV/AIDS myth brands you as an "AIDS denier" – a vicious, derogatory term thrown about like a linguistic hand grenade in an attempt to instantly halt any intelligent conversation about HIV and AIDS.

This leads us to the incontrovertible fact that in today's society, you either agree with the conventional AIDS propagandists, or you're a "crazy conspiracy kook." Don't question. Just believe what the "officials" tell you. There's no open-mindedness for those who might actually think for themselves (gasp!) instead of just swallowing the monumental myths as if they were scientific fact. Which begs the question: What's the point of having a **scientific** method if the **scientists** aren't going to follow it?

Bottom line: HIV tests are a crock of crap. AIDS isn't caused by HIV, but AIDS is real, and it's easily treatable. But you've got to fix the gut, the intestine, the bowel and the parts that are leaking into the blood. On the other hand, destroying your intestine is something that will certainly kill your T-cells and allow all of the fungal and bacterial illnesses that affected the original AIDS patients to occur. What a strange coincidence.

I like the way Liam Scheff put it: "*We don't live in a world plagued by HIV infection, but a world in which many people are ill for many reasons: poverty, pharmaceutical poisoning, street drug abuse, toxic environmental poisoning, pure starvation, filthy parasite-ridden water, and fear.*" And that fear is propagated by the mainstream media, the Medical Mafia, and the AIDS industry.

"If there is evidence that HIV causes AIDS, there should be scientific documents which either singly or collectively demonstrate that fact, at least with a high probability. There is no such document."

~ Dr. Kary Mullis, Biochemist, 1993 Nobel Prize for Chemistry

RESOURCES

Websites
http://www.collective-evolution.com/2011/12/19/hiv-myth-hiv-causes-aids/
http://www.harmonikireland.com/hiv-hoax/

Movies
"House of Numbers"
http://www.youtube.com/watch?v=_p-ttLfkZHQ
"HIV is a Myth"
http://vimeo.com/13562122

Books
Official Stories (Liam Scheff)
AIDS: The HIV Myth (Jad Adams)

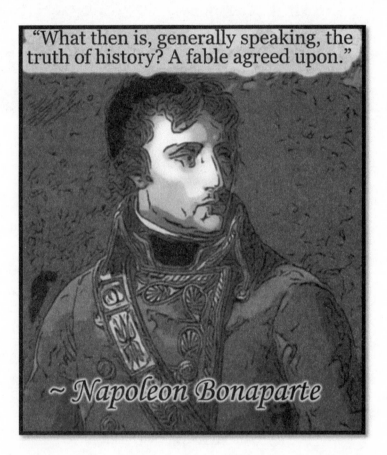

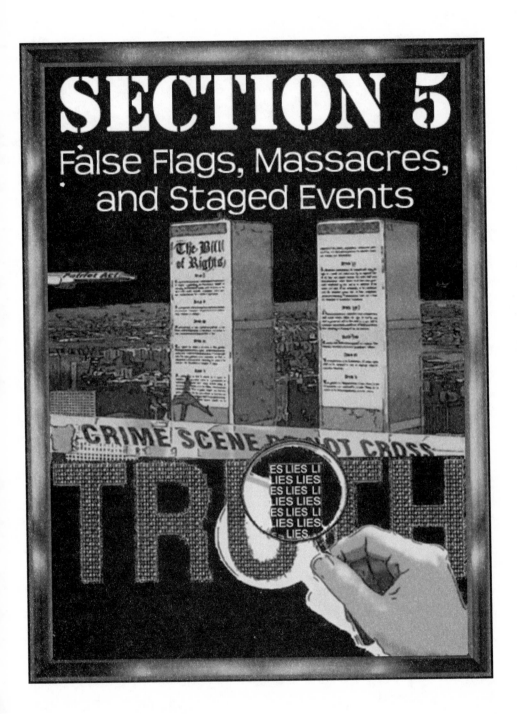

SECTION 5
False Flags, Massacres, and Staged Events

Chapter 21

~ HISTORY OF FALSE FLAGS ~

MONUMENTAL MYTH

Governments are compassionate and caring toward common citizens. A government would **never** attack its own citizens and then blame another country (or entity) as a pretext to invade the other country, demonize the entity, or to curtail liberty for its own citizens.

CAN YOU HANDLE THE TRUTH?

Wikipedia defines false or black flags as *"covert operations designed to deceive the public in such a way that the operations appear as though they are being carried out by other entities."*

Remember the Hegelian Dialectic which I mentioned earlier in the book? You know – *"thesis, antithesis, synthesis"* (aka *"problem, reaction, solution"*) – where a problem is manufactured usually with a ready-in-the-wings antithesis (reaction) so that the resulting synthesis (solution) can take society further toward a knee-jerk direction that it doesn't really want to go. This is the premise behind false flags, which serve as a fake, hostile action by some sinister (yet vague) enemy, requiring some bold, new reaction by the all-caring, loving, protective government. Typically, the actions – new laws, restrictions, warnings or declarations (of war) – have been written long ago.

Most importantly, false flags allow beleaguered, often inept "leaders" to go before the public and pretend to be strong and "leaderly" to the terrorized masses. Allegedly under attack by the ambiguous boogie man and victimized by the continuous doses of propaganda spewed forth by the bobble-head "reporters" on TV, the people seek the solace and protection of their fearless leader and their government. Do I sound cynical? OK, maybe I am. But the truth is that **it's all an act** – scripted from the very beginning – from the first explosion to the close up on the fearless leader by the TV news camera, focusing on their determined expression, the victims, the flags, and the national seal in the background. Whatever weakness the bumbling idiot leader displayed in the weeks, months or years beforehand, can be brushed aside with a few, well-prepared, scripted speeches.

History is replete with examples of "false flag" attacks.

For instance, in AD 64, Nero set fire to Rome and then blamed the Christians. He then proceeded to burn, crucify, dismember, and feed them to the lions.

On February 27, 1933, after Hitler came to power, the Nazis burned down the Reichstag (Parliament) building and blamed it on the Communists to justify a "temporary" suspension of civil liberties to cope with the terrorist threat. This is how Hitler became dictator. The "temporary" suspension lasted until Germany was in ruins. Just three weeks later, the Nazis passed the Enabling Act which gave Hitler the authority to pass laws without the approval of Parliament. Then, in Operation Himmler, the Nazis faked attacks on their own people and resources which they blamed on the Poles, to justify the invasion of Poland.

The US Navy's own historians now admit that the sinking of the *USS Maine* in 1898 (which was justification for the US entry into the Spanish-American War), was caused by an internal explosion of coal rather than an attack by the Spanish. But, hey, that didn't stop the USA. Never let a good opportunity for war go to waste!

And then there was Pearl Harbor. A BBC special found it likely that America knew of the Japanese plan to attack Pearl Harbor — down to the exact date of the attack — and allowed it to happen to justify America's entry into World War II. You see, we had broken the Japanese "purple code" up to 2 months prior to the attack on Pearl Harbor. Moreover, with the McCollum Memo of 1941, the White House apparently had launched an 8-point plan to provoke Japan into war against the USA. President Roosevelt, over the course of 1941, implemented **all eight** of the recommendations contained in the McCollum memo. Following the eighth provocation, Japan attacked. Surprise, surprise.

Just like the "bully" at school, if you push the "weak kid" long enough, if you tantalize him and mock him, eventually the fear turns to anger, he gets furious and retaliates. When Japan attacked, Americans were told that it was a complete surprise, an "intelligence failure," and the USA entered World War II. Complete surprise my ear! We literally begged the Japanese to attack us!

Moreover, declassified US government documents show that in the 1960s, the US Joint Chiefs of Staff signed off on a plan code-named "Operation Northwoods." The plans, which had the written approval of the Chairman and every member of the Joint Chiefs of Staff, called for innocent people to be shot on American streets; for boats carrying refugees fleeing Cuba to be sunk on the high seas; for a wave of violent terrorism to be launched in Washington, D.C., Miami, and elsewhere. People would be framed for bombings they did not commit; planes would be hijacked and blown up (using an elaborate plan involving the switching of airplanes), and then the Cubans would be blamed and their country invaded. The operation was not carried out only because the JFK administration refused to implement these Pentagon plans, which was one of the reasons JFK was killed, as we learned in a previous chapter.

In the Gulf of Tonkin incident, North Vietnamese torpedo boats allegedly attacked the *USS Maddox* in the Gulf of Tonkin, off Vietnam, in a pair of assaults on August 2nd and August 4th of 1964. It was the basis for the Tonkin Gulf Resolution, which committed major American forces to the war in Vietnam. The resolution passed the House of Representatives unanimously, and passed in the Senate with only two dissenting votes.

Here's the problem: It was pure fable, pure fiction, a myth, a tall tale. Invented as a pretext for war and delivered in a one-two punch, the Gulf of Tonkin incident never happened. The US government admitted this in declassified documents. The "attack" was fabricated. War ensued.

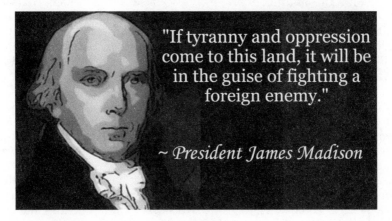

"If tyranny and oppression come to this land, it will be in the guise of fighting a foreign enemy."

~ *President James Madison*

In 1967, during the six day war between Israel and the Arab nations, the *USS Liberty* was sent into the Mediterranean Sea for "intelligence reasons." The American flag aboard the *Liberty* flapped clearly in the breeze. On June 8th, in an attack lasting more than two hours, the *Liberty* was bombed, rocketed, napalmed and torpedoed. Three unmarked Israeli aircraft, accompanied by three torpedo boats, conducted the brutal assault. As valiant crewmen fought the flames and rushing sea water, their life rafts and lifeboats were deliberately destroyed by Israeli gunfire. The *Liberty* continuously called for help to the two aircraft carriers nearby. Some fighter jets were scrambled, but were recalled by the White House. In response, the Admiral of the Fleet called the White House to determine exactly why the rescue fighters were recalled and why the naval commanders should be denied permission to defend the *Liberty*. It has been said that LBJ told the Admiral: "*I want that g*ddamn ship on the ocean floor.*"

On that day, 34 Americans were killed, and 171 were wounded. There is no question the Israelis not only intended to sink the *Liberty* but also to kill the entire crew so that no living witnesses could emerge to point the finger at them. Fortunately, there was an Egyptian ship nearby, and as a result, the Israelis didn't sink the ship. The *Liberty* survivors were told to "*shut up*" and anyone who talked was threatened with court-martial. "*If anyone asks,*" the sailors were told, "*tell them it was an accident.*" The survivors were dispersed worldwide so that no two men were sent to the same place. More than forty-five years later, we know that this was without a doubt a "false flag" operation. LBJ had an inside deal with Israel for this attack. Egypt was blamed for the attack, which gave the USA an excuse to enter the war and take over the Middle East.

Another false flag: 9/11. Yes, we'll talk about that in a few moments. Don't get too squirmy in your chair. I know it's uncomfortable. But please focus on the facts. Do you remember what happened right after 9/11? You know, the anthrax scare – when those letters which contained anthrax along with notes purportedly written by Islamic terrorists were mailed to members of Congress? Well, I'll bet you didn't know that the anthrax was a "weaponized" anthrax strain from the top US bioweapons facility in Fort Detrick? Indeed, top bioweapons experts have stated that the anthrax attack may have been a CIA test "gone wrong."

Huh? "Gone wrong" is an understatement. How about "false flag" to scare Americans into more overarching government control to "keep them safe"? Never mind that the only Congress members mailed anthrax letters were key Democrats, and that the attacks occurred one week before passage of the freedom-curtailing PATRIOT Act, which seems to have scared them and the rest of Congress into passing that act without even reading it. And though it may be a coincidence (certainly it must have been a coincidence), White House staff began taking the anti-anthrax medicine before the anthrax attacks occurred.

This all sounds nuts, right? Completely crazy! You've never heard of this "false flag terrorism," where a government attacks its own people then blames others in order to justify its goals? And you are skeptical of the statements discussed above?

Please take a look at this quote by Hermann Goering, Nazi leader and close confidante of Adolph Hitler.

> "*Why of course the people don't want war ... But after all it is the leaders of the country who determine the policy, and*

> *it is always a simple matter to drag the people along, whether it is a democracy, or a fascist dictatorship, or a parliament, or a communist dictatorship ... Voice or no voice, the people can always be brought to the bidding of the leaders. That is easy. All you have to do is to tell them they are being attacked, and denounce the pacifists for lack of patriotism and exposing the country to danger. It works the same in any country."*

Please get your head around the fact that we live in the matrix. At least it's a propaganda matrix. Big lies substitute for the truth. Stories are made-up. Political scoundrels promote them. Terror threats are manufactured. States of emergency are declared. Pretexts are needed for militarism, imperial wars, and homeland repression. False flags provide the necessary "ammo" to fool the public. If and when people learn they were duped, it's too late to matter.

It's an American tradition. Incidents are strategically timed. Innocent victims suffer. So does everyone living under heightened national security state conditions.

Rule of law principles are discarded.

Unobstructed domination alone matters.

Wars on humanity follow.

Monumental myth-makers and lying liars facilitate them.

Media whores and "press-titutes" repeat them.

False flags play their part.

RESOURCES

Websites
http://www.wanttoknow.info/falseflag

Video
"Jesse Ventura On False Flags"
http://www.youtube.com/watch?v=Bk6XwjLxb58

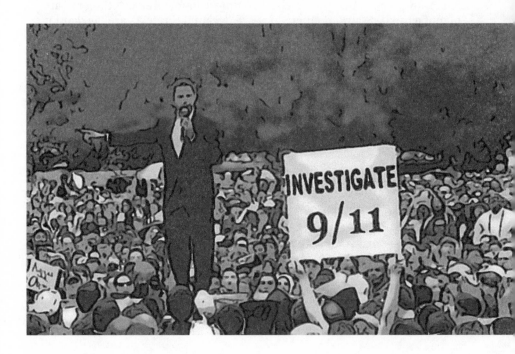

Chapter 22

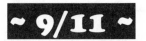

MONUMENTAL MYTH

"On the morning of September 11, 2001, 19 men armed with box cutters directed by a man on dialysis in a cave fortress halfway around the world using a satellite phone and a laptop directed the most sophisticated penetration of the most heavily-defended airspace in the world, overpowering the passengers and the military combat-trained pilots on 4 commercial aircraft before flying those planes wildly off course for over an hour without being molested by a single fighter interceptor.

These 19 hijackers, devout religious fundamentalists who liked to drink alcohol, snort cocaine, and live with pink-haired strippers, managed to knock down 3 buildings with 2 planes in New York, while in Washington a pilot who couldn't handle a single engine Cessna was able to fly a 757 in an 8,000 foot descending 270 degree corkscrew turn to come exactly level with the ground, hitting the Pentagon in the budget analyst office where DoD staffers were working on the mystery of the 2.3 trillion dollars that Defense Secretary Donald Rumsfeld had announced "missing" from the Pentagon's coffers in a press conference the day before, on September 10, 2001.

Luckily, the news anchors knew who did it within minutes, the pundits knew within hours, the Administration knew within the day, and the evidence literally fell into the FBI's lap. But for some reason a bunch of crazy conspiracy theorists demanded an investigation into the greatest attack on American soil in history." – James Corbett (the *Corbett Report*)

CAN YOU HANDLE THE TRUTH?

It was a dramatic, cinematic event. Everyone remembers where they were when the 9/11 event happened. I call it the 9/11 "event" instead of the 9/11 "attack" because I am not convinced it was indeed a terrorist attack, as there are just too many anomalies. Remember Lieutenant Columbo? The murderers always believed they got away with the perfect crime, except that they always make mistakes, since it's virtually impossible to think of everything, all the finest and most intricate details of the crime. When Columbo started to sniff around the crime scene, he'd slowly realize there were inconsistencies, and it was these inconsistencies that ultimately and inevitably led him to the truth and helped him answer the question of "who dunnit."

So, "who dunnit" ... when it comes to 9/11? Bin Laden, of course! At least that's the official myth. If you remember, even as the World Trade Centers were burning, a stream of disinformation laying down the key official 9/11 myth was being actively being put in place via the mainstream media. We all remember the myth: the impact of the planes weakened the structures, the "intense" fires caused the collapses, and Bin Laden was the only possible suspect.

What I want to do in this chapter is to list a multitude of anomalies that just don't make sense. Let's not focus on whether or not the buildings fell from fire, controlled demolition, or whatever. Let's focus on facts. One fact is that accepting the official story of the 9/11 attack requires one to accept a long series of anomalies, amazing coincidences, physical impossibilities, and contradictions, many of which defy the laws of the universe, the laws of physics, the laws of probability, and quite frankly, many of them just defy common sense.

Liam Scheff, my friend and colleague, painted a vivid picture of what really went down on 9/11 in his book, Official Stories. Since it was a huge inspiration to me, especially for this chapter, I'll be quoting from it throughout.

Anomaly #1 – The Prelude, "War Games" and Put Options

On the very morning of 9/11/01, no less than fifteen war games and terror drills were being conducted by several US defense agencies, including one "live fly" exercise using real airplanes. The Head of the Joint Chiefs of Staff on 9/11 (Air Force General Richard B. Myers) admitted to four of the war games in congressional testimony. These war games focused on hijacked aircraft by military fighters, which, as part of the war games, were sent hundreds of miles over the Atlantic Ocean (chasing "ghosts") rather than intercepting actual hijacked planes.

Operation Northern Vigilance redeployed northeast sector air defense resources to northern Canada and Alaska. Operations Vigilant Warrior and Vigilant Guardian, which simulated airline hijackings and involved live radar "injects," may have confused military and civilian personnel monitoring aircraft. The National Reconnaissance Office (NRO), which monitors satellites and airborne objects, was evacuated while the attack unfolded because it was conducting a plane-into-tower crash drill. This is the reason why the satellite surveillance of 9/11 has not been made available. Allegedly there is none because, due to the NRO drill, all space based surveillance was conveniently disabled in time for the 9/11 attacks. The Tripod II bio warfare exercise, scheduled for 9/12/01, resulted in the deployment of FEMA to Manhattan before the attack. There were many other drills: Amalgam Warrior, Global Guardian, and as my mother used to say, "*oodles and gobs*" more. Check them out. Do a web search. They're there.

Just three months before 9/11 (in June 2001) there was another war game called Amalgam Virgo, which was a NORAD exercise involving a suicide pilot attacking a military installation in the USA. If you do a search for "Amalgam Virgo tactical exercises," you should be able to find the PDF. Check out the cover! (I posted it below.)

Do you recognize the picture? Of course.

It's the boogie man!

No, it's Freddie Krueger!

No, it's ... it's ... Osama Bin Laden! Wow, what a coincidence!

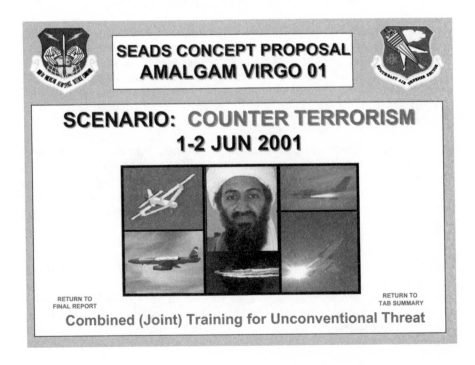

As a result of the war games happening simultaneously while 9/11 was unfolding, air traffic controllers and radar operators didn't know if what they were seeing on the screens were exercises or real events. According to Boston Air Traffic Control: *"We need someone to scramble some F-16s or something up there, help us out."* Northeast Air Defense Sector replied: *"Is this real world or an exercise?"* Boston reiterated: *"No, this is not an exercise. Not a test."*

As Liam wrote, *"No, the plastic-knife-hijackers didn't just get lucky. They were part of a program. 'The Combined Dark Lords of Banking and Chaos present: Day of Supreme Confusion!' How else can you get the US military to ignore an attack in North America? These kids sign up to kick ass and righteously shoot bad guys. You're telling me they just didn't give a crap because it was too early in the morning? Of course not. They were bound and gagged."*

An eminent mathematician worked out the probability of this coinciding with a real event; he actually arrived at a figure with 41 zeros behind it! A number that is greater than all the grains of sand of all the deserts in the entire world. Let me show you the actual number. It will blow your mind. 900,000,000,000,000,000,000,000,000,000,000,000,000,000 to 1 odds of the drills coinciding with a real event. Just think about it! And they want you to believe it was a coincidence! I'm **not** making this up.

And then there was Able Danger. Ever heard of Able Danger? Probably not. But I'm sure you know who the so-called "tactical leader" of the 19 extremist, fundamentalist Muslim hijackers was. C'mon. Think hard. It was ... Mohammed Atta. While Osama was controlling the entire terrorist operation from a remote cave somewhere in Afghanistan, Atta was his right hand man here in the USA. At least that's the official story. Atta's face became the symbol of Islamic terrorism.

Now, over a decade later, we know that Atta was connected to a top secret operation of the Pentagon's Special Operations Command (SOCOM) in the USA. According to Army reserve Lieutenant-Colonel Anthony Shaffer, a top secret Pentagon project (code-named Able Danger) had identified Atta and three other 9/11 hijackers as members of an al-Qaida cell more than a year before the attacks.

According to Shaffer, Able Danger was a highly classified operation tasked with *"developing targeting information for al-Qaida on a global scale"*, and used data-mining techniques to look for *"patterns, associations, and linkages."* The official 9/11 Commission, which according to its own declaration aimed *"to provide the fullest possible account of the events surrounding 9/11"* in its 567-page report, failed to mention Operation Able Danger or any other US-based SOCOM operations.

Hmmm ... no wonder I (and many others) refer to it as the 9/11 "Omission" Report.

And then there were the stock trades. Although uniformly ignored by the controlled mainstream media, there is abundant and clear evidence that a number of transactions in financial markets indicated specific (criminal) foreknowledge of the 9/11 events which occurred at the World Trade Center and the Pentagon. In case you aren't aware of the terminology, "put options" are stock trades betting on the value of stocks to fall. In the days preceding the 9/11 event, put options on American Airlines stock rose to **25 times** normal levels.

Coincidence? You tell me.

And then we had San Francisco Mayor Willie Brown who received a warning not to fly on 9/11, meanwhile Scotland Yard prohibited Salman Rushdie from flying that day. Oh yes, I almost forgot, numerous Pentagon officials canceled flight plans for 9/11.

Somebody knew about the attacks ahead of time ...

Anomaly #2 – NORAD, the FAA and PTech

It is standard operating procedure for North American Aerospace Defense Command (NORAD) to scramble jet fighters whenever a jetliner goes off course or radio contact with it is lost. Period. No debate. It's just what happens. Frequently. For instance, between September 2000 and June 2001, interceptors were scrambled 67 times. In the year 2000 jets were scrambled 129 times.

But routine interception procedures were not followed on September 11, 2001. Despite normal intercept times of between 10 and 20 minutes for errant domestic flights, the airliners commandeered on 9/11 roamed the skies for over an hour without interference, traveling hundreds of miles in the opposite direction of their flight plans.

There were three particular types of failures on 9/11.

Failures to Report – According to NORAD's timeline, the FAA reported errant airliners after inexplicable delays. The FAA took 18 minutes to report Flight 11's loss of communication and deviation from its flight plan. The FAA took 39 minutes to report Flight 77's deviation from its flight plan.

Failures to Scramble – Interceptors were only scrambled from distant bases after long delays. Despite the fact that Flights 11 and 175 were headed for New York City, no interceptors were scrambled from nearby La Guardia, or from Langley, Virginia. Despite NORAD's having received formal notification of the first hijacking at 8:38 AM, no interceptors were scrambled from Andrews to protect the nearby Pentagon until after it was hit at 9:37 AM.

Failures to Intercept – Once in the air, interceptors flew at only small fractions of their top speeds, assuring they would fail to intercept the airliners. According to analysis published at <u>www.911research.wtc7.net</u>, the two F-15s scrambled from Otis AFB to chase Flight 11 flew at an average of 447 mph, about **23.8%** of their top speed of 1875 mph. The two F-16s scrambled from Langley to protect the capital flew at an average of 410.5 mph, about **27.4%** of their top speed of 1500 mph.

I have a friend named Al who is a pilot. He told me the story about when he accidentally veered off course while flying his small jet plane. According to Al, who happens to be ex-military, it was less than 5 minutes before he had an F-15 on each wing. They actually fired a flare at him, basically warning him that if he didn't get back on course, they were going to shoot him down.

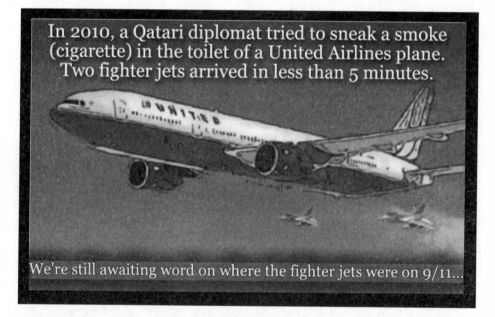
In 2010, a Qatari diplomat tried to sneak a smoke (cigarette) in the toilet of a United Airlines plane. Two fighter jets arrived in less than 5 minutes.

We're still awaiting word on where the fighter jets were on 9/11...

But four jets flew off course on 9/11 for well over an hour, yet not a single F-15 or F-16 intercepted them? Maybe they were all busy chasing after "ghosts" in the Atlantic? Maybe all the F-15 and F-16 pilots were in the snack room? Or perhaps the reason was more sinister.

On May 6, 2004, the *New York Times* printed an article stating that on 9/11, the FAA received an audiotape of an interview with six air traffic controllers who tracked two of the "hijacked" planes on 9/11. The recording was actually made within hours of the 9/11 event, so they were recounting events which had happened that same day. Now, here's where it gets interesting. The FAA official destroyed the tape! He didn't just crumble it up into a ball and then toss it into the trash bin. He cut it up into small pieces and then scattered the remnants into multiple trashcans in the building – just to make sure that nobody could ever piece it back together and listen to it. I'm not making this stuff up.

And then there was PTech. In early 2002, Indira Singh, risk-management architect, was innocently helping JP Morgan Chase update their security needs, when she accidentally discovered that an alleged Saudi terrorist (named Yassin Al-Kadi) was running a tiny software company out of his basement in Quincy, Massachusetts.

The company, named Ptech, supplied enterprise architecture which was able to analyze the critical data (in real time). But that's not all. They had carnivore software. You know, high end hacking type software used for *"borrowing without permission"* confidential information from a company. Singh was shocked to see PTech's client list, which included the USAF, the CIA, the FBI, the IRS, Department of Justice, Department of Energy, NATO, the Secret Service, the FAA, and even the White House!

Singh immediately called the Boston FBI office to notify them that a suspected terrorist had gained "backdoor access" to the highest levels of the US government. She was ignored ... month after month. No answer from the FBI. Singh was finally forced to question whether PTech was being protected. Growing increasingly nervous, Singh began notifying every local, state, and federal authority she knew. But not only did her screaming from the rooftops accomplish almost nothing, she even lost her job at JP Morgan Chase after her bosses there (who evidently enjoyed a considerable Saudi client base) told her to *"shut your mouth"* or end up 6 feet under.

By the way, what do you think is the most critical data for the FAA? Yeppers. The most critical data of all lies on FAA radar screens. Guess why the US military didn't intercept and shoot down the rogue hijacked planes? Because they were confused. Reports from 9/11 include "ghost" images on radar screens amongst other FAA anomalies.

Bottom line: due to the "war games" and "weirdness" on the FAA's screens, due in large part to Ptech, the FAA didn't know their backside from a hole in the ground.

Anomaly #3 – Box Cutters ... Really?

The official story is that the 19 Arabs hijacked four planes with nothing but box cutters and plastic knives. That's five "terrorists" per plane (except the plane in Pennsylvania, which had four). There were anywhere from approximately 35 to 70 passengers per plane, plus the crews. Why do I say "approximately"? Well, the names and numbers of passengers have been changed multiple times since 9/11. Seriously. Oh yes, the planes were piloted by at least one, and in one case, two former retired military (Air Force) pilots.

At least five years ago, I told my wife, Charlene, that any red-blooded American on those planes would have "butt-whipped" those emaciated Muslim "hijackers" before you could count to ten, and most likely the passengers would have sent them on their way to their 72 virgins. When I read Liam Scheff's book, Official Stories, I was delighted to find that at least one other person felt the same way that I did.

Despite the fact that Liam and I had never met at that point, we had both come to the same conclusion: that if you can muster up the courage to think rationally and unemotionally, you'll be able to see clearly that the purported events on the planes were farfetched and extremely improbable. If we place ourselves on the plane and in the fight, we can easily see that the "official story" is a "monumental myth." Let me paraphrase his arguments ...

Put yourself on one of the planes on 9/11. Five skinny Arab terrorists whip out their box cutters and begin screaming "Allah!" The plane is under attack. The scrawny Muslims are apparently attempting to break into the cockpit door and overtake two large, well-trained military pilots. And they're going to do it quickly enough and with enough "shock and awe" that the well-trained military pilots forget to transmit a hijack alert. Because, on 9/11, not a single pilot managed to find the three seconds necessary to key in their emergency four-digit "hijacking" code, which would have sent an instant, but silent alarm to the ground, causing the letters "HJCK" to appear on the monitors at air traffic control. I guess they were too petrified by the Muslims screaming *"Allah,"* waiving around their box cutters, and kicking on the cockpit door.

Remember. The hijackers didn't have any guns. **None.**

Every red-blooded American in the cabin with the most minuscule amount of testosterone and adrenaline would never have allowed them to carry out their dirty deeds and crash those planes. Three or four guys beat the crap out of the hijackers, while a few fellas and gals thrash another, while the others get walloped by another half dozen passengers, and so on. The worst thing that could possibly happen is that the "terrorists" might slice up your hands and forearms while someone behind them knocks their block off. The plane flies back to the nearest airport and the passengers and pilots drag the bloody, unconscious bodies of the hijackers to the authorities, where they take them to jail.

Then, as Liam wrote: "***Crisis averted.*** *Now the only thing you have to do is to keep the crowd from murdering the hijackers.*" Yes, after careful musing, it's likely that the hijackers would have quickly been on their way to receive their "72 virgins." No doubt about it. Well, no doubt about the fact that they would have been beaten to a pulp. The 72 virgins? Well, that's another story altogether.

Of course, no box cutters were found at any of the crash sites on 9/11.

Anomaly #4 – Cell Phones & Black Boxes

In 2001, cell phone calls from commercial aircraft much over 8,000 feet were essentially impossible. Between 2,000 and 8,000 feet, calls were "highly unlikely," while below 2,000 feet were only "unlikely." Moreover, even at 2,000 feet (and below), the handoff problem appears. Any airliner at or below this altitude, flying at the normal speed of approximately 500 mph, would encounter the handoff problem. An aircraft traveling at this speed would not be over the cell site long enough to complete the electronic "handshake" (which takes several seconds to complete) before arriving over the next cell site, when the call has to be handed off from the first cell site to the next one. This also takes a few seconds, the result being, in the optimal case, a series of broken transmissions that must end, sooner or later, in failure.

Qualcomm solved this problem ... **in 2004**. Three years after 9/11, Qualcomm Corporation issued a press release stating that they had developed a new technology that would finally make it possible to make cellular phone calls from commercial airliners. Using a technology called "Pico Cells," the system will work as a link between the airliner and ground towers. According to the 2004 press release, it was currently impossible to connect by cell phone in a plane that is above 4,000 feet.

Deena Burnett, widow of Flight 93 victim Tom Burnett, spoke of the four telephone calls she received from her husband aboard the doomed airliner on 9/11, all of which were received from his cell phone, one of which lasted 13 minutes. With the FAA statement that Flight 93 never went below 29,000 feet until its sudden fatal plunge, these two stories seem to be mutually exclusive.

Ted Olson, former US Solicitor General, told CNN that he received two phone calls from his wife Barbara Olson, a passenger on AA Flight 77.

Olson's story changed several times – sometimes he claimed that the calls from his wife were made from seat back phones and other times he claims that she used her cell phone. However, according to American Airlines, the seatback phones on 757s had been deactivated prior to 9/11/01. So, Barbara Olson didn't make the call from a seatback phone. So, it must have been a cell phone, right? But wait, cell phones didn't work at over 2,000 feet.

Interestingly, it was the FBI that revealed the evidence that decisively disproves Ted Olson's story. In the Zacarias Moussaoui trial in 2006, the FBI presented a report on the cell phone calls from all four 9/11 flights. Their report on Flight 77 shows that there was only one phone call from Barbara Olson, but that it was an unconnected call lasting zero seconds, probably due to the handoff problem discussed earlier. So Ted Olson either lied about receiving calls from his wife or was deceived into believing he received calls from her.

Because, on 9/11, either it **was** possible to make cell phone calls from a commercial jetliner in flight at cruising altitude ... or it **wasn't.**

According to Qualcomm, an industry leader in cell phone technology, it wasn't...

But if it was impossible to make cell phone calls on 9/11/01, which it most definitely was, then why were there so many reported cell phone calls from the planes? Ever heard of "*speech cloning*" or "*voice morphing*"? Yes, as far back as 1999, it was possible to "fake" a person's voice. In 1999, the Los Alamos Laboratory in New Mexico revealed their voice morphing technology. General Carl W. Steiner, the former Commander-in-chief of US Special Operations declared on tape: "*Gentlemen! We have called you together to inform you that we are going to overthrow the United States government.*" Of course, it wasn't Steiner, but it sure as heck sounded like him! Another example was Colin Powell saying, "*I am being treated well by my captors.*" Again, it wasn't really Powell, but the voice was virtually identical to his.

The fact of the matter is that prior to 9/11, with just a 10-minute recording of someone's voice, they were able, in almost real time, to clone that person's speech. Perhaps this explains why Flight 93 passenger, Mark Bingham, allegedly called his mother and then proceeded to call himself by his first **and** last name. "*Mom, this is Mark Bingham,*" he purportedly said. **Question:** Have you ever talked to your parents on the phone and called yourself by both your first **and** last name? Me either. Maybe it wasn't Mark Bingham, but it just *sounded* like him? Think about it.

Then we get to the "black boxes." All jetliners are equipped with flight data recorders (FDRs) and cockpit voice recorders (CVRs) contained in "black boxes" designed to survive the most severe crashes. To date, none of the contents of any of the black boxes have been released to the public, with the exception of a partial transcript of Flight 93's CVR, the contents of any of the black boxes remained unknown to the public until August of 2006, when the National Security Archive published long-hidden NTSB Reports including flight path and other studies of the commandeered flights, including FDR data from Flight 77 and Flight 93. Authorities had previously claimed that all but the voice recorder on Flight 93 were either not recovered or too damaged to yield data. It was widely reported in the media that the FDR for Flight 77 was found at 4 AM on September 14, 2001. However, the file containing the FDR data was dated over four hours earlier. In other words, we are asked to believe that the data from the FDR was downloaded prior to the FDR being found.

According to the federal authorities controlling Ground Zero, the black boxes from the two crashed 767s (Flight 11 and Flight 175) failed to turn up in the rubble taken from the site. No black boxes. **Gone. Vanished. Poof! Too bad.**

The 9/11 Commission Report backs the FBI's story, flatly stating: "*The CVRs and FDRs from American 11 and United 175 were not found.*" Despite the fact that New York City firefighter, Nicholas DeMasi, published a book (with other Ground Zero workers) in which he describes the recovery of the black boxes.

Anomaly #5 – the "Twin Towers"

The official myth about 9/11 tells us that the fire (from the planes and office furniture) caused the floors to heat and sag, which pulled these floors away from their metal trusses. The trusses, unable to handle the strain, broke and dropped the whole floor onto the floor below and the floor below and so on – known as the "domino" or "pancake" theory.

Now, this is where it gets really remarkable. Apparently, this eventually caused both Twin Towers to disintegrate into powder, dust, and twisted metal, without leaving behind their colossal metal cores. We're told that after the top floors began to fall, that collapse was unavoidable. **Really?** Hey, we should share this information with controlled demolition companies. They don't really need to wire the entire building after all. They just need to knock down the top floors and ... **poof!** ... the rest of the building will "mystically" collapse. It's magic! And you don't even need any pixie dust or fairies!

The crazy thing is that it's never happened before or since 9/11. Yep, the "Twin Towers" (WTC1 & WTC2) are the only buildings in recorded history to have totally collapsed due to fire along with some minor structural damage. Well, except for WTC7, which we will discuss later. Remember, not just one but **three** buildings in total collapsed due to fire and some minor damage. In comparison, on October 18, 2004, in Caracas, Venezuela, Parque Central East Tower, a 56-story building, caught on fire. The fire broke out shortly before midnight on the 34th floor, burned for over 17 hours and spread over 26 floors, reaching the roof. It did not collapse. After the fires went out, the building (albeit a burned out shell) was still standing.

Back to the Twin Towers. The plane crashes resulted in significant fires in both Towers, at least for the first few minutes after the crashes. The fires in the North Tower were considerably more extensive than those in the South Tower, and as time progressed the fires in the South Tower appeared to diminish greatly in severity. This was probably due to most of the jet fuel being exhausted within a few minutes of the impacts. Since kerosene (jet fuel) has a low boiling point and a low flash point, most of it would have evaporated and caught fire quickly.

As you watch the videos, notice the color of the smoke. Dark. Very dark. Dark smoke implies the presence of soot (uncombusted hydrocarbons) produced when a fire is oxygen-starved, or has just been extinguished. Not necessarily what you would expect to see right before a building collapses, is it? I mean, personally, I would expect to see raging 100 foot flames. But no, not with the Twin Towers. The fires were starved for oxygen. They were going out. Then ... **BOOM**! They collapsed. Out of nowhere. At free fall speed.

When you watch the videos of the Twin Towers collapsing, if you're honest, you will have to admit that the collapses both look like controlled demolitions: sudden onset accompanied by deafening bangs, visible explosions ringing their perimeters, energetic ejections of dust at regular intervals, demolition squibs on the floors below the collapse line, and copious production of dust. A controlled demolition will bring a building straight down, when all the integral supports are blasted away. Kind of like what we saw on 9/11. No, let me rephrase that. **Exactly** like what we saw on 9/11. A controlled demolition.

How long would a "non-explosive-triggered" collapse take? Some suggest 90 seconds for total collapse of such tall structures. But no. The Twin Towers fell as if in "free fall" taking only 11 seconds each. For this 11 second demolition to occur, all the internal supports would have to be blasted away; there were indeed reports of loud explosions throughout the building. Numerous New York City firemen, like Lou Cacchioli and Craig Carlsen, have testified that there were explosions: "*Bang, bang, bang, bang! ... just like a ... what do you call it when they bring a building down intentionally? A controlled demolition. Yeah. A controlled demolition.*" Multiple explosions. Dozens of witnesses.

The government's ludicrous "pancake/domino theory" states that one floor fell onto another, then another, then another, and eventually brought the towers down at near "free fall" speed. In actuality, this would have brought them down much slower than free fall speed, as each floor hit the next, they would have responded as if someone was applying brakes. As each floor hit the one underneath, it would have buffered it and they would have slowed down. The inertia and momentum would have been reduced, times by 110 floors, even though the weight would have been added every time one floor hit the next, this would still have made the towers fall a lot slower than their 11 second free fall.

As Liam Scheff points out in Official Stories, **WATCH THE VIDEOS!** It's the tedious, gut-wrenching research that you must do if you want to discover the truth about 9/11. Let me paraphrase his arguments. If you really watch with an open mind, there is no doubt that you'll be able to see what happened. No pancakes and syrup on these videos. Nothing but buildings being pulverized and disintegrated, forming a pyroclastic cloud, sort of like a volcano eruption. You'll see New York City being blanketed with toxic clouds of grey dust, making it look like the Moon's surface. The first responders were literally breathing asbestos, concrete, blood, bone, and guts.

Molten steel was seen to pour like a river out of the WTC as it burned, yet the fires inside were not hot enough to melt steel. Dr. Steven Jones, physicist and then professor at BYU, found a military grade explosive called Nano-thermite in settled dust of the WTC residue. Nano-thermite, which can be detonated easily by remote, heats to thousands of degrees instantly, will liquefy steel in a matter of seconds, and even burns underwater. On 9/11, it melted thousands of tons of steel, which ran down channels into the basement and low areas, forming pools of molten metal that persisted for over three months under a lake of water, at the base of the annihilated towers.

Dr. Jones collected samples from in and around the exploded WTC buildings, and residents trying to help even mailed him bags of the dust. Along with his international team of scientists, Jones published his findings (including the unexploded Nano-thermite chips, the debris, and other data proving that explosives were used) in a peer reviewed chemistry journal in March of 2009. To say, *"thanks for the diligent work,"* BYU promptly fired him. The Bush administration wanted nothing to do with his report. The mainstream media called him a traitor. I guess no good deed goes unpunished, eh?

But it wasn't just Bush. It's Obama too. The Obama administration has the evidence discussed in the Jones paper but has ignored the discovery of Nano-thermite in the rubble and refuse to discuss the evidence of explosions in the towers on 9/11. On May 18, 2009, during a trip to Los Angeles, Vice President Joe Biden was given a copy of Jones' paper and asked about the administration's position on the need for another investigation. Biden refused to answer the journalist's questions, but took the paper and immediately left the event.

According to the official myth, the molten metal was caused by burning office furniture. Seriously. They can't do any better than that? Was the originator of the official story smoking crack or dropping acid? You could burn office furniture for a million years and it would never get hot enough to melt steel. Molten steel has a temperature of 2500° but the hottest temperature could only be off the burning jet fuel, but that burns at a maximum of 1800° (700° cooler than was needed to melt the steel). 9/11 was basically a huge office fire yet it was as though it was a building ablaze in a war zone like Beirut or Dresden in WWII when they used phosphor bombs. Of course, most of the rubble, including the Nano-thermite laced residue, was quickly loaded on GPS-monitored trucks and shipped off to Asia. Seriously? Nothing like cleaning up the crime scene, eh?

Each tower was supported by a structural core extending from its bedrock foundation to its roof. The cores were rectangular pillars with numerous large columns and girders, measuring 87 feet by 133 feet. The core structures housed the elevators, stairs, and other services. The cores had their own flooring systems, which were structurally independent of the floor diaphragms that spanned the space between the cores and the perimeter walls. The core structures, like the perimeter wall structures, were 100% steel-framed. Some of the core columns apparently had outside dimensions of 36 inches by 16 inches. Others had larger dimensions, measuring 52 inches by 22 inches.

If the "pancake theory" is correct, then after 110 floors "pancaked," there should have been all of the core pillars still standing. Where did they go? Oh yes, the *9/11 Omission Report (err... ummm ... I mean the 9/11 "Commission Report")* denies their very existence, claiming the towers' cores were *"hollow steel shafts."* **Really?** That's not what the blueprints show. I think someone's head might be hollow, but not the Twin Towers.

Watch the videos. They're all over YouTube. They didn't collapse. The buildings were blown up. No doubt about it. That is, if you have your head out of the sand. In the words of my friend Liam Scheff, *"The only 'collapse' that occurred was that gravity pulled the exploding debris to the ground after it blew up. 'Collapse.' It's a word-game played against what we see with our own eyes. When a plane is blown out of the sky and falls to the ground, it hasn't 'collapsed.' It's been pulled to the Earth by gravity. When the Twin Towers were burst, shredded and pulverized in a shockwave and dispersed into thin air; just because the heavy bits fell down, doesn't make it a 'collapse.' These buildings were detonated, violently, sending four-ton steel girders 600 feet and embedding them into the face of a nearby skyscraper. They rained down molten, fiery debris on the smaller buildings in the complex – WTC 3, 4, 5 and 6 – which, despite having flaming girders dropped on them, still didn't explode or collapse in seconds; they stood and burned and took the beating. When the smoke cleared, they remained standing where they had not been forcefully crushed by girders. Why did the small ones survive worse punishment than their big brothers? Because their big brothers were blown up."*

He continues, *"The explosions in the towers vaporized over 1,000 people. Of the approximately 2,740 dead in the towers, only 293 bodies were found intact. One thousand people were just not there, because they were exploded into fragments so small they could not be gathered. Or they were heat-vaporized by the up to 2,500° thermitic fire. In total, cleanup crews found over 19,900 human fragments. One person's remains were counted among two hundred different pieces. Tiny shards of bone were still being found 5 years later on the rooftop of a neighboring sky-scraper, a football field's distance away. That's explosive firepower. That's a military-grade thermite explosive. The fires didn't destroy the buildings and neither did the impacts. The second tower to be hit had a smaller fire - a fire that was going out. This can be seen on video. But instead of going out, the whole building exploded downward and outward. The first tower hit burned hotter and longer. Its fires were more intense and more widespread, still contained to upper floors. Its fires were not going out when it fell - but it fell second. Why? My wager: The second tower hit had a weaker fire that was diminishing. A building "collapsing" with no fire would have dampened the believability for the audience. Before that could happen and the public could focus their shocked and awed eyes on the details, the building was detonated. So, the second hit was the first to be exploded."*

Anomaly #6 – Explosions and William Rodriguez

It's something you won't hear much about in the controlled mainstream media: a loud devastating explosion in the sub-basement of the WTC's North Tower **before** the impact of an airplane that hit between the 93rd and 99th floors.

That was the account of William Rodriguez, who was a 20-year employee of the WTC until the towers were destroyed on 9/11/01. He was later hailed as a national hero for pulling people out of the buildings and saving a number of lives that morning. He was believed to be the last person to escape the North Tower before it fell, and he was photographed with President George W. Bush. Now, the government doesn't want to hear anything he has to say.

When Bush shook hands with Rodriguez, he had no idea how damaging this WTC employee's account of 9/11 would be...

But Rodriquez isn't alone. There were over **100** reports of loud and powerful explosions around the very base of the Twin Towers shortly before they collapsed. Several times the buildings shook so badly that the evacuating staff inside thought it was an earthquake.

These reports were not from a couple of individuals but from a multitude of pedestrians, camera crews, journalists, firefighters, police, paramedics and evacuating office workers, many of whom have since died in accidents, by illness or suicide.

Lou Cacchioli, a firefighter in WTC 1, was one such person. Cacchioli found one of the only functioning elevators (one only going as high as the 24th floor), and he recounts what happened: *"Tommy Hetzel was with me and everybody else also gets out of the elevator when it stops on the 24th floor. There was a huge amount of smoke. Tommy and I had to go back down the elevator for tools and no sooner did the elevators close behind us, we heard this huge explosion that sounded like a bomb. It was such a loud noise, it knocked off the lights and stalled the elevator."*

He continues: *"Luckily, we weren't caught between floors and were able to pry open the doors. People were going crazy, yelling and screaming. And all the time, I am crawling low and making my way in the dark with a flashlight to the staircase and thinking Tommy is right behind me. I somehow got into the stairwell and there were more people there. When I began to try and direct down, another huge explosion like the first one hits. This one hits about two minutes later, although it's hard to tell, but I'm thinking, 'Oh. My God, these bastards put bombs in here like they did in 1993!' "*

Anomaly #7 – WTC Building 7 (The Third Building)

Did you know that three buildings fell on 9/11? The collapse of building 7 is the "smoking gun" of 9/11. WTC7 was a 47 story building that was **not** hit by a plane, yet it collapsed at near free fall speed around 5:20 PM on 9/11/01. According to NIST, the building *"collapsed by fires fueled by* *office furniture.*" No, I'm not kidding. Seriously. That's what they said. I wonder if he made this statement before or after his partial lobotomy.

The official report is that WTC7 fell in about 7 seconds at free fall speed. I'm sure it was just a coincidence that the building housed Mayor Rudy Giuliani's 23rd floor command center, the SEC and its then ongoing Enron and WorldCom investigations (which could now be buried – literally), the IRS, the Secret Service, and the largest CIA base outside of Langley, Virginia.

The collapse of WTC7 is a physical impossibility, it cannot be replicated experimentally, and it defies the laws of physics. Set aside politics, religion, and use the scientific method, then you'll see that WTC7 **must** have been a controlled demolition. In light of the free fall and the uniform acceleration of the towers, the only thing that makes sense scientifically is that they were blown up.

On February 9, 2009 in Beijing, China, the Mandarin Oriental Hotel, a 44-story building, was reportedly set ablaze accidentally by fireworks. The fire burned throughout the night and early morning for approximately 10 hours, with giant flames reaching 30 feet above the roof. Most of the building was gutted, yet there was **no** collapse. Seven of these "non-9/11" building fires burned well beyond three hours over multiple floors – some burned for 10 or more hours. None collapsed. In fact no steel framed high-rise outside the World Trade Center has ever suffered a complete collapse blamed on fire. The WTC1 and WTC2 fires burned for only 60 to 90 minutes. Yet, along with WTC7, the Twin Towers were completely destroyed – in just seconds.

I remember when I "woke up" about 7 years ago, I was talking to a friend of mine about 9/11. I saw his demeanor change when I began to share about the anomalies and series of odd events that were associated with the fateful day in 2001. After I began to ask him how it was possible for two 110 story buildings to collapse at free fall speed into the path of most resistance, he said, *"The Muslims did it."*

I tried to repeat the question to him, letting him know that I was **not** asking him **who** did it, but was just asking him to tell me **how** it was possible, in light of the immutable laws of physics, for 40,000 tons of steel to, in essence, disintegrate as the towers fell, resulting in the possibility of free fall collapse, without the aid of some sort of explosive devices. He then bellowed, *"You're a crazy conspiracy nut!"*

Ahhh ... good one ... his "mind control" had paid off. Rather than thinking critically and logically, he attacked me personally and dehumanized me by labeling and name calling. Right out of the playbook of Edwin Bernays (the "Father of Spin") in his best-selling book,

Propaganda. I'm sure Uncle "Siggy" (Sigmund Freud) was proud of his nephew Edwin.

Not deterred from my mission, I asked him, "*How many buildings fell in New York on 9/11?*" To which he responded, "*A bunch!*" **Really?** "*A bunch.*" That's the best answer you have?

Here's a guy who wants to kill all the Muslims for 9/11, a guy who tells me that I'm "crazy" and a "conspiracy nut" for trying to think logically about the events of 9/11, yet he doesn't even know that three buildings fell in New York. He just knows that "a bunch" of buildings fell.

Honestly, I didn't know that buildings came in "bunches." Apples maybe. Perhaps bananas. But not buildings. Anyway, the phrase, "*speaking out of ignorance*" comes to mind. He might as well have said, "*Don't bother me with the facts; my mind's already made up.*"

But my friend (ex-friend actually) isn't alone. A large number of folks still don't know that **three** (not two) towers fell in New York on 9/11. Perhaps that's because WTC7 wasn't mentioned in the 9/11 Commission Report. Yes, you read that correctly. They acted like it didn't happen. Do you think it has anything to do the irksome difficulties of trying to explain why 47 floors of a steel framed building that had **not** been hit by a plane and had only minor damage by falling debris and a few isolated fires (all of which were basically extinguished by late afternoon), plummeted at free fall speed, as if all of its vertical supports were suddenly destroyed? Kind of like you would see in a (gasp!) ... controlled demolition?

Have you heard of Barry Jennings? I betcha haven't. Among all the highly credible video and forensic evidence indicating that WTC7 was brought down by explosive controlled demolition on 9/11, the accounts of explosions related by eyewitness Barry Jennings are particularly persuasive. On 9/11, Jennings was the Deputy Director of the Emergency Services Department for the New York City Housing Authority. He and Michael Hess, the New York City Corporation Counsel, were rescued from WTC Building 7 before it collapsed at 5:21 PM.

On several occasions, Jennings stated that an explosion trapped them in WTC7 and that he continued to hear explosions, **lots of explosions**, throughout the building until they were rescued. Jennings talked about "*stepping over (dead) bodies in the lobby,*" despite the fact that the official story is that nobody died in building 7. The statements of first responders Craig Bartmer and Kevin McPadden have also been captured on video, and certainly corroborate the testimony of Barry Jennings.

In a YouTube video, which you can still watch, Craig Bartmer (a former New York City police officer and 9/11 first responder) stated about the collapse of WTC7: "*All of a sudden, the radios exploded and everybody started screaming, 'Get away, get away, get away from it!' And, I was like a deer in the headlights. ... And the whole time you're hearing, THOOM! THOOM! THOOM! THOOM! THOOM! So, I, I think I know an explosion when I hear it, you know? So yeah, I wanna know what took that building down. I don't think it was a fire, and it certainly wasn't a plane...It had some damage to it but nothing like what they're saying...Nothing to account for what we saw...I am shocked at the [official] story we've heard about it, to be quite honest."*

Regarding the collapse of WTC7, Kevin McPadden (an emergency medical technician and 9/11 first responder) stated: *"Yeah, there was like, there was a whole lot of commotion. The firefighters were picking up, and they were starting to roll out...The Red Cross rep was like, he goes over and he says [to us], 'You gotta stay behind this line because they're thinking about bringing the building down.'...He goes over and he asks one of the... firefighters what was going on...He came back over with his hand over the radio and [you could hear] what sounded like a countdown. And, at the last few seconds, he took his hand off [the radio] and you heard 'three-two-one,' and he was just saying, 'Just run for your life! Just run for your life!' And then it was like another two, three seconds, you heard explosions. Like,* **BA-BOOOOOM!** *And it's like a distinct sound ...* **BA-BOOOOOM!** *And you felt a rumble in the ground, like, almost like you wanted to grab onto something. That, to me, I knew that was an explosion. There was no doubt in my mind..."*

Tellingly, despite his prominence on national TV, Jennings was never called to testify before the 9/11 Commission, and his account was not included in the 9/11 Commission Report or the NIST WTC Reports. Similarly, the 9/11 Commission also completely ignored the firefighters' reports of explosions in the Twin Towers, as we've already seen. Sadly, Barry Jennings died on August 19, 2008.

Did you know that the BBC reported that WTC7 had collapsed ... **before** it collapsed? Yep. They did. It's on film. You can see it on YouTube. The time stamp is 21:54 (4:54 PM EST) when news of the Salomon Brothers Building (aka WTC7) is first broadcast, a full 26 minutes in advance of its collapse. The incredible footage shows BBC reporter Jane Standley talking about the collapse of the Salomon Brothers Building while it remains standing in the live shot behind her head.

The fact that the BBC reported on the collapse of WTC7 over twenty minutes in advance of its implosion obviously provokes a myriad of questions as to how they knew it was about to come down when the official story says its collapse happened accidentally as a result of *"fires fueled by office furniture."* Is it just me, or do you also almost crack up laughing every time you hear that?

When questioned about their bizarre act of "clairvoyance" (how they were able to report the collapse before it happened), the BBC responded, *"In the chaos and confusion of the day, we're quite sure we said things which turned out to be untrue or inaccurate."* **Hold on here!** How do "*chaos and confusion*" explain how the BBC reported on the "unexpected" collapse of a building before it happened? Do BBC reporters have access to a time machine?

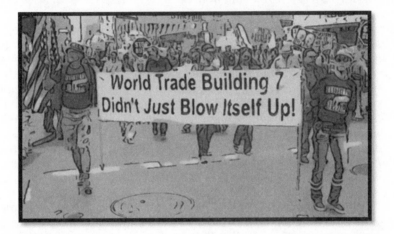

Of course they were told that WTC7 was coming down, just like the firefighters, police, first responders and CNN were told it was coming down. They had to have had a source for making such a claim. The BBC is acting like the naughty little boy who got caught with his hand in the cookie jar. I'm not saying that the BBC are "part of the conspiracy," but their repugnant proclivity to just repeat what authorities tell them without even a cursory investigation (with the building they are telling us has collapsed mockingly filling the background shot of the report), is a damning indictment of their "yellow journalism" when it comes to 9/11.

Did I mention CNN? Yes, I did. At 4:20 PM, CNN reporter Aaron Brown told the live audience that WTC7 *"had collapsed or is collapsing."* Even though the video showed the building still standing. He seemed to have no clue as to which building he was talking about. He was just reading the teleprompter. Like a good reporter should. He just read the teleprompter a bit too early. I guess he should have waited about an hour, or maybe they got the time zones mixed up. In any case, yes, the collapse of WTC7 was scripted. No doubt about it. That's how they knew to report that the building had collapsed.

Because it was supposed to collapse. It was probably supposed to have been hit by the airplane that got "off-script" over Pennsylvania. You know, Flight 93 – the one that was shot down – we'll get to that in a few minutes.

Oh yes, I almost forgot. Then there's Larry Silverstein, the billionaire owner of the WTC, who stated about WTC 7: "*I remember getting a call from the fire department commander, telling me that they were not sure they were going to be able to contain the fire, and I said, 'We've had such terrible loss of life, maybe the smartest thing to do is pull it.' And they made that decision to pull and we watched the building collapse.*"

Within the construction industry, to "pull it" means execute a controlled demolition. In other words, **to blow it up**. This means the building must already have been rigged up with explosives, as it takes weeks to set up something like that and Silverstein admitted he knew about it by his statement. But the US Department of State contends that Silverstein's "pull it" statement refers to withdrawing firefighters from WTC7. There is one huge greasy problem with that assertion, namely there were no firefighters in WTC7.

According to the FEMA Report on WTC7, "*No manual firefighting actions were taken by FDNY.*" The 11/29/01 edition of the *New York Times* said, "*By 11:30 AM, the fire commander in charge of that area, Assistant Chief Frank Fellini, ordered firefighters away from [WTC 7] for safety reasons.*"

By the way, just six weeks before 9/11, Silverstein took out a 99 year lease on the entire WTC complex which "fortuitously" covered acts of terrorism. He eventually made a cool $4.55 billion from the insurance settlement. But I'm sure he shared most of that with the 9/11 victims' families...

Anomaly #8 – The Pentagon

The official story is that the Pentagon was hit by a plane which disappeared into a hole (approximately 25 feet in diameter) at the base of the building, but left no mark on the lawn. If we do the math, assuming the entry angle of 75°, the 125 foot wingspan of the Boeing 757 would have made a hole about 175 feet wide (give or take a bit for the wings snapping off) in the Pentagon wall. This clearly did not happen.

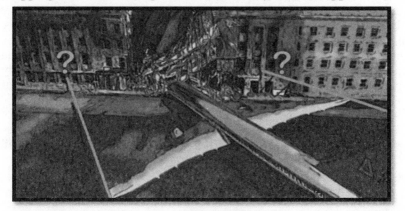

The skies around the Pentagon are amongst the most heavily defended in the USA, and the Pentagon also has the most cameras per square yard than any other Government buildings in the USA. No unknown aircraft are allowed within 50 miles of the Pentagon. **Period.** I've flown in that neck of the woods a few times on small propeller jets. Literally, you would be shot down if you didn't have permission to fly in that restricted airspace. The Pentagon has its own anti-aircraft missiles that should have fired to protect the building on 9/11. Only a military aircraft with a special IFF transponder (identifying it as a friend) would have been allowed to approach the Pentagon.

Jamie McIntyre, a CNN reporter on the scene shortly after the impact, stated that *"there's no evidence of a plane having crashed anywhere near the building."* Just to make sure that nobody learned the truth, the FBI seized all CCTV coverage (86 videos from office blocks, car parks, gas stations, hotels) of the Pentagon event and only released a crummy and doctored 5 frames of time lapse footage to the press. It showed an explosion but it did not show what exactly exploded! Hey FBI ... if you got nothing to hide, why are you hiding something? Just as dead men tell no tales, dead evidence tells none either!

Now let's talk about the purported pilot of Flight 77, Hani Hanjour. This is a man who, three weeks before 9/11, attempted to rent a Cessna at an airfield in Maryland. Suspicious of his dubious "pilot's license," officials at the airfield insisted he take a chaperoned test-flight before rental would be approved. He failed his test flight miserably. He could neither control, nor properly land the Cessna. In fact, the instructors at the airfield in Maryland said, *"It was like he had hardly even ever driven a car. He could not fly at all."* And yet, the official myth asks us to believe that Hanjour pulled off a stunt that would press the limits of even the most experienced aviation test pilot.

Every professional, highly experienced airline pilot has stated that they could not have flown a plane into the Pentagon with the given flight parameters – 400+ mph descending into a deep dive at 3,500 feet per minute and finishing with a tight parabolic hairpin turn through 270° – then flying at 20 feet above the ground to hit the Pentagon (without even disturbing the grass). I won't even get into the aerodynamic impossibility of flying a large commercial jetliner 20 feet above the ground at 400+ mph. A discussion on ground effect energy, wake turbulence, vortex compression, downwash reaction, and jet blast effects are beyond the scope of this section of the book. Let it suffice to say that it is **physically impossible** to fly a 250,000 pound plane 20 feet above the ground at 400+ mph.

In light of these facts, it's fair to say that the official flight path defies logic, lucidity, reason, and physics. But let's have some fun with it, shall we? Hanjour was about five foot nothing and weighed about a hundred and nothing. Not exactly NFL material. But let's go with the flow of the official myth. So, Hani "Tiny" Hanjour fights his way into the cockpit and wrestles control of Flight 77 from a massive 6'4" former Marine combat fighter pilot named Charles Burlingame, a man family members and colleagues say would never have given up his aircraft or the safety of his passengers.

After taking care of the co-pilot as well, "Tiny" Hanjour settles in and turns his attention to the bewildering array of gadgets and devices of a Boeing 757 instrument panel (a panel he was totally unfamiliar with) in an airplane traveling 500 mph. Then, in the words of Nila Sagadevan, an aeronautical engineer and pilot, without the help of any ground control or air-traffic controllers providing him information and/or settings, Hanjour (who could not control a tiny Cessna a few weeks earlier) *"would have to very quickly interpret his heading, ground track, altitude, and airspeed information on the displays before he could even figure out where in the world he was, much less where the Pentagon was located in relation to his position."*

Hanjour then flies into the most restricted airspace in the world without eliciting a single military intercept – despite the crash of two other known hijacked aircraft into the Twin Towers. Andrews Airbase with 3 squadrons of fighter aircraft is situated only eleven miles from the Pentagon, and there were 2 combat-ready fighter jets on 9/11. Yet, not one plane was scrambled from there to intercept the supposed plane that flew into the Pentagon.

Oh it gets better … and **more bizarre.**

With no idea how soon fighter aircraft would show up to shoot him down, Hanjour finds himself pointed in the ideal direction toward the East wing of the Pentagon, where all the top brass in the military are known to be stationed. But then he apparently changes his mind as to his heading, and pulls off that incredible, sweeping 270 degree descending turn at 400+ mph to approach the Pentagon from the opposite direction.

When he arrives at the Pentagon, he knocks over a couple of light posts and levitates over the lawn at 500+ miles per hour, finally managing to wedge the plane into the ground floor of the Pentagon, without even bothering the grass on the lawn. Now, that's impressive. Especially in light of the fact that if you parked a 757 next to the Pentagon and rested it on its engines with its landing gear retracted, the nose would be about fifteen feet above the ground (i.e. second floor). It would be impossible to make a hole in the bottom floor without plowing through dirt to get there.

At the Pentagon, witnesses stated there was not the expected amount of plane wreckage – undercarriage, wings and fuselage sections, engines, and seats were nowhere to be found. Only some small components were found with bits of landing gear, some engine parts and a bit of fuselage with other bits of twisted metal. This is not consistent with airplane crashes where the area of impact is literally strewn with debris, bodies, and body parts. It was reported that 189 people were killed in the attacks on the Pentagon, with 184 bodies recovered, yet official reports say the intensity of the explosion and resulting fire was so great that it totally incinerated and vaporized the plane, hence not much wreckage. Wouldn't human bodies also have been incinerated?

Could Flight 77 (and all the aircrafts in question on the morning of 9/11) have somehow been overridden, or swapped out (as with the plan in Operation Northwoods) and then guided remotely by sophisticated navigation systems? The technology does exist. Was it a Global Hawk (remote control drone UAV) that was flown into the Pentagon? Could it have been packed with explosives and then remotely flown right into the Pentagon? The landing gear and engine parts found in the Pentagon actually matched up to the ones used on this craft. Just asking. Think about it.

And in another of the wildly unbelievable coincidences that have proved commonplace in the narrative of 9/11, the former CEO of the world's leading remote aviation technology company (System Planning Corp) is Dov Zakheim. In May of 2001, four months before 9/11, Mr. Zakheim was appointed Undersecretary of Defense and Comptroller of the Pentagon.

In the words of Lt. Columbo, "*One more thing sir.*" Then Secretary of Transportation, Norm Mineta, testified to the 9/11 Commission that on the morning of 9/11, he arrived at the Presidential Emergency Operating Center (PEOC) at 9:20 AM and that Vice President Cheney was already present with his staff. Mineta testified: "*During the time that the airplane (Flight 77) was coming into the Pentagon, there was a young man who would come in and say to the Vice President, 'The plane is 50 miles out; the plane is 30 miles out.' And when it got down to, 'The plane is 10 miles out,' the young man also said to the Vice-President, 'Do the orders still stand?' And the Vice President turned and whipped his neck around and said, 'Of course the orders still stand! Have you heard anything to the contrary?!'*"

What orders? Think about it. The orders to **not** shoot down the plane headed for the Pentagon. That's the only thing that makes sense, isn't it? Well, Norman Mineta's entire testimony before the 9/11 commission was removed. **Bye bye. Gone.** Just like he never said it. It was removed from the text and the video record.

But it's still available on YouTube and other online video services. Thanks to the folks that recorded the C-Span hearings and uploaded the videos.

Otherwise, we wouldn't even know that it ever happened. Oh yes, when questioned about this, representatives at the National Archive stated that the video may have been lost because of a "snafu." Those pesky "snafus" ... I tell you. They always appear at the worst times!

And finally, for the icing on the cake ("the gravy" if you're from Texas, or if you're Creole, the "lagniappe") – on September 10, 2001, then Secretary of Defense, Donald Rumsfeld, admitted: *"According to some estimates we (the Pentagon) cannot track $2.3 trillion in transactions."*

After 9/11, nobody was asking about the $2.3 trillion any more...

Anomaly #9 – The "Crash" of Flight 93

The official myth tells us that Flight 93, the fourth jetliner commandeered on 9/11, was the only plane where the passengers actually made an effort to resist the skinny Muslim hijacking terrorists. The brave ringleader, Todd ("Let's Roll") Beamer and his no-nonsense call to arms became a defining battle cry in America's "war on terror."

They tell us that Flight 93 eventually crashed into a field in Shanksville, Pennsylvania at 500+ mph and apparently totally vaporized on impact, leaving no dead bodies or plane wreckage.

Really? In the words of Elmer Fudd, *"Good heavens. It disintegrated!"*

Of the four aircraft "hijacked" on 9/11, the exact fate of Flight 93 after its two-hour journey is proving difficult for US officials to explain.

In the NBC and Fox News television footage from 9/11 we hear:

- NBC Reporter: *"The debris here is spread over a 3 to 4 mile radius which has now been completely sealed off, and is being treated according to the FBI as a crime scene. This is one of those cases where the pictures really do tell the story ... one of the most horrifying aspects of this is how little debris is visible ... that's all you see, just a large crater in the ground, and just tiny, tiny bits of debris ... the investigators out there, and there are hundreds of them, have found nothing larger than a phone book."*
- Fox Reporter: *"I've seen the pictures, and it looks like there's nothing there except a hole in the ground."*
- Fox Affiliate Photographer: *"Basically that is right ... The only thing you could see was a big gouge in the earth, and some broken trees."*
- Fox Reporter: *"Any large pieces of debris?"*

- Fox Affiliate Photographer: *"There was nothing that you could distinguish that a plane crashed there ... nothing going on down there, no smoke, no fire ... you couldn't see anything, you could see dirt, ash, and people walking around."*
- Fox Reporter: *"How big would you say that hole was?"*
- Fox Affiliate Photographer: *"From my estimate it was 20 to 15 feet long ... 10 feet wide."*
- Fox Reporter: *"What could you see on the ground other than dirt, ash?"*
- Fox Affiliate Photographer: *"You couldn't see anything ... just dirt, ash, and people walking around."*

Indeed the Flight 93 crash site looks remarkably different from other plane crash sites, such as Pan Am Flight 103 or Delta Flight 191.

Just check out the photo below.

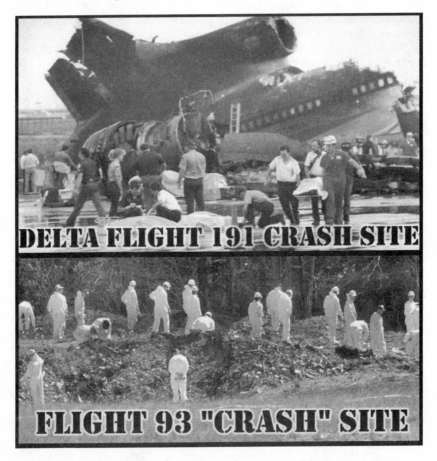

There were little bits of metal strewn over a four mile radius, but none bigger than a phone book size? **Seriously?** I guess this was yet another "first" that happened on 9/11 – this being the first time in the history of aviation that a whole plane has vaporized on impact along with the entire crew and passengers. Wow. I guess the immutable laws of nature, physics, and science are a little bit different in the rural areas of Pennsylvania.

Oh yes, the FBI says 95% of the plane was recovered, but we've never seen pictures of this recovered debris. Hmmmm … perhaps they're "hiding" with the 86 videos of the "plane" hitting the Pentagon?

Actually, one version of the official myth is that Flight 93 totally vanished because the ground was very soft from past mining operations, with one version even stating that the plane completely disappeared into an abandoned mine shaft! But, hey, wait! I've seen the news reports when a group of miners get trapped in a mine shaft. They always bring out the bright lights and heavy equipment and dig, dig, dig, 24/7, in the hope that, by some miracle, someone might have survived.

Did that happen with Flight 93? Nope. Just think of the spectacular television coverage had such a "rescue attempt" been undertaken. Why didn't they search for possible survivors? Think about it.

They even trimmed the burnt trees and shrubs to make sure that they could not be subjected to chemical analysis to determine whether the damage had been caused by jet-fuel based fires. Subsequent studies by the EPA of the crash site have confirmed that there was no residue from the jet fuel that would have been pervasive had a Boeing 757 actually crashed there. Research on the "crash sites" thus appears to be pure dynamite in blowing the "official narrative" of Flight 93's plight right out of the proverbial water.

What did the first responders see? Wallace Miller, Coroner of Somerset County (which includes Shanksville) and one of the first to arrive at the "crash" scene, said of the area, *"This is the most eerie thing,"* he says. *"I have not, to this day, seen a single drop of blood. Not a drop."* **No bodies, no wreckage, no engines, no wings, no tires, no nothing.**

And then there were more local officials who stated that crash debris was spread over a wide area. According to the *Pittsburgh Post-Gazette*, state police Major Lyle Szupinka *"confirmed that debris from the plane had turned up in relatively far-flung sites, including the residential area of Indian Lake"* (over six miles away).

Eyewitness accounts corroborate physical evidence that portions of the plane were destroyed in the air, consistent with a missile strike from a nearby military plane.

These accounts support the following elements:

- A white jet in pursuit of the jetliner
- Peculiar engine sounds before the crash
- Sounds of explosions before the plane fell from the sky
- Appearances that the plane suddenly began to drop vertically

Was the plane shot down? During a 2004 Christmas Eve interview with Brigadier General James Marks, Secretary of Defense Donald Rumsfeld stated: "*the people who attacked the United States ... **shot down** the plane over Pennsylvania.*" The Pentagon says Rumsfeld "*simply misspoke.*" Oh yeah, I believe that. He was mistaken. Confused. Sure thing, Donald. Whatever. Of course, the initial media reports regarding Flight 93 also indicated that it was **shot down** by the US National Air Guard. Do a search for "*Fox Flight 93 Shot Down*" and you can watch the YouTube video.

Fox News first aired the news report on 9/11/01 around 4:30 PM and then they aired it again around 10:30 PM that same evening. A service-woman (Lt. Colonel Phyllis Phipps-Barnes from DC Air National Guard) confirms this fact to the Fox reporter. The report specified that Flight 93 exploded in the air (while still at a high altitude) and its debris were scattered at a distance of at least 6 miles. Keep in mind that the Fox report is not like the infamous "slip of the tongue" by Donald Rumsfeld. This is a public news report (i.e. legally admissible evidence). You can go to court with it if you want. Check out www.911thology.com.

There was more weirdness. Mark Bingham allegedly called his mother, Alice Hoaglan, from Flight 93. She recounted for reporters her final call from her son: "*Mom, this is Mark Bingham. I just want to tell you that I love you. I am on a flight from Newark to San Francisco. There are three guys on board who have taken over the plane and they say they have a bomb. You believe me don't you, Mom?*"

Before my mother died, I probably talked to her on the phone at least 2,000 times over the course of 36 years. Perhaps more. Not one time did I ever say, "*Mom, this is Ty **Bollinger** ... you believe me don't you, Mom?*" Ummmm ... that's just weird. It's unnatural. Sons don't use their first **and** last name when talking to their mother. And they don't ask their mother, "*...you believe me, don't you.*" This is just strange, weird, odd, bizarre, absurd, outlandish, whatever you want to call it. This is like a bad script from a "B" movie. My guess is that it wasn't Mark on the phone...

Two more questions: Why did Air Traffic Controllers in a Nashua Telegraph article report an F-16 was circling Flight 93 and was in visual range at the time of the crash? Why does the US government still deny this? Then, on April 28, 2009, Pilots for 9/11 Truth released Air Traffic Control transcripts that revealed that Flight 93 was actually airborne **after** its alleged crash. What does this mean? You tell me.

The important point here isn't the alleged shoot down. Most people would agree that under the circumstances (if the plane was **actually** hijacked by "terrorists" and heading for WTC7 or perhaps the White House) it was the best course of action. The point is that we are seeing clear evidence of the manipulation of information being fed to the public regarding 9/11.

Physics, simple physics, says the official Flight 93 "crash story" is **impossible**. There are more holes in this story than there is bird poop on the pier!

My question: What else is the government hiding about 9/11?

Anomaly #10 – Osama

Within hours of the 9/11 events, Osama bin Laden was identified (without evidence) as the architect and mastermind of 9/11. On the following day, the "global war on terror" had been launched. And the mainstream media disinformation campaign went into full gear.

Who was Osama Bin Laden? He was a member of a very powerful and wealthy Saudi Arabian family. In the 1980s, he was an Afghani freedom-fighter and friend of the USA. Then, by the late 1990s, he was one of the main "terrorist" enemies of America, with ties to al-**CIA**-duh (err ... ummm ... I mean ... al Qaeda).

The fact is that the US government trained, armed, funded and supported Osama bin Laden and his followers in Afghanistan during the cold war. Al Qaeda was created by the CIA in their offices in Washington D.C. with a huge investment of $3,500,000,000 (yes, that's 3.5 billion) of American taxpayers' money. But don't expect the controlled mainstream media "stenographers" to deviate from their Pentagon generated scripts and connect the dots regarding the "in-your-face" link between the CIA and al-Qaeda "terrorism." Right up until 9/11/01, al Qaeda was ours; we created it, we trained the terrorists, and we used them! Research it yourself.

Now, concerning 9/11, Osama Bin Laden categorically stated that he did **not** do it. Let's hear what the "dastardly" Bin Laden said about 9/11 right on September 28, 2001: *"I was not involved in the September 11 attacks in the United States nor did I have knowledge of the attacks. There exists a government within a government within the United States. The United States should try to trace the perpetrators of these attacks within itself."* Typically, terrorists can't wait to take the credit for blowing stuff up – it's good for their ego, street credibility, and for their movement. Had Osama Bin Laden been the "mastermind" behind the largest attacks in history on American soil, don't you think he would have been proud of it? A major victory against the "infidels," a major notch in his belt, a huge triumph! But, no, he denied it instead.

Oh I can hear it now – *"But Osama **did** claim responsibility in … you know … that video."* Ah, yes, there was that good ole' bizarre, peculiar video that the FBI "found" in Afghanistan. Well, that video definitely did show someone posing as left-handed Osama (who was right-handed, with darker skin, different bone structure, and a wider nose) and claiming responsibility. Check out the photo below. Apparently living in caves and eating scorpions and lizards does a body good. Osama looks younger, healthier, with better complexion, and even looks like he's put on 20 or 30 pounds. Hey, maybe we all should move to the nearest cave. But even though it looks bogus and smells like a fraud (heck, it totally reeks of fakery), since the government told us that was Osama, I guess it was. They wouldn't lie, would they? Naw....

*"Will the **real** Osama please step forward?"*

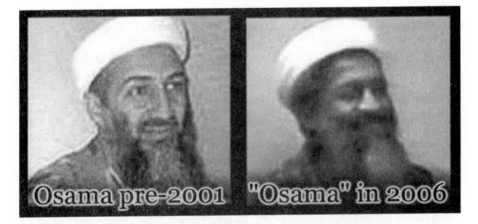

And then we have the Marfan syndrome issue. You see, Osama had Marfan syndrome. In 2002, Dr. Steve Pieczenik (a State Department official in three different Presidential administrations and an award-winning Harvard Medical School VIP) asserted that Bin Laden had been "dead for months," and that the government was waiting for the most politically expedient time to roll out his corpse. Pieczenik said that Osama Bin Laden died in 2001, *"Not because Special Forces had killed*

him, but because as a physician I had known that the CIA physicians had treated him and it was on the intelligence roster that he had *Marfan syndrome*," adding that the US government knew Bin Laden was dead before they invaded Afghanistan.

"*Huh? Didn't SEAL Team 6 kill him in 2011?*" Well, that is the official myth. But I don't believe it. I want to see the body. Because I have a hard time believing that they killed "America's Top Terrorist" but didn't bother to show anyone the body, choosing rather to dump it in the ocean and "feed the fish." In stark contrast to Obama's declaration that Osama was "buried at sea," US Navy Sailors on the *USS Carl Vinson* have stated on record that they did **not** witness Osama's "burial at sea."

My good buddy, Liam Scheff gives us his angle: "*...they dumped it at sea, if you recall. Too gruesome for gentle America to bear, on the news after 'Survivor,' 'CSI,' and the 'Bachelorette.' Too provocative for the world to tolerate. But they showed us Saddam's sons shot to death and Saddam himself dangling from a rope around his neck, like an animal strung up for show. They showed us Gaddafi, a bloody corpse dragged through the streets like Hector behind a chariot. They showed us people leaping to their deaths from the top floors of the towers. Did you know that hundreds of people died fleeing for the roof exits, only to find they were bolted shut? Yes, that happened too. So, no, I don't believe that he died in 2011.*"

Someone is lying about Osama's death.

Did Barry Soetoro (aka Barak Hussein Obama) chop down the cherry tree? There are many high ranking officials who think so, and at least one of those who spoke of this in public, Benazir Bhutto, was assassinated shortly after saying it. Oh yes, Hollywood chimed in with the blockbuster propaganda film ("Zero Dark Thirty") in support of the US government's monumental myth about Osama's death. Now, everybody's "*happy, happy, happy*" – except for those of us who actually want to learn the truth. By the way, no one in Abbottabad or Pakistan actually believes the fictional bin Laden raid drama either.

What does this mean? It means that the entire mythical account of Bin Laden's alleged assassination put out by the Obama administration is an act of mass public deception. Oh, the members of SEAL Team 6 were definitely shooting at someone, but it just wasn't Obama. Did I say Obama? I meant Osama. Silly me. And by the way, Obama has benefited immensely from cultivating a "tough guy" image out of the legendary raid.

And I almost forgot. Most of SEAL Team 6 was killed in August of 2011 when their Boeing Chinook helicopter (with the call sign *Extortion 17*) was shot down during landing in Afghanistan. At least that's the official story. We're told that all 38 people on board (including 25 American special operations personnel) were killed. The US government claims that the bodies were so badly burnt that they were forced to cremate them immediately. Hmmm … that's weird … sounds like they were on some sort of deadline to make them disappear? In any event, regardless how what really happened, there are no survivors, no bodies, no photos, and no real evidence available that prove the US government's "creative" version of events. There's nothing like getting rid of the eyewitnesses and evidence, eh? How convenient for the government.

For those who really want the truth, it's crystal clear that Osama was dead long before 2011. According to French intelligence reports, CIA agents visited Bin Laden at the American Hospital in Dubai in July 2001, two months before 9/11. It was also widely acknowledged at the time that Bin Laden needed a kidney dialysis machine because of renal health problems. On January 28, 2002, CBS News reported that Bin Laden was having kidney dialysis treatment the night before 9/11.

Here's another interesting quote: *"Usama bin Laden has died a peaceful death due to an untreated lung complication."*

Who made that wacky statement? Let me give you a clue. *"Fair and Balanced"* – does that help? Yes, that would be Fox News on December 26, 2001.

Want another thought-provoking quote? *"The reason why 9/11 is not mentioned on Usama Bin Laden's Most Wanted page is because the FBI has no hard evidence connecting Bin Laden to 9/11."*

What ignorant paranoid "nutter" said that? That would be Rex Tomb, Chief of Investigative Publicity for the FBI. Yes indeed. Not your typical tinfoil hat wearing loon. And Mr. Tomb isn't the only one saying this.

Then, in a 2006 interview with Tony Snow, another "conspiracy theorist" made a wacky, zany statement: *"…we've never made the case or argued the case that somehow Osama bin Laden was directly involved in 9/11."*

Who was the wacko? Who was that nutty kook? It was … drum roll … Vice President Dick Cheney!

And then there was Edmonds … Sibel Edmonds … the FBI translator who reported that US alphabet agencies maintained "intimate relations" with bin Laden and the Taliban *"all the way until that day of September 11."* Edmonds discovered a network of drug trafficking and money laundering, funneling money to the very "terrorists" alleged to have perpetrated 9/11, and even implicated members of Congress. As a result, she received an enormous raise and was promoted.

Oops ... rewind. **My mistake**. As a result, she was fired by the FBI and "His Highness" (Attorney General John Ashcroft) placed her under a gag order, which prevented her, under penalty of treason, from testifying or speaking about what she knew.

And then there was O'Neill ... John O'Neill ... the FBI Deputy Director and counter-terrorism expert, who was trying to "follow the money" in an effort to identify terrorist networks. After being thwarted by his own superiors in the FBI, O'Neill was reassigned to head of security for the Twin Towers. His first day on the job was 9/11/01, which was also his date of death.

Just days after 9/11, wealthy Saudi Arabians, including members of the bin Laden family, were whisked out of the USA on private jets. No one will admit to clearing the flights, and the passengers weren't questioned. Quite an odd way to treat the family of the person who was deemed to be the *"biggest terroristic threat to America"* eh?

So, here is what you need to believe about Osama:

- Despite the fact that he adamantly denied involvement ...
- Despite his Marfan syndrome ...
- Despite the kidney dialysis ...
- Despite the bombs being dropped all over his "hideouts" for over a decade ...
- Despite his altered facial features on the video and the fact that he appeared to be growing younger ...
- Despite the fact that our own government said he wasn't involved with the attacks ...

... Osama Bin Laden **was** the mastermind behind 9/11 and **was** killed in a valiant military raid in 2011.

This is what happened because the government said so! Don't question it. Go back to sleep. Turn back on the TV. Suck your thumb. Whatever makes you feel warm and fuzzy. Don't rock the boat. Don't be a "dissenter."

Anomaly #11 – Bush

Remember the video of President Bush when he was told about the second plane hitting the Twin Towers? He was at a school reading a story about a pet goat to a classroom of children. He remained sitting there, book in hand for several minutes, doing absolutely nothing, looking rather befuddled and uncomfortable – a strange reaction to just sit there, doing nothing, from a President who has just been told his country is apparently under attack from terrorists. An expected reaction would have been to stand up, dismiss the class, walk out of the school straight away and head back to base in Air Force One to coordinate movements.

Why didn't the highly trained men of the Secret Service (whose job it was to protect President Bush at the school) quickly whisk him away for his own safety? Wouldn't their first priority be to protect the President, just in case there were planes heading for the school?

Now, here's where it gets interesting. President Bush has stated on **two** separate occasions that on the morning of 9/11, he saw a plane hit World Trade Center 1.

The first occasion was on December 4, 2001, at a town hall meeting, aired live on CNN. Someone asked, "...*how did you feel when you heard about the terrorist attack?*" Bush answered, "...*you're not going to believe what state I was in when I heard about the terrorist attack. I was in Florida. And my chief of staff, Andy Card – actually I was in a classroom talking about a reading program that works. And I was sitting outside the classroom waiting to go in, and I saw an airplane hit the tower – the TV was obviously on, and I use to fly myself, and I said, 'There's one terrible pilot.' And I said, 'It must have been a horrible accident. But I was whisked off there – I didn't have much time to think about it, and I was sitting in the classroom, and Andy Card, my chief who was sitting over here walked in and said, 'A second plane has hit the tower. America's under attack.'*"

The second occasion where Bush mentioned this was at a town hall forum in California on January 5, 2002. Bush told the crowd, "*I was sitting there, and my Chief of Staff – well, first of all, when we walked into the classroom, I had seen this plane fly into the first building. There was a TV set on...*" You can still find the quote on www.whitehouse.gov.

Whoa! Hold on a second! There is a problem with the above statements. Can you guess? Yep, I think you got it. There was **no live video footage** of the first plane hitting the tower. There couldn't be. Video of the first plane hitting the tower did not surface until **after** the second plane had hit WTC 2.

So, Bush told us a whopper lie ... twice! Liars always get their stories mixed up, don't they? *"Would you like some fries with your whoppers, Mr. Bush?"*

Oh yes, this section wouldn't be complete without mentioning Securacom. I'm sure you've heard of them. What? You haven't? OK, well, Securacom was the company that provided security for the entire World Trade Center. Remember the Twin Towers collapsing at free fall speed?

How would that have been possible without explosions removing the resistance below the fall line?

"But that would mean that the buildings were wired for demolition well in advance of 9/11 right?" You got it. And here's a tidbit of fascinating info that the mainstream media didn't tell you. In the weeks (and months) preceding 9/11, there were dozens WTC office workers who reported power outages, evacuations of entire floors, and the sound of massive machinery being moved around on vacant floors. Guess who had keys to every floor of the buildings? Oh yeah, you're hot as a firecracker! Securacom did. But what does this have to do with President Bush? Well, guess who ran Securacom? A man named Wirt D. Walker III was the CEO. *Walker?* Like George Herbert **Walker** Bush? Yep. Wirt is the nephew of "Bush 41," cousin of Marvin Pierce Bush, who was on the board of Securacom, and just happens to be the brother of George Walker Bush, otherwise known as "W."

I wonder what George, Marvin, and Wirt would say if we asked them about Securacom's relationship to the events of 9/11. Maybe they should be forced to testify. Of course, if the "testimony" were anything like George's testimony before the 9/11 Commission, then it would be virtually worthless.

You see, the 9/11 Commission (i.e., the group tasked with fabricating the "official myth") was full of Bush supporters, oil men, neo cons, and family insiders. George and Dick (Bush and Cheney) were asked to give their testimonies separately. Kind of like the way that police question suspected criminals in different rooms, so they can't collaborate on their fabricated stories and are more easily caught in a lie. Guess what? George and Dick said, "**No.**" And as Liam stated, *"Their testimony was done in secret, not filmed or recorded, as per their demands. And get out the clothespins for your nose – they were not under oath. Why? Because they were both dirty."*

Something smells fishy in Denmark.

A Few More Anomalies

- The DIA destroyed 2.5 TB of data on Able Danger, but that's alright because it probably wasn't important.
- The SEC destroyed their records on the investigation into the insider trading before the attacks, but that's fine because destroying the records of the largest investigation in SEC history is just part of routine record keeping.

- NIST has classified the data that they used for their model of WTC7's collapse, but that's acceptable because knowing how they made their model of that collapse would "jeopardize public safety."
- The FBI has argued that all material related to their investigation of 9/11 should be kept secret from the public, but that's OK because the FBI probably has nothing to hide.
- No video of any of the 19 hijackers at any of the three originating airports of the four flights has been made public, except for a video allegedly showing hijackers of Flight 77, but that's OK because the government told us that they did it and the government wouldn't lie to us.
- At least seven of the alleged hijackers have turned up alive since the attack. (Abdulaziz Alomari, Saeed Alghamdi, Salem Al-Hamzi, Ahmed Al-Nami, Waleed Alshehri, Abdulrahman al-Omari, and Ameer and Adnan Bukhari). But that's no big deal, because they're lying "terrorists" and nobody should believe them. They probably faked their own deaths.
- No crime scene investigators were requested or even allowed to inspect the WTC site known as "Ground Zero." But that's no big deal, because it was only the biggest crime ever perpetrated on American soil and the government said there was nothing to see at Ground Zero. Plus, investigating the crime scene might "endanger our safety."
- One of the alleged hijacker's passports just happened to be found in all the WTC rubble. Oh yes, it was in immaculate condition. But that's normal when planes explode to jettison paper items without even a burn mark. Plus, from what I understand, most passports are "crash proof."

Seriously ... did an 8 year old make up the official myth about 9/11? Perhaps it resulted from collaboration between an infant, a crack head, and someone tripping on LSD? That would explain it, wouldn't it?

9/11 Summarium

James Corbett said it best: *"Preserve the crime scene. Follow the money trail. Establish the motive. Look for those with the means to pull off the crime. Any criminal investigator will tell you that these are the most basic principles of any investigation. But none of them were followed on 9/11 ... Fundamentally, 9/11 was a crime. It was a particularly horrific crime, one that played itself out like a high-budget Hollywood block-buster over the course of three terrifying hours on live TV, but a crime nonetheless."*

According to Canadian economist, Michel Chossudovsky, *"The tragic events of 9/11/01 constitute a fundamental landmark in American history. A decisive watershed. A breaking point. An era of crisis. A far-reaching overhaul of US military doctrine was launched in the wake of 9/11."*

The filth who planned 9/11 (no, I'm not talking about Osama) knew that it would evoke such a visceral response of hatred and anger and tears that all logic, lucidity, clarity, sanity, and restraint would give way to sanctimonious, irrational revenge. They counted on it! They wanted it! They needed it.

And they got it!

They got the event they needed to unite Americas with the common goal of *"go kill 'em all – all the terrorists."* Who is "they"? The Project for a New American Century (PNAC) was a neocon "think tank" riddled with soon-to-be members of the Bush administration. Their primary goals were *"massive expansion of the US military"* and *"increased centralized power for the CIA, FBI, and NSA."*

One major obstacle was that, before 9/11, over 90% of Americans were against wars of aggression in the Middle East. In its own words, what this country needs is a *"catastrophic and catalyzing event,"* kind of like a *"new Pearl Harbor."* Voila! Along came 9/11. After 9/11, all they had to do was tell the media whores who the "bad guys" were and then they ran with it. If you dared to question the official story, you "hated America" and were a traitor. Bush told us that *"you're either with us or you're with the terrorists."*

The rest is history.

The events of 9/11 set in motion endless wars of aggression under the humanitarian cloak of "counter-terrorism." Sadly, 9/11 was also a stepping stone towards the relentless repeal of civil liberties, the militarization of law enforcement, and the inauguration of "Police State USA." You see, without an "outside enemy", there could be no "war on terror." The entire national security agenda would collapse like a deck of cards. The war criminals in high office would have no leg to stand on.

And, yes, they are war criminals who should be prosecuted for crimes against humanity. And their story stinks to high heaven. But don't just listen to me. There are literally **thousands** of military, public officials, ex-CIA, architects, engineers, and pilots that are questioning the "official myth" about 9/11. Just visit www.patriotsquestion911.com if you dare.

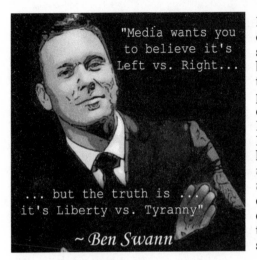

"Media wants you to believe it's Left vs. Right...

... but the truth is ... it's Liberty vs. Tyranny"

~ Ben Swann

Please don't believe the lies and disinformation that you are spoon-fed from the propaganda box. And please try to see that the "left vs. right" is a false paradigm. There is very little difference between most Democrats and Republicans. If I had a nickel for every time I've heard this pile of dung: *I won't vote for an Independent – it's a wasted vote.*" What a load of crap. How about voting your conscience? How about doing the **RIGHT** thing rather doing something that is "less wrong"?

Meanwhile, the US government is busy at work behind the scenes stripping us of our Constitutional rights under the guise of protecting us from the "terrorists." This is not a "left vs. right" issue. It's a "liberty" vs. "tyranny" issue.

But using false flag terror as an excuse to increase tyranny is nothing new. In the words of Alexander Solzhenitsyn - "*A state of war only serves as an excuse for domestic tyranny.*"

The purpose of 9/11 was manifold:

- To spread fear.
- To distract the public about critical missing Pentagon trillions.
- To create a new "power elite" in as few hands as possible.
- To crack down on civil liberties
- To increase "police state" activities
- To create a wider swath of powerful new "enemies" and shadowy groups able to attack us here in America.
- Then to create a powerful pretense to attack the new "enemies" and gain possession of their resources.

That's right ... 9/11 was used as the pretext for war in Afghanistan, Iraq, for the PATRIOT Act, the Homegrown Terrorist Act, the NDAA, the drones patrolling the skies of the USA, etc. Basically the pretext for the obliteration of the Constitution and urination on the Bill of Rights!!

After 9/11, the mesmerized "sheeple" were plunged even deeper into their "double think" and "cognitive oblivion," since 9/11 was trauma based programming. But there's good news! Refreshing news! In the end, 9/11 caused a bud to bloom in the portion of the population that is still sane, who have resisted the mainstream media's lies, propaganda, and allure.

Those with "eyes to see" eventually realized that 9/11 was undoubtedly a contrived media circus – the mother of all "false flags" – glaring "PR theater."

Too scary? Can't believe it? Please don't crawl back into the box. Despite what the mainstream media tells you, ignorance is **not** strength.

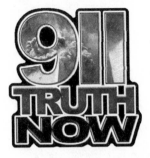

RESOURCES

Websites
www.911research.wtc7.net
www.patriotsquestion911.com
http://www.911truth.org/
http://www.ae911truth.org/
http://pilotsfor911truth.org/
http://911scholars.org/
http://www.scientistsfor911truth.org/
http://rethink911.org/
http://www.mo911truth.org/
http://www.corbettreport.com/911-a-conspiracy-theory/

Movies
"Loose Change 3rd Edition"
http://www.youtube.com/watch?v=YsRm8M-qOjQ
"9/11 Mysteries"
http://www.youtube.com/watch?v=2O7LwySqtr4

Books
Official Stories (Liam Scheff)
9/11 – Ten Years Later (David Ray Griffin)
The New Pearl Harbor Revisited: 9/11, the Cover-Up, and the Exposé
(David Ray Griffin)

"If we remain silent when our popularly elected government violates the laws it has sworn to uphold and steals the freedoms we elected it to protect, we will have only ourselves to blame when Big Brother is everywhere. Somehow, I doubt my father's generation fought the Nazis in WWII only to permit a totalitarian government to flourish here."

~ *Judge Andrew Napolitano*

Chapter 23

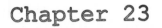

MONUMENTAL MYTH

The Branch Davidians, a cult led by David Koresh, lived at Mount Carmel Center ranch in the community of Elk, Texas, nine miles northeast of Waco. The group was suspected of weapons violations and a search and arrest warrant was obtained. On February 28, 1993, the Bureau of Alcohol, Tobacco and Firearms (ATF) attempted to raid the ranch. An intense gun battle erupted, resulting in the deaths of four agents and six Branch Davidians.

Upon the ATF's failure to raid the compound, a siege was initiated by the Federal Bureau of Investigation (FBI), the standoff lasting 51 days. Eventually, the FBI launched an assault and initiated a tear gas attack in an attempt to force the Branch Davidians out. During the attack, a fire engulfed Mount Carmel Center and over 80 men, women, and children (including David Koresh) died. In 2000, an official government investigation concluded that cult members themselves had started the fire at the time of the attack.

CAN YOU HANDLE THE TRUTH?

I went to college in Waco, Texas at Baylor University, graduating in 1991. I had never heard of the Branch Davidians while I was in Waco. Two years later, on April 19, 1993, that all changed, when agents of the ATF, FBI, CIA (and several other clandestine alphabet agencies) decided to make an example out of the Davidians by attacking their commune and murdering helpless women and children with bullets, battle tanks, flame-throwers, and poisonous gas. Nearly 100 innocent people lost their lives as a result.

What makes this a tragedy of the most terrible proportions is that the Davidians had done nothing to provoke this attack by the US government. Sadly, twenty years later, the 51 day siege is now nothing more than a series of fading memories and vanishing images in the minds of most Americans.

What's the truth about what really happened? Were the Branch Davidians a "cult"? Were they "dangerous"? Was Koresh a dastardly devil?

The mainstream media did their job well, painting the Davidians and their leader as a "Jonestown-like suicide cult" headed by a psychopathic, power-hungry megalomaniac and self-proclaimed "messiah." We were told that they abused (and raped) the children, had a tremendous arms cache, wanted to take over Waco, and were planning on committing mass suicide. Heck, I think I even heard that they hated baseball, apple pie, and their own mothers! Well, maybe not, but you get the gist of the propaganda that was spread about the Davidians by the mainstream media's teleprompter readers. Of course, the purpose of all the distortions and defamations was so that we would all cheer when we saw the Branch Davidian compound burning to the ground on April 19, 1993. We were supposed to say, *they deserved it* when we learned that 80+ children, women, and men died in that inferno.

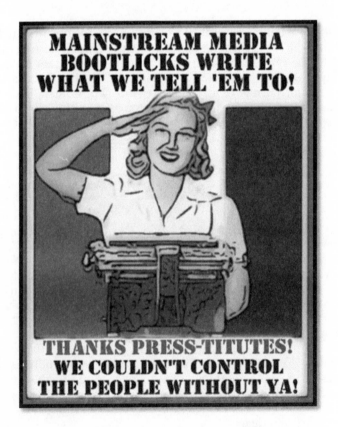

Were the Branch Davidians "Dangerous"?

The reality is that people in Waco, including many of my friends who were attending Baylor at the time, describe the Branch Davidian community as a group of ordinary people and as caring, pleasant, and compassionate. The Branch Davidians got along well with the nearby community. Many of the 100+ people who lived on the ranch in Mt. Carmel held normal jobs, just like everyone else.

No, I absolutely refuse to refer to it as a "compound." That's more of the brainwashing terminology to demonize the Davidians. It was a commune where multiple families lived. Nothing more...

A little known fact is that several Davidians were highly educated in theology, religion, and law. Many were school teachers, college professors, and computer programmers. They eventually built the building with their own hands that was destroyed in the 1993 siege. They had some religious beliefs that made them different from other churches, but, then, many of the so-called standard churches differ from each other. Their religious differences were certainly no excuse for the US government to destroy their home and their lives, especially without a trial. The consensus amongst those that knew them was that they were not dangerous.

And neither was David Koresh, although he was demonized by those who committed the atrocity. Bob Ricks, the man in charge of the Waco massacre, stated that David Koresh was a *"classical sociopath."* Attorney General Janet Reno called him *"a dangerous criminal."* Fort Worth News columnist Bill Thompson called him *"a vile mass murderer,"* and Bill Clinton referred to him as *"dangerous, irrational, and probably insane."* These people practice what Vladimir Lenin advised: *"Call your enemy what you are, and always tell the exact opposite of the truth."*

Contrary to the image of a reprehensible, treacherous, sociopathic "gun nut" with a "messiah complex" – a picture propagated by the controlled mainstream media in an effort to justify the immorality and unconstitutionality of the siege – official ATF records prove that David Koresch was rather harmless. It was common knowledge that Koresh came into town (Waco) regularly and he gladly obliged when law enforcement asked him to come to town. As a matter of fact, the ATF agents invited him to go shooting with them just 9 days before they raided the commune. Koresch supplied the ammunition. The BATF agents allowed Koresch to try out their weapons.

Does this sound like a man who was one of "America's Most Wanted"?

Were They a "Cult"?

In 1893, the Seventh-day Adventist church split off a small sect called "Branch Davidians." In 1935, a group of Branch Davidians moved to Waco, Texas. Fast forward almost sixty years to 1993 – during the raid, news reports incessantly referred to the Davidians as a "cult." **But why?** Were the bobble-head bleached blonde TV anchors also theologians? Did they actually understand the intricacies and nuances of the Davidian's theology and eschatology? Or, on the flip side of the coin, were they given a "script" to disseminate to the masses? A script which pejoratively referred to the Davidians as a "cult" in order to demonize them and eventually justify the massacre?

Just so you know, the words "cult" and "sect" are used any time the government or news media want to cast suspicion on or discredit a particular church group. Throw in a few articles in the local newspaper, and you have a concerted propaganda effort to demonize. For instance, the *Waco Tribune-Herald* ran a two part smear piece against Koresh on February 27, 1993, the day before the raid, and on the morning of entitled, "The Sinful Messiah."

One of the reasons that derogatory label (i.e. "cult") stuck to the Davidians was that film clips were widely broadcast in which David Koresh was shown saying, *"You better watch out – I'm God."* In his article entitled "Holocaust at Waco," Gary Null provides the rest of the story: *"What wasn't revealed was that this segment was actually part of a longer film clip. A reporter from an Australian network had been asking Koresh about accusations made by an ex-Branch Davidian leader that he, Koresh, had gotten the former leader's 70-year-old mother pregnant. In reply to this obviously around-the-bend assertion, Koresh had said that if he could get a 70-year-old woman pregnant, then you'd better watch out, because he is God. It was a joke. In the uncut film segment, laughter is heard in the background. In the clip, Koresh's remark was taken out of context and played as if it were a serious statement. This deceptive use of a piece of film was enough to paint Koresh as a nut."*

Bill Cooper, a former member of the Office of Naval Intelligence, also has looked into the Waco affair. Cooper offers an interesting perspective on the idea of cults. *"The definition of a cult is extremely difficult to pin down,"* he says. *"It depends largely upon who is labeling something as a cult. If you really want to get honest with all of this, all of our forefathers who left Europe to come to the United States to escape religious persecution belonged to cults. You could say that this nation was built by cultists ... The truth is that we have protection in this country under the Constitution to practice whatever religion we wish, as long as we're not harming anyone else in the practice of that religion.*

The truth is that the members of the Branch Davidian religion, their church, were adults and had the right to believe and practice whatever they wished." The First Amendment to the Constitution guarantees the right to worship God according to the dictates of one's own conscience, but the government completely ignored this right in the massacre at Waco.

Were the Children "Abused" and/or Raped?

Apparently the FBI received a tip from the Easter Bunny or Keebler Elf, or maybe Santa Claus and his helpers, that the Davidians were raping the children. Nothing like an "insider" to provide important information, eh? Well, the FBI eventually admitted that they made up the rape allegation.

How nice, FBI. We appreciate you being honest (for once), but don't you think it's a little late? Over 80 men, women, and children were burnt to a crisp and poisoned with toxic gas, partly due to this bogus, fabricated allegation. Shame on you! The allegations of child abuse came from one man who was, in essence, a disgruntled former member of the Branch Davidians. In any event, the government has never presented any evidence that any child was ever abused at the Waco commune.

"But They Had a Huge Cache of Illegal Guns, Didn't They?"

Ummm … no, they didn't. At least, not according to the local sheriff. You see, on multiple occasions, the sheriff had investigated the allegations that the Davidians possessed illegal weapons and were engaging in illegal activities with those weapons. Heck, the sheriff had even confiscated all their weapons and inspected them, but then returned them all when they were all deemed to be legal. There were no illegal weapons, nor illegal activity concerning those weapons, whatsoever. **Period.** In fact, on a per capita basis, the Davidians had less than half the number of weapons possessed by the average citizen of the state of Texas.

Yes, the fact is that the Davidians had only a few dozen firearms. But here's something very disturbing. According to Dave Hall, a reporter and the manager of KPOC-TV, *"We saw evidence the ATF admitted that they had let their weapons mingle in with the weapons that were taken into evidence [at the trial].... That was put in the court records. So the evidence that was admitted in court in the trial period was contaminated. Why the judges let it happen, I do not know."* Let me translate this for you: The ATF "planted" their own guns and "integrated" them in with the Davidians' weapons to make it appear that they had a large cache of weapons, when, in fact, they didn't.

The Siege on Mt. Carmel

The siege on the Davidians began on February 28, 1993. Instead of simply knocking on the front door, almost one hundred government agents stormed the commune to arrest David Koresh. Koresh went jogging quite frequently, and the government could have arrested him during those times, but they weren't interested in simply arresting Koresh. The government **wanted** a confrontation. They **needed** a confrontation. But they didn't get one. You see, contrary to the official "fairytale," the Davidians were actually peaceful folks who didn't want to fight. But that didn't matter to the US government, as **un**threatened ATF and FBI agents opened fire with automatic weapons at the front door and the walls, knowing that there were innocent women and children inside. No crimes had been committed by David Koresh or the members of his group. None. Zilch. Nada.

I've seen a couple of documentaries in the siege – "Waco: the Big Lie" and "The Waco WTF" – both of which portray a very different picture of the siege than the official narrative. In the video, the ATF can be seen firing at the Branch Davidians with automatic weapons, but the Davidians do not return fire. According to Dave Hall, *"For nine to 12 minutes, these people were being attacked, unannounced, with bullets flying indiscriminately through that building. They were calling for help from the sheriff's department ... Wayne (a Davidian) is telling the 911 operator that there are men out there shooting at them. He was asking them to get the police out to call these people off of them ... We have reporters that have told us that the ATF did not announce themselves until well into the shooting. And judging from the 911 tape, we come to the conclusion that, at the very least, they were under attack for nine minutes by over 100 men, and possibly as much as 15 minutes, before firing back."*

One more interesting tidbit: in the beginning, the Davidians did **not** know that they were being attacked by ATF agents, because the letters "ATF" are on the back of the uniforms and not the front! What would you do if you were being attacked by dozens and dozens of men in black suits with no identification? You'd be freaking out, and so would I. And so did the Davidians! Adding to the insanity was a helicopter gunship firing down on the roof of the house! Please tell me why it was necessary for the ATF to execute this ruthless military-style assault which killed six Davidians in the initial hours of the raid. Please tell me why, if it was so urgent for them to get to Koresh, that the ATF didn't just call the sheriff. I mean, he had been out to Mt. Carmel on numerous occasions and had never had any problems. By the way, ten days after the raid, ATF agent Roland Ballesteros made two statements to the Texas Rangers that the ATF shot first and made no announcement that they were federal agents.

As I mentioned previously, it is well-documented that David Koresh had left the commune many times while under the surveillance of the ATF. Agent Robert Rodriguez told Dave Hall that the reason Koresh was not arrested when he was observed leaving was that they had a search warrant, but no arrest warrant. But when Hall checked at the courthouse in Waco, he found that the warrant was, in fact, an arrest warrant. Hmmm ... sounds like the ATF couldn't keep their story straight. Tends to happen when you're ... **lying**! Oh yes, the night before the raid, one of my best friends saw Koresh at a restaurant in Waco. If they wanted him so badly, why didn't they just arrest him then? I'm sure he was under surveillance. Think about it.

According to chilling eye-witness testimony from Clyde Doyle, a Branch Davidian that wasn't murdered during the siege, *"David (Koresh) advised everybody to stay cool and to go back to their rooms. He would go and talk to (the agents) at the front door. I then went back to my room, which was in the front of the building on the first floor, up towards the north end. Within a minute or so, I heard his voice at the door saying, 'Hold on a minute. There are women and children here. We need to talk about this.' Before he could get the last words out of his mouth, shots came from the outside."*

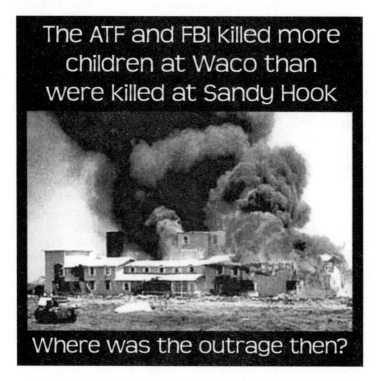

Where was the outrage then?

Doyle then recounts seeing multiple Davidians (including David Koresh) shot, laying in pools of blood, screaming, panic, machine gun fire from the outside, shots raining down from the helicopters above, and absolute pandemonium. He describes seeing a woman who had been shot in her bed while nursing a baby and an elderly man who was gunned down while eating a piece of toast.

"I never saw anybody shoot back," Doyle says, *"...although I'm not saying that they didn't. From all the evidence presented, I believe there were a few people who grabbed some weapons. I believe they retaliated because Perry and David had both been shot at the front door without being armed. I guess some people took the stand that they were defending the women, the children, and their teacher. You might say it was in self-defense, or as a reaction to seeing people gunned down for no reason."*

Dead Federal Agents

In "Waco: The Big Lie," Linda Thompson's video footage raises other vital questions. Search for it on the internet and watch it. I've saved it to my hard drive just in case it mysteriously "disappears." Anyway, in the video, it's apparent that there is a group of four agents climbing ladders to reach a first-floor roof. Once there, they break into a second-floor window, apparently after throwing some kind of smoke bomb into the house, then three of the agents enter through the window. The Branch Davidians do not fire upon the agents. Then, the fourth man seems to throw a grenade and then fire a machine gun into the room. Is the fourth man attacking his fellow agents? The three agents who entered that window died in the assault. By the way, those agents had all been bodyguards for Bill Clinton from the time of the Democratic convention until he became President. Hmmm ... I wonder what they knew.

Let me point out that this video footage was provided to local news affiliates. How do I know? I am close friends with a man who used to be program director of a television station in Dallas. He's actually a very good buddy of mine. Now, in 1993, his station was provided with the footage that I described in the previous paragraph. But here's the anomaly. They "doctored" the footage before they ran it on TV, removing the footage of the ATF agents throwing a grenade into the room. Then, they aired the film as "live" footage! Even though it was **not** live, and despite the fact that it had been **edited**! My friend said that he stepped down after this incident, as he would have no part in the fabrications regarding the Waco siege.

The FBI took charge of the siege a few days after the initial assault, and during the remainder of the assault, the media was kept three miles from the Mt. Carmel commune. Each morning, a press conference was held and the FBI spokesman told the nation what was purportedly happening. *"This is our story and we're sticking to it!"* Anyway, I have a very close friend who is a pastor, and he was present many days during the 51 day siege. His daily ritual consisted of bull horning the federal agents, for hours on end, saying *"Shame on you!"* When the agents would hear him, they would look down at the ground and their shoulders would drop, kind of like when you catch a child "in the act" and he knows he's busted. In the words of my friend, *"They wouldn't look me in the eye they were so visibly ashamed. It was very telling and dramatic … almost surreal."*

According to Gary Null, *"During the 51 days between the initial AFT raid and the final holocaust at the compound, the FBI cut off all utilities and sanitation. Phone lines to everyone but the FBI were severed, and radio communications were jammed. Government loudspeakers blared nonstop with such sounds as chants by Tibetan monks, jet planes, Nancy Sinatra singing 'These Boots Are Made for Walking,' and the cries of rabbits being slaughtered. Tanks fired percussion grenades. Stadium lights kept the house illuminated around the clock. Black helicopters flew overhead. Linda Thompson notes that around the 40th day of the siege, Koresh indicated that the children and babies were out of milk. Yet relief efforts to bring baby food to the compound were turned back. The authorities were supposed to be concerned about the children inside the compound; in fact, that was the main rationale for the government's actions. So why were its agents trying to starve the children?"*

In the words of Texe Marrs, *"During the 51-day siege, the FBI perverts camped outside the Branch Davidian church/home were told to be 'as bad as you wanna be.' Almost on a daily basis, they would come close to the Branch Davidian compound, so close they could see frightened men, women, and children watching from the windows. The drunken, sadistic FBI would shamelessly drop their pants and underwear and, with gales of satanic laughter, grab and fondle their naked genitals, shoot their fingers, and moon the watching Branch Davidians. I repeat: The federal agents fondled themselves in the belief that children were watching! On one occasion, the FBI took the dead body of a hapless Branch Davidian they had machine gunned when they caught him just outside the church/home building. They mutilated it and then draped the desecrated body over a fence in plain view of the compound's inhabitants."* This is based on eyewitness testimony. During the siege, the FBI acted like a bunch of gangsters, delinquents, pedophiles, and perverts.

According to the FBI, they were constantly "urging" the Davidians to surrender. Yet Linda Thompson reports that an FBI spokesman announced on April 17th that *"anyone who came out would be considered a threat to the ATF agents and would be shot. Shots and percussion grenades were fired at a person who tried to leave through a window that day."*

The Davidian "Holocaust"

*"Torch the Mother f****rs. Do it today!"* That was the direct order given to Janet Reno's Justice Department by Hillary Rodham Clinton from the East Wing of the White House. On April 19th, the day of the nauseating "holocaust" at Mt. Carmel, beginning at 6 o'clock in the morning, CS gas (a type of toxic tear gas which is banned under the Paris Convention on chemical warfare) was pumped into the Davidian building. It's been well established that CS gas can combine with other compounds to form the deadly hydrogen cyanide gas.

According to investigators, the deadly gas was pumped into the building until noon, when government tanks hit the compound with a big injection of an atomized mixture of orthochlorobenzylidene malono-nitrile and ethanol. The mixture was heated so that it would release hydrogen cyanide and carbon monoxide into a vapor. Autopsies indicate that large numbers of people were already dead from hydrogen cyanide gas before the fire. People died from cyanide poisoning within four to five minutes. The government's use of CS gas inside the building is one of the most disturbing aspects of the entire tragedy. CS gas is never supposed to be used inside a building, since it can create fires and produce cyanide.

"But why didn't the Davidians run outside to get some fresh air once they were effectively being tear gassed?"

Good question. More on that in a moment...

Around noon, a fire broke out in the building. How? The video footage shows a tank with an extension that looks like a blazing blowtorch pushing into the house, then pulling out. Also, ATF agents are shown jumping from the burning building, and it looks as if they are removing fire-repellent clothing as they head away from the building. The FBI would not allow firefighting crews to approach until the conflagration had reached a point where everyone could be assumed dead or fully incapacitated. There was a bunker a short distance from the house connected by an underground passageway, but a tank maneuvered repeatedly back and forth across the entrance, collapsing it.

Clyde Doyle describes his experience. *"Shortly after noon, somebody came running into the church saying the building was on fire ... I went through the doorway, still on the stage but around the back of this partition. The tanks had knocked a fairly large hole in the south wall of the chapel behind this partition. It had a lot of rubble in front of it. People began to gather in that area, not knowing what to do. They would ask, 'Where's the fire? What's going on? What should we do? Should we jump out?' More and more people crowded into this narrow area. I was closest to the opening."*

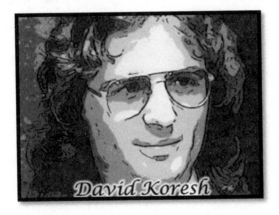

David Koresh

The Paul Wilcher Report

A considerable amount of the information in the following section of the book was extracted from a report (based on eyewitness testimony) prepared by attorney Paul Wilcher and presented to Attorney General Janet Reno on May 21, 1993. The members of the very assault team mentioned in the aforementioned report had been in contact with Wilcher (via a third party) and, even though these were hardened professional killers, what they had been ordered to do and actually did at Waco had deeply disturbed them. This is very compelling, so sit up, grab some nuts, refill your coffee, and pay attention.

According to Steve Barry, retired Army "Special Forces" and a top expert in the field of military special operations, on the morning of April 19th, there was a 15 man Delta Force commando team (a select group of the CIA's top professional killers) assembled in Waco. The plan was to massacre the Davidians and then *"make it look like a mass suicide."* These are the actual words of the Delta Force team as communicated to Wicher. No kidding.

According to Barry, "two bricks" (four-man teams) were involved in the actual attack. He said assigned to them, supposedly in an advisory capacity, were members of the British SAS ("Special Air Service"), an elite British special operations force. Barry said the Delta Force team received its orders from ... guess who ... President William Jefferson Clinton.

Barry said that during the siege at Waco, first lady Hillary Clinton operated a "crisis center" at the White House. Serving with her was another former member of her Little Rock law firm, White House Deputy Counsel Vincent M. Foster, who was later found dead under shadowy circumstances in a Virginia park across the river from Washington D.C. We'll get to Vince's "suicide" later in the book. Foster's widow, Lisa, later stated that his depression at the time of his death *"was fueled by horror at the carnage at Waco for which the White House had given the ultimate green light."* Foster was also preparing a "Waco report" when he died. This has been confirmed by veteran British journalist, Ambrose Evans-Pritchard, in his book, The Secret Life of Bill Clinton.

Back to the happenings of April 19th. The Delta Force team was all dressed in **black** — black pants, black shoes, black jackets, black gas masks, and black gloves — very poetic for a "**black** op" eh? And they were dressed to look like all the other FBI officers on the ground, probably even wearing jackets with FBI insignias on them. As I've already detailed, the federal agents used CS gas, which is a type of virulent tear gas. As a matter of fact, it was so virulent and irritating that even in an outdoor fresh air situation, it was guaranteed to cause people to flee from its presence simply in order to be able to breathe. However, at Waco, it was being used in a closed, indoor, living quarter's situation where almost 100 men, women and children were trapped inside. So let's go back to the question, *"Why didn't anyone flee the building?"* I mean, the logical expectation would have been that everyone who could walk would have immediately fled outside, right? Just to be able to breath. But strangely, not a single person came out of the compound. Not even after 6 hours of continuous exposure to tear gas.

Why? Why did not a single person, not one man, woman or child, flee the building for fresh air? The official narrative is that David Koresh and his "cult" members had stockpiled and outfitted themselves with gas masks. This is another lie. The truth is much more disturbing and sinister. According to the testimony, the CS gas was merely a "cover" for what was actually propelled into the compound – a neurotoxic nerve gas – which instantly paralyzed and rendered totally helpless and defenseless all of the men, women and children inside the building – except for those nine people who were later rescued and were on the 2nd and 3rd floor with their windows wide open on both sides and who were thus spared the deadly effects of this tear gas/nerve gas combination. For all the others, they could no longer coordinate their muscles in the effort required even just to get up, much less flee to the life sustaining fresh air outside, only a few feet away.

According to the Delta Force testimony, after this deadly tear gas/nerve gas combination had had time to do its debilitating and paralyzing work on all the men, women, and children in the building, one "brick" (four-man team) made its entry into the building after being dropped on the roof by helicopter. However, before they entered the building, all four men had received shots of atropine (the antidote to the nerve gas) so that they would not be paralyzed.

One of the first things the Delta Force team did was enter into the so-called "communications center" where they found, and quickly subdued and killed, David Koresh, with a single shot to the middle of the forehead, about an inch above the eyes, fired from a distance of about four inches away. In a May 18, 1993 article in *The Washington Post*, the forensic pathologist, Dr. Cyril Wecht of Pittsburgh, said that the gunshot wound in the middle of Koresh's forehead was *"not typical of suicide."* No wonder! It was **not** suicide. This was a premeditated, carefully planned, cold-blooded mass murder.

Withdrawing from the building, having massacred an untold number, the next step was to do as Hillary ordered – torch whole complex and leave it in ashes, all the way down to concrete and dirt. The Delta Force testimony confirms that they placed a few canisters of "Willie Peter" (White Phosphorus) in strategic locations throughout the compound in order to start the fires. These canisters were all equipped with delayed timing devices, all set to go off simultaneously around 11:45 AM, which is exactly when the fires were actually sighted by outside observers on the scene.

White phosphorus is one of the most fearsome incendiary devices imaginable, and is therefore a favorite of the CIA's "black op" teams. It ignites instantly, immediately burns with white hot intensity, and consumes, beyond all recognition, everything in its path. It also conveniently destroys all possible forensic evidence and covers the trail of assassins, thereby allowing the government to later claim that the massacre was merely a "mass suicide" or a "tragic accident."

According to Wilcher's report, all four members of the "black op" Delta Force team that committed the atrocities at Waco were sickened by what they were ordered to do and what they actually did to the innocent Davidians. In their own words, it was all *"too easy"* – the people inside the compound (as a result of the nerve gas) simply *"never had a chance."* And those consigned to this horrible fiery fate – being burned alive – included men, women, and children. Pictures from the massacre showed small children, burned black, with their backs arched backward in what had to have been a most horrible death.

Do you get this? Do you understand the magnitude of this information? It means that the US military, the FBI, and Department of Justice (directed by the CIA) used nerve gas on innocent civilians (including women and children) in our own country and then proceeded to murder them in cold blood! This clearly rises to the level of "war crimes" against a civilian population during peace time – an unspeakable human rights violation.

Didn't the Obama administration almost push the USA into World War III due to the allegation that Syrian President, Bashar al-Assad, used chemical weapons against his own people, namely women and children? Apparently, it's OK for the US government to use chemical weapons against its own citizens. Of course, if you read the chapter on fluoride, you will remember that the US government has no qualms about dripping sodium fluoride into the water supply of most municipalities across the USA, and sodium fluoride is a chemical weapon. So I guess we shouldn't be surprised.

The Crime Scene – Destroying the Evidence

Let's not forget about the destruction of the crime scene. A telling fact is that (in similar style to the rubble of the Twin Towers being shipped to Asia) the crime scene at Mt. Carmel was razed. On May 12th, less than a month after the final day of the siege, the ATF destroyed everything that remained of the Branch Davidians' building and bulldozed the entire site. Isn't that odd? I mean, usually, after a disaster, authorities take pains to preserve evidence so that it can be studied to fully understand what happened. So why would they immediately level the evidence at Waco? And why would Texas state fire marshals be refused access to investigate the fire scene? It couldn't be that they were attempting to get rid of any "clues" that would shed light on what really happened? Naw! The government would never do that. They love us. They care for us.

Oh yes, much like the 86 "confiscated for your protection" videos of the supposed plane crash into the Pentagon on 9/11, according to the FBI, there were four video cameras pointing at the Davidians' front door that could tell you everything that happened that day. *"But why haven't we seen the videos?"* Good question. I'm glad that you are wearing your "thinking cap." Are you ready for this? The FBI claims that all four videos disappeared. Vanished! Poof! Gone! How convenient. Those pesky video tapes! They like to grow legs and get up and walk away...

Then, in the spring of 1998, under the Freedom of Information Act, the public gained access to the Waco investigation "evidence lockers" and some more shocking information. The evidence gathered (under the supervision of federal officials) contradicted the FBI's congressional testimony, raising serious and disturbing questions about events surrounding the siege at Mt. Carmel and the deaths of the Davidians. **Bottom line:** The FBI was lying and they got caught.

A disturbing constitutional aspect of the events at Waco is that helicopters from the Texas National Guard were supplied, along with military tanks and manpower from Ft. Hood, for a police action against civilians. This violates "Posse Comitatus." It is also illegal in Texas, since Texas law forbids the use of the National Guard in police action against a citizen of the state, except when drugs are involved in a criminal action. Apparently the ATF fabricated a drug charge to gain the use of the helicopters. Later, Texas Governor Ann Richards stated publicly that she had been lied to by the Department of Justice.

Why Did This Nightmare Happen?

Linda Thompson's opinion is that *"Waco was merely one of the first tests of using federal law enforcement with military, and using military tactics. The government proved it could use the major media to tell the government's version of the story to the public. It was a victory for mass propaganda. They murdered 96 people in front of our eyes on national TV, and the public bought it."*

Amazingly, many people still believe that David Koresh and the Branch Davidians were responsible for the deaths of the 80 men, women and children who died in the inferno at Waco on April 19, 1993. **This is a lie.** The guns they had were legal. The local sheriff investigated and found no basis for complaints against them. These were law-abiding American citizens, even if they thought differently to most other folks. They trusted the US Constitution to ensure their political rights, but they were **massacred** by agents acting under the authority of the US government. Twenty-one children died at Waco. Anyone who accepts without question the official version of the government's war against the Branch Davidians has, in reality, already surrendered.

Oh yes, I almost forgot about Paul Wilcher. Remember that on May 21, 1993, just one month after the massacre at Waco, Wilcher presented the infamous report to US Attorney General Janet Reno? Guess what? On June 23rd, his badly decomposed body was found in his apartment in Washington D.C. Upon discovery, his apartment was sealed and searched and all documents removed. That indeed might have been the end of the matter but Wilcher had given a copy of his 100-page report to Sara McClendon, a senior White House correspondent, shortly before his death. Otherwise, we would never have known about the Delta Force "black op."

Wilcher had made one critical mistake. He presumed that Janet Reno and Bill Clinton were innocent and not involved in the massacre. **It was a mistake that was to cost him his life.** Then, in 1999, the four members of the "black op" team all mysteriously died in "training accidents." Wow! How convenient for the government. Waco has one final, absolutely unsettling message to the people of America: *"It is useless to resist ... Don't confront your government, or you'll be dealt with."*

"But that could never happen to my church." **Really?** OK, please go back to sleep. Stick your head back in the sand. Grab the clicker. Turn on the NFL. Fantasize about the cheerleaders. Watch MSNBC.

It could never happen to you. Nothing to see here. Move along...

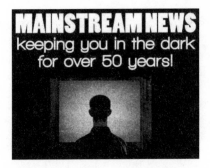

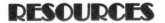

Websites
http://bigeye.com/pentwaco.htm
http://vaticproject.blogspot.com/2012/09/attny-paul-wilcher-report-waco-untold.html
http://www.serendipity.li/waco.html
http://www.apfn.org/old/wacopg.htm
http://scribblguy.50megs.com/waco.htm

Movies
"Waco – A New Revelation"
http://www.youtube.com/watch?v=UGT1F0jYhFw
"Waco – The Rules of Engagement"
http://www.youtube.com/watch?v=QRCokWb2UiY
"Waco – The Big Lie"
http://www.youtube.com/watch?v=-wUucANBY_8
"Waco II – The Big Lie Continues"
http://www.youtube.com/watch?v=ABiCv_KP1BA

Books
Massacre at Waco, Texas (Clifford Linedecker)
A Place Called Waco: A Survivor's Story (David Thibodeau)

Chapter 24

~ OKLAHOMA CITY ~

MONUMENTAL MYTH

It was April 19, 1995 – exactly two years from the date of the Branch Davidian inferno in Waco – and a flawless, sun-drenched Oklahoma morning in springtime. Against a perfect blue-sky background, a yellow Ryder Rental truck carefully made its way through the streets of downtown Oklahoma City (OKC). Just after 9 AM, the truck, driven by disgruntled US Army veteran and "government-hating" wacko, Timothy McVeigh, acting in concert with another "nut job" right-wing extremist, Terry Nichols, pulled into a parking area outside the Alfred P. Murrah Federal Building and the two men exited the truck and casually walked away.

Unbeknownst to the innocent folks in downtown OKC, there was an ANFO (ammonium nitrate/fuel oil) bomb in the back of the truck. A few minutes later, at 9:02 AM, the truck's deadly 4,800-pound cargo exploded with enough force to blow off the front side of the nine-story federal building, collapsing floors and burying victims, both adults and children, under masses of concrete, glass, and steel. The result was 168 dead, including 19 children, and more than 800 injured.

About 90 minutes later, McVeigh was stopped by an Oklahoma state trooper for driving a vehicle without a license plate, who then arrested him on a firearms charge. Two days later he was charged in the bombing. Terry Nichols was arrested in Kansas, and formally charged with the bombing a few weeks later. Timothy McVeigh was executed June 11, 2001. In 2004, after being tried in state court in Oklahoma on 160 charges of first-degree murder, Terry Nichols was found guilty of all charges, but the jury deadlocked on the death penalty, thus sparing his life.

According to the press, the OKC bombing was a result of right-wing politics, "paranoia," and revenge, as the two wackos did this to avenge the attack on the Branch Davidians. The bombing left the American people fearing a new "terrorist" enemy: the home-grown, militia-loving, anti-government, right-wing "extremist."

CAN YOU HANDLE THE TRUTH?

The truth about OKC involved not only a terrible human tragedy but also a story of government conspiracy, media complicity, and destruction of evidence, intimidation, and torture. Virtually all Americans would agree with the notion that any government which conspires and carries out unspeakable atrocities, mass murders, and indescribable human rights violations upon its own citizens (in the process violating its own laws and the laws of God) – that government is an outlaw and should be ousted and its leaders brought to justice.

Is the above representative of the old Soviet Union? Red China? Cuba? Iran? Probably all Americans would conclude one or more to be true. But I warn you here and now, with proofs herein that it also applies to the USA. Incredible? Yes, but more to the point, so frightening as to shake one's entire belief structure. Get ready to have your world rocked as we examine a few aspects of the official narrative that just don't make sense and, if viewed with an open mind, will most certainly lead the reader to conclude that the US government was complicit in the OKC bombing.

So, please grab a soda and donut .... sorry .... grab a cup of organic green tea and a piece of watermelon, and get ready to have your mind blown. And please ... keep an open mind. We're here to discover the truth and jettison the lies. Sometimes that's uncomfortable, I know, but please try.

Timothy McVeigh – A Patsy?

Timothy McVeigh was a disenchanted, government-hating, right-wing extremist, militia-loving, nut-job who "did" OKC to get back at the Feds for Waco. At least that's what we heard (and still hear) from the "repeater" teleprompter reading, controlled mainstream media.

It's well documented that before McVeigh was released from the Army, he was invited to join "Special Forces" in 1991. The official narrative is that he didn't pass muster in Special Forces and was released from the Army. But after the bombing, while in prison awaiting execution, McVeigh told a fellow prisoner a different story – a story of being involved with "black ops."

This story is supported by the testimony of both Terry Nichols and McVeigh's younger sister. Nichols, in 2006, stated that that in November 1992, McVeigh told him he had been recruited by the Army for a "black op" (i.e. undercover mission). This is also the exact time, according to other defense records which reveal that McVeigh was suddenly able to pay off all of his credit card bills after he had accumulated an enormous debt while gambling on football games.

Following his "release" from the Army, according to McVeigh, his first task was to go home and act "disgruntled" and "unhappy" with the army. He did a nice job at this task. His next task was to get involved in right-wing rhetoric and ideology and then await further instructions. In 1993, McVeigh went to Waco to observe the raid on the Branch Davidians. This is well documented. His photograph was taken in Waco to prove his "interest." He now had the perfect cover for his future involvements with anti-government militants.

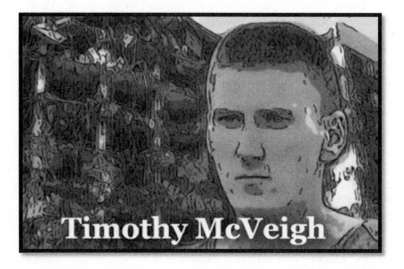

Timothy McVeigh

Film producer, Christopher Emery, began researching the OKC bombing back in 2000, even moving to Oklahoma from New Mexico in 2003 so he could be close to witnesses and other sources of information. The result of all these years of work is a remarkable piece of investigative journalism and documentary filmmaking called *A Noble Lie*. The film does the work that the controlled mainstream media refused, and still refuses, to do. According to Emery, rather than being a radical government-hater, McVeigh was actually a CIA sharpshooter and assassin who had been involved in covert government drug trafficking operations. He had been decorated several times, even receiving one commendation while he was in prison for the bombing. "*McVeigh was a very cunning, very talented sharpshooter,*" Emery says, "*He was a puppet, a showpiece for the official narrative.*"

According to McVeigh's last cell-mate, David Hammer, McVeigh worked directly for the Feds; his role was to infiltrate the burgeoning "patriot movement" and posture himself as an anti-government extremist to build up this false persona. McVeigh himself confided to his first lawyer that he had been recruited by the government and that his job was to "*search for neo-Nazis and other problem troops*." In other words, the public persona of convicted bomber, Timothy McVeigh, as an anti-government right-wing radical extremist, was a complete fabrication, a hoax, a myth.

Let's see if we can dissemble the myth. According to the official OKC narrative, McVeigh attacked the government in response to Waco. But wait! Not a single BATF or FBI agent was killed or injured and every badge carrying federal agent was mysteriously absent from the Murrah Federal Building on the morning of the attack. That's weird? Almost like they had been tipped off or something ... we'll come back to that ...

Rewind to April 17th, two days before the OKC bombing, when Timothy McVeigh allegedly picked up the Ryder truck at Elliot's Body Shop in Junction City, Kansas. McVeigh had been filmed by a security camera at a nearby McDonald's 24 minutes before the time stamped on the truck rental agreement, wearing clothes that did **not** match either of the men seen at Elliott's. It was pouring rain at the exact time McVeigh supposedly picked up the truck; there is no plausible explanation of how he traveled the 1.25 miles from McDonald's to Elliot's, carless and alone as he claimed, without getting soaked in the rain. The three people interviewed (employees of Elliot's) all agreed that the two men who rented the Ryder truck were wearing dry clothing.

According to Stephen Jones, who has seen the interview transcripts, it took 44 days for the FBI to "convince" the car rental agency owner that "John Doe #1" was Timothy McVeigh. And, no, the owner did not testify in court. I guess the Feds were afraid to put him on the witness stand for fear of what might happen under cross-examination. Also, this might explain why the initial description of John Doe #1 (which was circulated by the FBI) referred to a man with "pock-marked skin, fairly stocky" standing about 5'10", whereas McVeigh was about 6'3" tall, thin as a rail (160 pounds), and had a smooth complexion.

Were McVeigh and Nichols involved? I think there is no doubt that they were. But they weren't alone. According to Nichols, McVeigh believed he was being "manipulated" by FBI agent, Larry Potts, who was no stranger to anti-government confrontations, having been the lead FBI agent at Ruby Ridge in 1992, and was also involved in the Branch Davidian siege in 1993.

Speaking of the FBI, they were unable to provide any forensic evidence linking McVeigh to the Ryder truck or the explosives. "*An FBI fingerprint expert conceded today that no fingerprints of Oklahoma bombing defendant Timothy J. McVeigh were found on a rental receipt for the Ryder truck used in the blast, inside the Ryder dealership, inside lockers the government believes were used to store explosives used in the bomb, or on the Ryder truck key found in an Oklahoma City alley after the bombing,"* the *Washington Post* reported on May 16, 1997.

While in prison, McVeigh was visited at least 18 times by a psychiatrist named Dr. Jolly West. Dr. West was the chairman of the department of Psychiatry at UCLA, but his real job was as a CIA asset, in charge of the MK Ultra Mind Control program. Dr. West had also paid visits to Sirhan Sirhan, another supposed "lone nut" gunman, accused of killing Robert Kennedy, but in reality a product of the CIA mind control program, set up as the "patsy." Dr. West was also the psychiatrist employed by the government to evaluate the "mental condition" of Jack Ruby after he shot Lee Harvey Oswald. As I've mentioned previously, when Ruby was interrogated, he told the FBI that there was a huge conspiracy surrounding the JFK assassination and he could only expose it if they moved him to a safe place – which they refused to do.

Multiple Bombs?

When the Murrah Federal Building blew up, it was declared that one man was primarily responsible, Timothy McVeigh, and his weapon of choice was declared to be an ANFO bomb. But according to Department of the Army and Air Force Technical Manual No. 9-1910, entitled *Military Explosives*, an ANFO bomb requires very low humidity, yet McVeigh and Nichols allegedly cooked up their bomb on the muggy banks of Geary Lake in Kansas. In addition, the official narrative is that 4,800 pounds of explosives virtually leveled the building, but retired Air Force Brigadier General Benton Partin (an explosives expert) proved that it was nigh impossible for a 4,800 pound ANFO truck bomb to have done this tremendous amount of damage.

According to Partin, former commander of the Air Force Armament Technology Laboratory, and a 25-year expert in the design and development of bombs, *"When I first saw the picture of the truck bomb's asymmetrical damage to the Federal building in Oklahoma, my immediate reaction was that the pattern of damage would have been technically impossible without supplementary demolition charges at some of the reinforced concrete bases inside the building, a standard demolition technique ... Reinforced concrete targets in large buildings are hard targets to blast. I know of no way possible to reproduce the apparent building damage through simply a truck bomb effort."*

General Partin also conducted scientific analysis which revealed that core columns were blown out and the extensive damage to the building was completely inconsistent with the explanation of a single and relatively weak fertilizer truck bomb. However, his request to have the bomb site preserved in order to examine the possibility of a second explosion was ignored by the government. Sam Cohen is an explosives expert who spent 40 years working with nuclear weapons and was one of the designers of the neutron bomb. He thinks the official OKC story stinks to high heavens. According to Cohen, "*I believe that demolition charges were placed in the building at certain key concrete columns and this did the primary damage to the Murrah Federal Building. It would have been absolutely impossible and against the laws of nature for a truck full of fertilizer and fuel oil – no matter how much was used – to bring the building down.*"

Joe Harp, a man with military explosives experience, stated in an affidavit there "*was a strong sulfur smell in the air that was very reminiscent of the gas-enhanced 'Daisy cutter' bombs I am familiar with from my tours of duty in Vietnam ... It was not an ANFO smell.*" In May 1995, former Senior Special Agent in Charge of the FBI in Los Angeles, Ted Gunderson, produced an evaluation of the bombing that revealed two distinct seismograph events. Dr. Raymond Brown, a senior geophysicist, analyzed the seismograph data and concluded there was a bomb **inside** the Murrah federal building.

Geophysicist Charles Mankin, Director of the University of Oklahoma's Geological Survey, also said two explosions occurred, the second coming approximately eight seconds after the first. The US Geological Survey decided not released this data. But that's nothing to be concerned about, because the Feds probably have nothing to hide, and releasing conclusive proof that there were two bombs detonated would "endanger national security."

The best documentary on OKC is most definitely *A Noble Lie*. Without a doubt. Watch it online. Do your research. The film conclusively proves that the blast damage at the Murrah Federal Building could not have come from the truck bomb that McVeigh is alleged to have placed there. Debris was blown **out** from the building, travelling hundreds of feet against the force of the blast. If the truck bomb had done all the damage, the force would have blown debris **into** the building. The film also provides proof that there was more than one blast, with timed charges, planted in the building, set to go off over a period of several seconds.

What about the initial newscasts? What did they say? Were there multiple bombs? Here are several samples of "live" news broadcasts documenting the OKC bombing.

> "*The first bomb that was in the federal building did go off ... the* **second explosive** *was found and defused. The* **third explosive** *that was found and they are working on it right now...*"
> ~ CNN transcript

*"... both the **second and third explosives**, if you can imagine this, were larger than the first. ... It is just incredible to think that there was that much heavy artillery that was somehow moved into the downtown Oklahoma City federal building."*
~ CNN transcript

*"A **second bomb** has been found inside the federal building, it was an explosion at 9 o'clock this morning that did that damage you are looking at now blowing off the entire North Face of that building. A second bomb was found in the east side of the building. A second bomb has not exploded."*
~ KWTV live coverage

*"The Justice Department has reported that a **second explosive** device has been found in the Oklahoma Federal Building. I'd like to tell you in addition to that, **two different explosive devices** were found in addition to what went off, a total of three."*
~ CNN transcript

A Department of Defense Atlantic Command Memo issued 36 hours after the OKC event reported that a *"second bomb was disarmed [and] a third bomb was evacuated."* This was confirmed by a US Forces Command Daily Log that stated at least two additional bombs *"were located [in the] vicinity [of the] explosion site. Evidently intended for the rescuers."* Oklahoma Highway Patrol radio logs also reported secondary bombs at the site.

There were others. Like Jane Graham, who worked on the 9th floor and survived the blasts. In an affidavit, she indicated that she saw two men who were caught on camera walking away from the building with walkie-talkies after the bombing. She had noticed these men in the building prior to the bombing wearing maintenance uniforms, but she didn't recognize them as employees. She also said that there were definitely two distinct events that occurred, and that the second blast was very loud and powerful. She also talked with the FBI about these incidents, but they showed little interest, only asking if she could positively identify either McVeigh or Nichols.

Oh yes, there were several other witnesses who saw a bomb squad at the scene **prior** to the bombing. Heck, it was even on TV! During a live-feed video interview, an Assistant Fire Chief on the scene stated that the bomb squad was at the Murrah building at seven o'clock that morning, two hours before the bombing took place. What were they doing there two hours before the bombing?

Were there multiple bombs? Of course there were. So why does the official myth contradict this known fact?

Where were the Feds? Where are the Tapes?

The Bureau of Alcohol, Tobacco, and Firearms (ATF) had offices in the Murrah Federal Building. On the day of the bombing, none of the ATF agents came to work that morning. The ATF agents, who had children in the day-care center, did not drop their children off that day. There were no ATF agents or their children on the casualty list of the OKC bombing.

How did they know? ATF employees who worked in the Murrah Federal Building received messages on their pagers prior to the bombing telling them not to go to work! That's how. Somebody knew ahead of time and tipped off the Feds. No doubt. Several individuals received prior warning that the bombing was about to take place. Bruce Shaw, who rushed to the Murrah building to find his wife who was employed there with the Federal Credit Union, testified that an ATF agent told him that ATF staff had been warned on their pagers not to come to work that day.

Did you know that there were almost two dozen surveillance tapes which captured the explosion? The only problem is that on all of the tapes, the video mysteriously fails to show the moments just before the truck bomb exploded. It's almost as if they have been edited. Sort of like the FBI doesn't want us to see what happened right before the blast. According to Salt Lake City attorney Jesse Trentadue, who obtained the tapes through a FOIA request as part of his investigation of the bombing, all of the tapes feature blanks just before the bomb went off at 9:02 AM, but *"the interesting thing is they spring back on after 9:02 ... The absence of footage from these crucial time intervals is evidence that there is something there that the FBI doesn't want anybody to see."* According to the FBI, the tapes were not edited. The fact that over 20 different videotapes all have a mysterious "black out" just prior to the blast is just a peculiar coincidence, a quirk, a fluke, pure happenstance. Really?

Mysterious Deaths of Eyewitnesses

Within minutes of the blast, all available on-duty and off-duty police, fire, and medical personnel from throughout the OKC metropolitan area responded to the scene. Citizens and rescue crews teamed up to ensure the injured were treated and transported as quickly as possible. Among the very first to arrive on the scene were OKC police officers, Terrance Yeakey, Gordon Martin and Ken Griffin, a number of Oklahoma City firefighters, Dr. Donald Chumley, and General Services Administration planner Michael Lee Loudenslager.

Coincidentally, these men all died mysterious deaths.

In this section of the book, I'm going to focus on the deaths of Terrance Yeakey, Dr. Donald Chumley, and Michael Lee Loudenslager.

Terrance Yeakey

Well-liked, and well-respected, Terry Yeakey was an upbeat, devoted, articulate and thoughtful young OKC police officer whose goal was to join the FBI. In 1986, Yeakey had enlisted in the Army and became a military policeman. He joined the OKC police in 1990 and served in the Persian Gulf. In 1991, Yeakey married Tonia Rivera, his college sweetheart, and although the marriage didn't last, reconciliation was in the works. They had two girls and two boys.

Yeakey, a giant of a man with a heart as big as his 6'3", 275 pound frame, was on duty the morning of April 19, 1995. Within two minutes of the explosion, he was at the Murrah Federal Building. By all accounts he was among the first uniformed police officers to arrive. Disregarding his own safety from falling debris, Yeakey began to rescue the injured and carry them to safety, running back and forth into that concrete mess of bricks and mortar all day long continuing beyond exhaustion, far into the night. In a cadre of heroes that day, Yeakey's performance was outstanding. He worked for 48 hours without sleep.

It had immediately become obvious to Terry Yeakey that a number of things about the bombing just didn't add up. If this were **really** a terrorist bombing, then why were police lines already up behind the building when he first arrived, within a mere two minutes after the fact? And where had all of those the ATF and FBI agents come from so quickly, arriving from outside of the building (most relatively unharmed) when he had only just gotten there himself? And most importantly, if this were the result of a sting operation gone bad, then why hadn't the building been evacuated beforehand?

The last person he carried out of the Murrah Federal Building was a man that weighed 300 pounds, and Yeakey fell two stories through a hole in the floor and injured himself. They wanted to admit him to the hospital, but Yeakey declined, because he (and a number of others at the bomb site) had already been threatened with death by federal agents to *"keep their mouth shut"* about everything they'd seen and heard there that morning.

He called his ex-wife, Tonia, and asked her to come and pick him up at the hospital. After she arrived, Yeakey got in the car and in tears he told her, *"It's not what they're saying it is, Tonia. It's not what they're saying it is. It's all a lie. It's all a lie. It's not true. It's not what they are saying. It didn't happen that way."*

Yeakey was subjected to daily harassment and intimidation from his fellow officers because he refused to go along with the official story. He spent weeks and months investigating and attempting to discover the truth about what really happened that day. On numerous occasions, he was told to *"drop it or you'll wind up dead."* He was afraid of what he had stumbled upon as a result of his eyewitness account. He was plagued by chronic back pain from the fall during the rescue. He suffered from insomnia and nightmares.

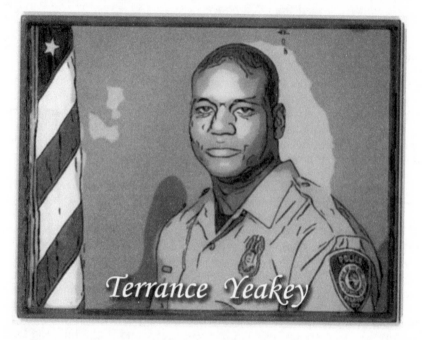

In a letter that he wrote to Ramona McDonald, a victim of the bombing who was questioning the federal government's official story, Yeakey told her, *"I think my days as a police officer are numbered ... Knowing what I know now, and understanding fully just what went down that morning, makes me ashamed to wear a badge from Oklahoma City's Police Department ... You and your family could be harmed if you get any closer to the truth."*

Terry Yeakey was scheduled to receive the Medal of Valor from the OKC Police Department on May 11, 1996. He never got it. He was murdered on May 8, 1996. Early that morning, Yeakey told a friend that the FBI was following him. At approximately 6 PM that evening, Yeakey's abandoned car was found. According to the Sheriff, there was so much blood inside it ran out the door. There was also a razor blade lying on the dash. The seats had been completely unbolted, the floorboards ripped up, and the side panels removed. Witnesses said it looked like someone had butchered a hog on the front seat, but Yeakey was nowhere to be found.

His body was eventually found over a mile from the blood-soaked car, but there was hardly any blood. He had been handcuffed, hog-tied, dragged and brutally beaten. Rope marks extended to the back side of his neck. His wrists, arms and throat were slashed, and he was shot in the head - execution style. Blood, which was not his, was also found on his shirt. Yeakey's car was never dusted for prints and no autopsy was ever conducted.

Without performing an autopsy, OKC's Chief Medical Examiner, Dr. Larry Balding, quickly ruled the death a "suicide." No, I'm not kidding.

Seriously, according to the official story, while still inside his Ford Probe that he had parked on a lonely country road, Yeakey slashed himself 11 times on both forearms before cutting his throat twice near the jugular vein. But that's not all. Then, after losing somewhere between two to three pints of blood, Yeakey supposedly got out of his car, and, apparently seeking an even more private place to die, he crawled 8,000 feet through rough terrain, crept under a barbed wire fence, waded through a culvert, then lay down in a ditch before shooting himself in the head with a small caliber revolver, which over 40 law enforcement officers couldn't find.

But miraculously, after an FBI helicopter landed at the scene carrying FBI Agent Bob Ricks, Yeakey's weapon was suddenly and unbelievably (literally) discovered within five minutes. Oh yes, I almost forgot, there were no powder burns on his body, which indicates that a silencer was used. I guess he wanted to make sure that he didn't disturb anyone when he committed "suicide."

C'mon. Give me a break. They actually expect us to believe this enormous load of excrement which they call the official story?

Suicide? Right! If you believe that Yeakey committed suicide, then let me tell you a "whopper" of a tale about a man (dying of renal failure and on dialysis in a cave half way across the world) who coordinated the hijacking of airlines in the USA where hijackers used box cutters ... (you get my point) ...

Yes, there was a giant government cover-up at OKC. Terry Yeakey became aware of that fact long before the rest of us. He discovered it during the first hours of rescue. **And he paid for that discovery with his life.**

Make no mistake about it, Terry Yeakey died in the line of duty – a "line of duty" which began when he got out of his patrol car at the Murrah Federal Building just minutes after the bombing, and began to selflessly help others. Terry Yeakey was an American hero.

Dr. Donald Chumley

One of the first doctors at the scene of the bombing was Dr. Don Chumley who operated the Broadway Medical Clinic located about half a mile from the Murrah Federal Building. Shaun Jones, Dr. Chumley's stepson, was assisting him.

Jones recalled the scene: *"Chumley, who was working with Dr. Ross Harris, was one of the few doctors who actually went into the Federal Building while the others waited outside. He had helped (get) many people (out), including seven babies, whom he later pronounced dead."*

According to Michelle Moore, who has investigated the bombing, Dr. Chumley was asked to bandage two federal agents who falsely claimed to have been trapped in the building. Since they were clearly not injured, Chumley was offended and refused to participate in their charade. When the agents asked another doctor at the scene, Dr. Chumley intervened, threatened to report them. Chumley was a man of integrity and character and, when asked to participate in a dubious and outright deceptive act, he steadfastly refused.

Chumley worked side by side with Officer Terry Yeakey during those first hours and days of rescue. Like Yeakey, he also had defied the federal officers at the scene who reportedly attempted to have him falsify reports. Something was terribly wrong. Both men realized it, and over the next months, both began to assemble evidence.

Dr. Chumley was an experienced private pilot with an instrument rating and over 600 hours flying time. His skills were never in question. Yet he died in a plane crash only five months after the OKC bombing. Chumley was flying his Cessna 210 when it suddenly, and without explanation, went into a nosedive from an altitude of 6,900 feet, plunging into a field near Amarillo, under "mysterious circumstances."

Chumley was killed instantly. Interestingly, the FAA investigators found **nothing** mechanically wrong to cause such a bizarre accident and the accident remains unsolved.

Besides being at the Murrah Building on the morning of the OKC bombing, Dr. Chumley and Terry Yeakey had one other thing in common: Each of them, at the time of his premature death, was attempting to compile and deliver evidence concerning the bombing itself, along with proof that Michael Loudenslager had been alive and well after the bombing.

Speaking of Loudenslager...

Michael Lee Loudenslager

In the aftermath of the bombing, the name Michael Loudenslager holds particular significance in the hearts of many folks in and around OKC. Why? Because of the forewarning he gave to a number of those families who had children in the Murrah Federal Building's day-care center.

In the weeks preceding the bombing, Michael Loudenslager had become increasingly aware that large amounts of explosives and missiles were being stored in the Murrah Federal Building and as a result he strongly urged a number of parents to take their children out of the Murrah Building. Other employees became concerned with an increased amount of missiles being brought into the building (by the DEA and ATF) and, as a result, a grievance was filed by the building's security director, whose wife ran the day-care center. As a result of his concern for the children and dedication to protect the occupants of the federal building, the security director received "praise and a raise."

Oops ... sorry ... rewind ...

As a result of his concern for the children and dedication to protect the occupants of the Murrah federal building, the security director was **fired.** *"Thanks for the 'heads up' ... now get your stuff and get out!"*

Then, after some remodeling work had been done to the day-care center, the security director's wife notified Fire Marshals that the work had been completed (as was required by her license). However, Fire Marshals were denied access by federal agents and were instructed to leave. And then, the day-care operator was **fired.** Second verse, same as the first: *"Thanks for the 'heads up' ... now get your stuff and get out!"*

After hearing rumors about an imminent bombing, Michael Loudenslager and the day-care center operator began speaking with parents, many of whom chose to remove their children. Due to their warnings, there were far fewer children were in the day-care center on that horrible Wednesday morning than there otherwise would have been.

On the morning of the bombing, Loudenslager was in court. Shortly after the bombs exploded, he was among those who were actively helping in the rescue and recovery effort, where he was seen by many folks. During the course of the early rescue efforts, however, Loudenslager was seen and heard engaging in a loud, livid exchange with someone there. This argument was seen by dozens of people, including police officers.

Therefore, when it was reported that Loudenslager's body had been found inside the Murrah Building at his desk on the first floor, supposedly a victim of the 9:02 AM bombing, those police and rescue workers were a bit bewildered, to say the least. The problem with the official story is that Loudenslager already been seen alive and well by numerous rescue workers at the bomb-site after the bombing, where he was actively engaged in the urgent task of rescuing critically injured victims.

Yes, he is officially listed as one of the 168 bombing fatalities. But Michael Loudenslager was murdered at the site, sometime after the bombing. Was he murdered and placed at his desk? Or, was he simply murdered and said to have been found at his desk? We may never know. The murder of Michael Loudenslager is unquestionably one of the most important sidelights of the OKC bombing.

What about the witnesses that saw Loudenslager alive and well after the bombing? Like Jack Colvert, Jackie Majors, and Buddy Youngblood? Sorry. They're all dead. Just like Dr. Don Chumley and Officer Terry Yeakey. As are about thirty other folks who either knew too much or asked too many questions.

"Move along now ... nothing to see here."

Who and Why?

Remember the Latin phrase, *"cui bono?"* which simply means *"who benefits?"* This is the very first question to be asked in any investigation.

So, *"who benefited from the OKC bombing?"* Well, since you asked ...

President William Jefferson "Bill" Clinton attributed the revival of his popularity after the 1994 election debacle to the bombing of the Murrah Federal Building in OKC. Relaxing on Air Force One after the election, he told reporters it was the Oklahoma bombing that proved the turning point in his "political fortunes." After the bombing, Clinton made great "political hay" of the tragedy by drawing parallels between the anti-government extremists behind the plot and the anti-big-government Republican revolution that had swept Congress. After the bombing, Clinton prodded Congress to move swiftly on his anti-terrorism legislation (Omnibus Counterterrorism Act) and avoid political "endless quibbling" over details.

The purpose of the OKC bombing was to get Congress to pass the anti-terrorism bill without debate, because if a debate had taken place, the issues of constitutional liberties and the creation of a domestic "police state" would have been raised. But the criminals in D.C. prefer that the police state be implemented without the public noticing by creating a climate of national hysteria using a staged terrorist attack, aka "false flag." Guess what? The Omnibus Counterterrorism Act sailed through with no debate or discussion.

In addition to the to the passage of the anti-terrorism bill, the aftermath of the bombing led to the demonization of the "patriot movement" which was spreading like wildfire as opposition to federal government abuse grew following the events at Ruby Ridge and Waco.

The bottom line is that millions of Americans realize that Timothy McVeigh did not act alone, nor did his truck bomb wreak the destruction and take all the lives in the Murrah Federal Building. When the Feds tore that building down and buried the evidence of internal explosions, and began to interfere with the grand jury, the fix was apparent to all who cared to see.

The OKC bombing was yet another "false flag" attack perpetuated by the government "to gain a political end" ... and that end was to demonize political opposition, especially "patriots" and "extremists."

Timothy McVeigh was another Oswald, another James Earl Ray, another ... **patsy.**

RESOURCES

Websites
http://whatreallyhappened.com/RANCHO/POLITICS/OK/ok.php
http://www.the-office.com/okc-witnesses.htm
http://www.rense.com/political/bombing1.htm

Movies
"A Noble Lie" http://www.anoblelie.com/
"The Government Cover Up of the Oklahoma City Bombing"
http://www.youtube.com/watch?v=DiF31q8kxhA
"OKC Bombing: Forerunner to 9-11"
http://www.youtube.com/watch?v=x6NfZa4daO4

Book
The Final Report on the Bombing of the Alfred P. Murrah Building
(Charles Key)

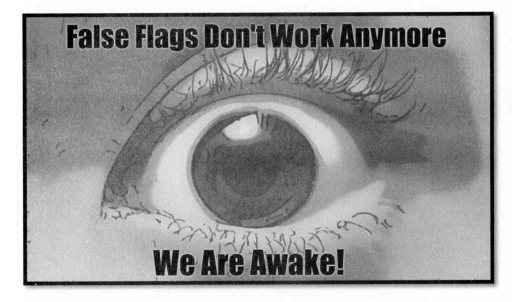

Chapter 25

~ BOSTON MARATHON ~

MONUMENTAL MYTH

The official story goes like this: On April 15, 2013, two radicalized Islamic Chechen terrorist brothers, Tamerlan and Dzhokhar Tsarnaev, unleashed weapons of mass destruction (pressure-cooker bombs containing bits of metal, nails, and ball bearings) at the Boston Marathon, killing four and wounding 264 in an unthinkable scene of *"bodies flying into the street … so many people without legs … and blood everywhere."*

CAN YOU HANDLE THE TRUTH?

Fifty years ago, Lee Harvey Oswald was framed for the assassination of JFK. The same US "National Security State" that executed JFK still rules America today, using identical tools of murder and deception. At the 2013 Boston Marathon, it appears that we have two more "Oswalds" – Tamerlan and Dzhokhar Tsarnaev. Why do I say this? The two alleged "terrorists" had no history of public violence, criminal activity, bomb-making, or terrorist affiliations. Even though they had been "radicalized" into terrorist forms of Islam, they nevertheless walked through the event openly, without disguising or hiding their faces. They both carried backpacks containing bombs, but somehow they managed to set off the bombs and still leave the marathon with their backpacks. They had achieved a blow against the "Great Satan," but they remained in town after the event, going to a party with friends. They didn't escape to New York City, where they could have booked passage to any city in the world.

Think about it: you just blew up bombs at the Boston Marathon. You're restless, disorganized, appalled, and overjoyed … all at the same time. You're paranoid because there were cameras everywhere. You're certain that the Feds are on your trail. So, what do you do? You … stay in town and hang out with friends? Huh? You … go to a party and manage to convince everyone that nothing's wrong? **Seriously?** We're asked to believe that the two "genius idiot terrorists" stayed, partied and seemed in good spirits after the bombing? At least, until guns were pointed at their heads, at which point, they ran. Hey, if they were going to run, why not run when the getting was good? Why not leave town immediately?

Why not call the "terrorist cell" leader and get directions for your next move? No, they decided to go party. Yeah right. Smells like "BS" to me.

These boys didn't really fit the typical "terrorist" profile. Dzhokhar, the younger brother, "tweeted" Jay-Z lyrics, but not a word about guilt, Allah, the infidel, or any other "identifying" mark of a "terrorist." Tamerlan, the older brother, who was reported as both being "*run over by his brother*" and also "*shot by police*" was reported dead, but then a man (identified as Tamerlan) was arrested and forced to strip naked before entering the police car.

Adding to the intrigue, an eye-witness identified Tamerlan as being "*run over by a police SUV and then shot by police multiple times.*" Dzhokhar allegedly hid in a boat where he scribbled a confession on the boat interior and was eventually seen by the boat owner who then called SWAT or the police or the FBI, depending upon which version of the story is being told. According to the official narrative, he then allegedly shot himself in the mouth. Did I miss anything?

Oh yes, I almost forgot. Then the mayor of Boston (Thomas "Mumbles" Menino) allowed the US Constitution to be "suspended" in the city so that the military, under the guise of "police," could enter homes and terrorize citizens, without warrants, without recourse, and without penalty. The right of Miranda and a fair and unbiased trial by peers was waived by the court, despite the fact that the alleged terrorists were American citizens, whose friends and family, almost to a person, boldly denied that the accusations were true, or expressed immense shock at the accusations.

In this chapter, I include numerous photographs because, unlike many of the other chapters in this book in which I use cartoonish photos and artwork, the photographs at Boston are a crucial piece of evidence. In 2013, everyone has hand-held devices, cameras, iPhones, etc. The photographic evidence will hopefully assist you in "connecting the dots" and determining what really happened at Boston, because it proves, beyond a shadow of a doubt, that the official story surrounding the Boston bombing is a myth, a fable, a hoax, a fairytale ... right up there with "Jack and the Beanstalk" and "Snow White" and "Rumpelstiltskin."

So let's look at more than a few anomalies and pesky "glitches" that surround the official mythology that is the Boston bombing!

The Drills

Remember what was happening on 9/11? You know ... the drills ... the "war games"? Well, guess what? There were drills taking place in Boston, too. Not just any drills, but drills that involved bombs. What a coincidence! University of Mobile cross country coach, Ali Stevenson, an eyewitness and participant in the Boston Marathon, confirmed that drills were taking place the morning of the Boston Marathon; drills complete with bomb squads and rooftop snipers.

In an interview with Anthony Gucciardi of www.storyleak.com, Stevenson detailed what went on before the race began: "*At the start at the event, at the Athlete's Village, there were people on the roof looking down onto the Village at the start. There were dogs with their handlers going around sniffing for explosives, and we were told on a loud announcement that we shouldn't be concerned and that it was just a drill. And maybe it was just a drill, but I've never seen anything like that — not at any marathon that I've ever been to. You know, that just concerned me that that's the only race that I've seen in my life where they had dogs sniffing for explosions, and that's the only place where there had been explosions.*"

On the morning of the explosions, the *Boston Globe* tweeted "*Officials: There will be a controlled explosion opposite the library within one minute as part of bomb squad activities*" and also "*BREAKING NEWS: Police will have controlled explosion on 600 block of Boylston Street.*" See the screen capture below.

Tweets

The Boston Globe @BostonGlobe   8m
Officials: There will be a controlled explosion opposite the library within one minute as part of bomb squad activities.
Expand

The Boston Globe @BostonGlobe   8m
BREAKING NEWS: Police will have controlled explosion on 600 block on Boylston Street
Expand

Photos released after the bombing shoot holes in the official story as they depict both middle-eastern **and** Caucasian men with large black backpacks (with unique insignias), hats with strange skull emblems, and tan boots, behaving suspiciously immediately before **and** after the explosions. Check out the image on the following page.

As Anthony Gucciardi has documented, two individuals identified in the images are likely to be employees of Craft International (a Blackwater-style private paramilitary security firm). However, the media and "authorities" have ignored the presence of what appears to be current or former military professionals standing just a few feet from the site of the explosion wearing backpacks similar to those used in the attack talking into their cell phones. My questions: Why was Craft International there? Who hired them? What was their mission? What's in those black backpacks, fellas? Hot dogs and chips? Tea and strumpets?

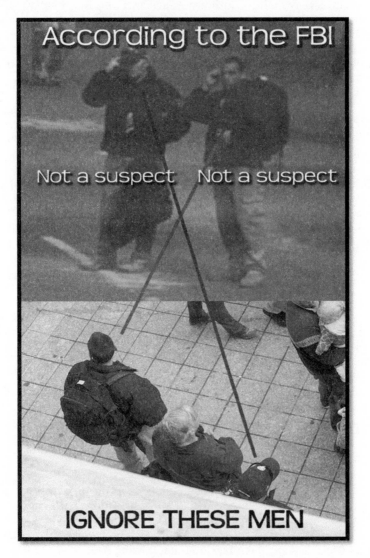

As I browsed through thousands of photos from Boston, I located three more private military operatives with the exact same dress: tan combat boots, black jackets, black backpacks, and tactical communications gear.

Here is a picture of three of these men reacting to the explosions.

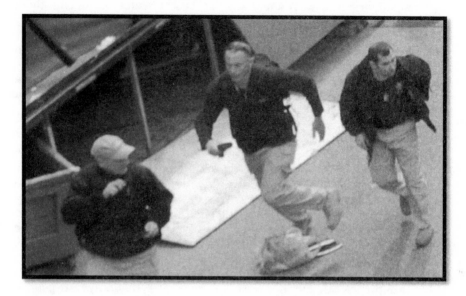

What do these photos indicate? You tell me. At the very minimum, they show me that there were, indeed, drills happening concurrently with the actual event. No, you idiot, this isn't "conspiracy theory." How are photos of **actual** people at the **actual** event part of some vague conspiracy theory? The answer is that they aren't. Period. In real police work, they're called "evidence," and the people in these photos should be persons of interest. Oddly enough, they aren't. The fact is that the entire controlled mainstream media (and law enforcement agencies) never investigated these men. They acted like they were nothing more than "Casper the Friendly Ghost" and didn't really exist. In my opinion, **that** is the real conspiracy theory!

The "Damage" and the "Pressure Cooker" Bombs

The official story is that there were *"bodies flying into the street ... so many people without legs ... and blood everywhere."*

However, the detonation of the first bomb, near the Lens Crafters shop, lacked the force to damage, or to displace, the nearby wooden fence and the barrier of blue steel scaffolding that separated the sidewalk from the street. As a matter of fact, the bomb didn't even damage the blue fabric screen that covered the street side of the blue scaffolding. None of the international flags that lined the street were damaged, nor displaced, by the blast. This is bizarre since the "pressure cooker" bombs allegedly contained bits of metal, nails, and ball bearings that should have frayed the blue fabric into shreds and left the flags threadbare. But, no, there was no evidence of a bomb exploding, at least not from the flags and fabric that were within a few feet of the blast site. At the second bomb's blast site, the white upholstered chairs on the Forum Restaurant's patio showed no signs of damage, and there were no bloodstains on the white upholstery. The green metal Post Office collection box located next to the blast site at the second bomb site showed no damage. Zero. None. Not a dent. Not a scratch.

Alright, this is really sounding weird. Totally inconsistent with reality. For instance, this past July 4th, we set off some firecrackers in the back yard. There was a cardboard box sitting about 10 feet away from the firecrackers. After we had exploded a few firecrackers, I noticed that the box looked like it had been shot with several dozen BB's. There were tiny holes, apparently from the miniscule bits of material that are jettisoned when a firecracker explodes. But in Boston, the official story is that the pieces of metal, nails, and ball bearings caused only negligible peripheral damage?

Seriously? OK. Maybe they were "magic bombs" that only hurt people, and not inanimate objects. Makes sense. Yeah, "magic bombs" ... created by leprechauns and elves at the North Pole with Santa (and Mrs.) Claus and Rudolph.

How many people were injured from the "magic bombs"? Officially, the US government and the controlled mainstream media claim that 264 people were injured by the two bombs. However, the photographs and videos of the immediate aftermath of the detonation of the two bombs show only about 50 people in close proximity to the first bomb site (near the Lens Crafters shop) and not more than 20 people in close proximity to the second bomb site (near the Forum restaurant). Let's see, I was never really that good at math. How many is that? OK, 50+20 = 70.

So the photographic evidence shows around 70 people near the two blast sites. Check out the photo on the next page. Count 'em yourself. It actually appears like far less than 70 people, but let's just say there were 70 for the sake of argument. Now, many of those people, at least half, were **not** bleeding, and they did not appear to be injured, after the blasts. So that gives us 35 "possibly injured" folks.

The photographs and the videos do not show nearly enough people in the near vicinity of the two bomb sites immediately after the blasts to account for the figure of 264 wounded. I'm not saying people weren't hurt. I'm just saying that the photographic evidence indicates that the "official numbers" may be greatly exaggerated.

Oh yes, I almost forgot. They were "magic bombs." Duh!

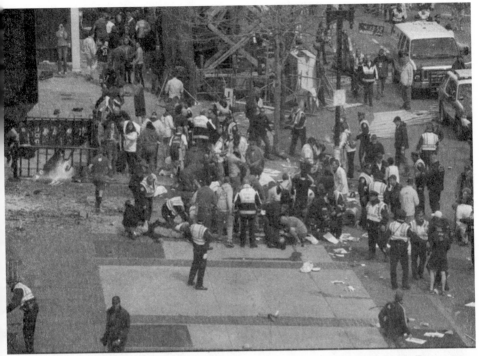

Above - outside Lens Crafters   Below - outside the Forum

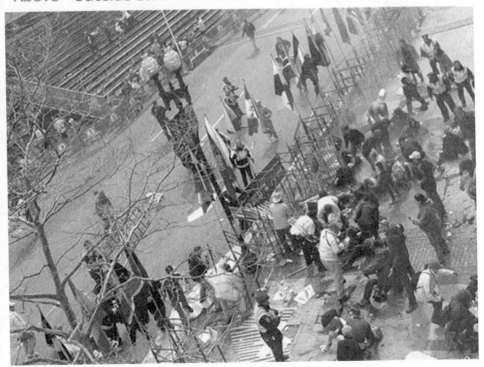

The Crime Scene and "Victims" – Lost Limbs & Blood?

The official story is that some of the victims had legs completely blown off by the bombs. But the photographic evidence is murky, at best.

The amputation of human limbs requires a great deal of concussive or cutting force, which was not demonstrated by either bomb, as I have already demonstrated by the lack of damage to surrounding fabric and flags. Heck, the explosion of the first bomb barely ruffled the blue fabric screen on the nearby fence! Almost like they were "flash-powder bombs," which create an impressive "theatrical" bright flash and a lot of smoke, but they lack any substantial concussive force.

"But I saw the man with his legs blown off. It was on TV." Maybe, maybe not. That man's name is Jeff Bauman. I'm sure you remember the photos of Mr. Bauman laying in the street with his legs blown off, right before he was carted off in a wheelchair (how nifty, they had a wheelchair handy) by the heroic man in the cowboy hat. Except, well, I don't mean to be insensitive, but the photos just don't seem very realistic. I mean, where is the blood? His legs were allegedly blown off, which would have resulted in not just one, but **both** femoral arteries being severed. Now, there was blood (or fake blood) on the ground, all over the ground actually, but there was hardly any blood (actually **no** blood) coming from his stubs. We'll come back to the fake blood ...

Seriously folks, the femoral arteries are extremely powerful. Without tightly tied tourniquets, there would be massive, colossal, gigantic, enormous amounts of blood. That is, until he bled to death. And "bleeding out" is worse with blunt force trauma (like shrapnel) because flesh is torn rather than cut, exposing more arterial and vascular tissue. Now, the femoral artery blood flow is around 600 ml/minute, and an average person has 5000 ml of blood.

This guy has **two** severed femoral arteries, which means he'd be "stone cold dead" in **three** minutes, with half of his blood gone in 90 seconds! If he really had both femoral arteries severed, there should be blood **everywhere**. I mean all over him. He would be literally drenched in blood, kind of like he just bathed in blood. And you would also see what's called "arterial spurting" from the injury. But I've seen literally dozens of photos of Mr. Bauman, and I still have yet to see a single photo of blood pumping, splattering, and/or spurting from one of his femoral arteries. Within 90 seconds, he would most likely vomit (after turning ghost white from shock), turn delirious, and then pass out.

Oh yes, he would also need an enormous volume of saline to replace the lost blood to keep his blood pressure up to prevent imminent cardiac arrest. Maybe he had a bag of saline solution in his pocket, just in case...

"But the man in the cowboy hat applied a tourniquet, didn't he?"

Well, actually, in this case, the alleged "tourniquet" was a mere piece of thin cloth. It was not a medical tourniquet, by any means. And if you notice in the photos, it's not even tied off! It's sort of "suspended" via gravity. I don't think that the tourniquet would have successfully stopped blood from dripping from his finger if he's pricked it with a needle, much less stop the flow of blood from an arterial sever. There's no pressure applied. There's no knot with a turn stick for leverage. You can clearly see a gap in the nonexistent wrap job on his left inner thigh.

And lest I forget, the tourniquet was only on **one** of his legs! Mr. Bauman supposedly had **both** legs blown off. What about the other (partial) leg? Let's just say that the loose tourniquet actually was successful at stopping the blood flow from one of his severed femoral arteries. Why wasn't the other leg bleeding profusely? Before we answer that question, let's go back to the technical details. There's a video (still available on YouTube) of the initial bomb being detonated. At the 7 second mark, the bomb (flash-powder bomb?) "explodes." Around the one minute mark, you can see the man in the cowboy hat for the first time, but he has not yet made it to assist Mr. Bauman, whose legs were reportedly blown off from the blast. The last time you see the man in the cowboy hat is at the 2:35 mark. Guess what? He has still not made it to help Mr. Bauman. That's 148 seconds from the time of explosion. By that time, Mr. Bauman would have lost over 75% of his blood volume and would be pale as an albino ghost, passed out on the ground, literally 30 seconds from losing all his blood, and would likely already be dead.

But the official story is that the "hero" in the cowboy hat applied the tourniquet and saved Mr. Bauman's life. And that's what we're supposed to believe. Although I'm not sure how that's possible since as I just illustrated, Mr. Bauman would have been dead before the man in the cowboy hat ever found him lying on the ground. Yet, in all the photos, the color in Mr. Bauman's hands and lips shows good circulation. Kind of like he really hadn't lost any blood? Weird, eh? Almost like he was an actor or something? Naw. The government would never lie to us.

In the words of Lt. Columbo, *"...one more question, Sir."* Check out the photo (on the next page) of the loose flaps of "skin" hanging from one of Mr. Bauman's stubs. No skin in the universe (except maybe George Hamilton's) is that thick. I'm not kidding. Those flaps make no sense and have never before been seen in human anatomy. And why, in every photo, is Mr. Bauman "holding on" to his stubs? I mean **every** photo. Without exception. He's holding on to his stubs. Is he trying to make sure that the "fake gore" prosthetic limb doesn't slip off? Just asking. Think about it.

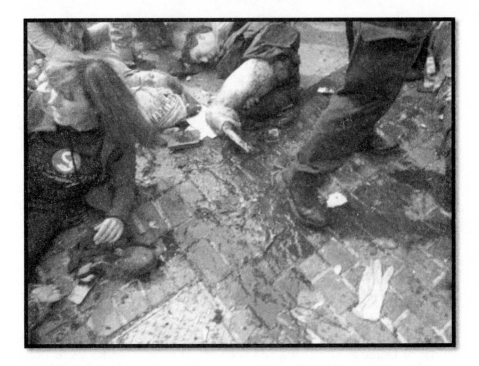

In the photo above, it appears that Mr. Bauman is "bleeding out" badly, but his stub remains clean, and there is no torn flesh! And the blood – the bright red blood in every photo – it almost looks like red paint. I've seen blood at the scene of accidents, and it is much darker color than the "blood" we see on the ground in Boston. The fact is that there is ample photographic evidence of fake theatrical blood that was splashed from bottles and packets on and around the alleged. Just do a quick search for, "*Fake Blood Boston Marathon*" and you'll be able to see dozens of high resolution, full-color photos with bright red blood.

Was the oxygen content of the earth's atmosphere different in Boston? What caused the "blood" to be so bright? I know, I know, the oxygenated blood spurting from arteries tends to be a brighter red color than blood expelled from impact wounds. But I've never seen any blood this bright red color before. What does it mean? You tell me. Think about it. And please don't give me the "*It really happened*" or "*I know (so-and-so) who was there, get a life, you're so cruel*" arguments. I'm just asking you to actually think and not just believe what you're told.

OK, let's go back to the **quantity** of blood issue rather than dwell on the **color** of the blood, shall we? At the top of the next page is a photo of the man in the cowboy hat pushing Mr. Bauman's wheelchair. Check it out.

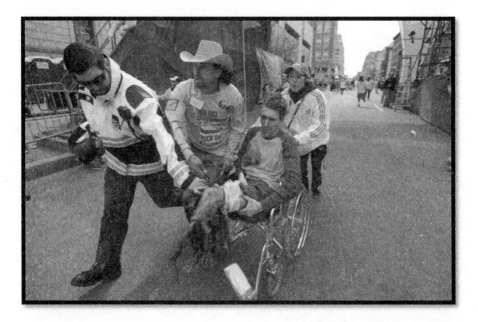

Look closely ... **very** closely. Approximately 100 yards behind them is the scene of the explosion. Even though, by some estimates this is over 5 minutes from the time of explosion and Mr. Bauman would have bled to death several minutes beforehand, it appears that he is still alive (looking calm and composed with a very healthy complexion, by the way) and they are eagerly rushing to the ambulance. Why he's sitting up (rather than turned upside down with his stubs above his head to prevent blood loss) is beyond me. Well, I guess they weren't too concerned about the blood loss, because, if you look closely at the pavement behind them, conspicuously absent will be one substance that should have been quite noticeable: **blood**. I don't see any blood ... anywhere. I mean, c'mon, two severed femoral arteries and there is not a single drop of blood for 100 yards! Not a drop! And I'm not exaggerating. I'm sure you can find a high resolution version of the above photo online. I did. And I looked and looked but never could find any blood.

There were other anomalies with the "blood" and the "injuries," but I'm not going to devote any more time to this topic. I think I've covered it adequately and need to move on. But if you're interested, just do a search for Nicole Gross, Sydney Corcoran, and Karen Rand, just to name a few "*oddities*" and "*things that make you go hmmmm.*" Check out the photos of the old lady in the wheelchair whose wearing a red shirt and black coat. You'll be able to see that immediately after the explosion, she's sitting on the ground with **no** blood on her left hand or face or legs. **None**. I mean, she's got zero injuries. But then, somebody helps her into a wheelchair, and ... voila! ... the photos indicate that she is bleeding from the face, left hand, and legs. Weird. More "magic" going on in Boston, apparently. First we had "magic bombs" and now we have "magic blood" that only starts to pour out of wounds when the "victim" is ready for the photo op. Was David Copperfield there? I'll give it a rest, but this is only the tip of the iceberg when it comes to anomalies and incongruities after the explosions.

The "Backpacks"

OK, this chapter wouldn't be complete without analyzing the backpacks. I mean, after all, the Tsarnaev brothers transported the "pressure cooker bombs" in their backpacks, right?

Below is an FBI image (from ABC News) of one of the backpacks after it exploded. Notice the color. **BLACK.** Why does it matter? Read on ...

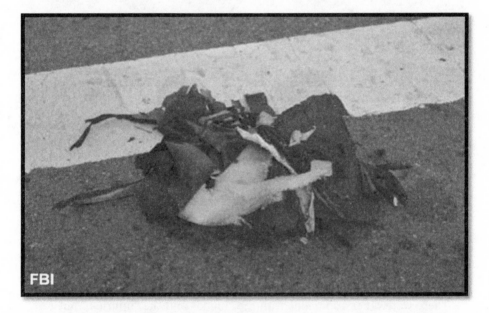

A few pages back, you saw a photo of two men carrying black backpacks who apparently worked for Craft International. Remember that photo? You know, the one where the FBI says *"These are not suspects; ignore these men"*? So, what I've done is placed the photos side by side at the top of the next page. Do you see the white insignia on the man's backpack (circled in yellow) in the image on the left? It sure looks to me like this backpack has the same insignia as the exploded backpack on the right. I've also circled the insignia in yellow. **Do you see what I see?**

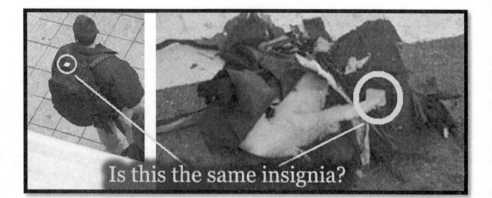

Is this the same insignia?

Oh yes, I also wanted to include a photo of the "terrorist" brothers. I know that these pictures aren't that great, and if you're reading the printed book, then they're in black and white. But full color photos are available online and I've saved them to my computer (and backup hard drive) just in case they may "disappear" in the future. Why do I mention color photos? Because the FBI report with accompanying photos indicates that the backpacks which carried the bombs were **black**. Check out the photo below of the Tsarnaev brothers. Do you notice anything odd? I've helped you out with the captions. That's right; their backpacks are the wrong color. They should be black. But they're not! Hmmmm ...

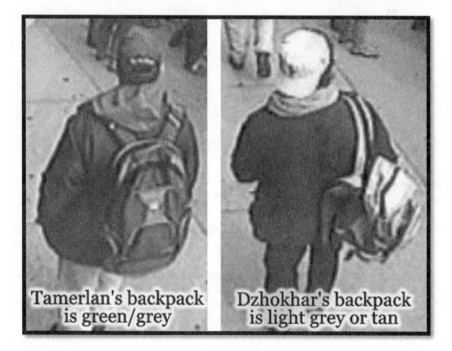

Tamerlan's backpack is green/grey

Dzhokhar's backpack is light grey or tan

Again, I'm not "nit picking" here. This is called "gathering evidence." And one of the strangest pieces of evidence is the photo of the same Craft International dude (with his black coat, camo pants, and tan shoes) running away from the explosion ... without his backpack! Where is it?

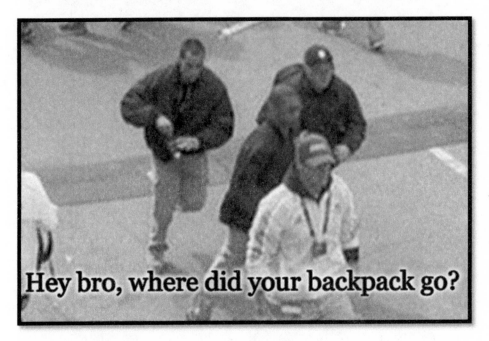

Hey bro, where did your backpack go?

The FBI came on national TV the night of the bombing and said, "*The only photos that should officially be relied upon in this investigation are before you today.*" In other words, "*Shut up slaves, these are the only suspects, because we say so!*" I guess they hadn't expected the thousands of cameras that would be taking (damning) pictures of the event. Damning pictures for the official story that is. Liberating pictures if you want to know the truth. I guess it all depends on perspective, doesn't it?

The FBI Catches the "Dynamic Duo"

So, after the FBI told us not to pay attention to the photographic evidence but merely swallow their "load of putrid crap" story, they needed our help to figure out "*who dunnit.*" Imagine that. "*We don't know who did it, but we're sure that the photos we allow you to see will nail those responsible for this dastardly deed. No, don't look at any photos other than what we spoon feed you, and, by the way, we need your help to identify the 'terrorists' in the select photos we forced down your throat.*"

I'm serious as a heart attack. At the April 18th press conference, the FBI spokesperson declared that they were *"working methodically and with a sense of urgency to identify those responsible for the bombings ... we are enlisting the public's help to identify these suspects ... We are releasing photos of these two suspects."* How did they know to focus on the brothers Tsarnaev? The official story from the FBI was that they had *"singled out these men based only on the video images."*

Quick question FBI: *"What about the Craft International dude who was photographed running away from the bomb scene without his backpack, which, by the way, matches the backpack used in the bombing?"* Oh yes, I almost forgot. Those photographs were **not** allowed to be used as evidence – they weren't "FBI approved." Now, let's get back to the officially sanctioned fairytale. So, the public was led to believe that the FBI had no knowledge at this time of who the men were, not even what their names were. We were led to believe that there was no prior connection between the FBI and these completely unknown (to the FBI) individuals.

Except for one big, fat, nasty, hairy detail: It turns out (based on a CBS News story a few days after the FBI press conference) that the FBI knew both of the Tsarnaev brothers very well. As a matter of fact, in 2011, the FBI had actually interviewed Tamerlan in his home and warned him that they were "watching him." Yes, they knew where he lived. Heck, they even had his phone number. So, why didn't they just go arrest him at his house, without further incident? Why did they release the photos, pretending (like a game of "Charades"), that they needed help to identify the brothers, whom they already knew? Could it have been because they wanted to flush them out and create a giant manhunt? Think about it. This proves that the FBI was lying to the public, to cover up the fact that the Boston bombing fits into the pattern: whenever a "terrorist" event happens (or almost happens) in the USA, it **always** involves individuals with a prior relationship with the FBI. How strange is that?

What happened after the press conference is quite bizarre, according to the official story. Once the FBI released the photographs of the brothers on Thursday night (April 18th), Tamerlan and Dzhokhar Tsarnaev sprang into vindictive action. They allegedly shot and killed an MIT campus police officer, then they carjacked a man ("Danny") in a black Mercedes SUV. According to the Feds, the Tsarnaevs used the Danny's ATM card to withdraw $800 from ATM machines. Then it gets kind of weird, actually it's already weird, but it gets weirder. The brothers Tsarnaev either dumped Danny at a gas station or allowed him to escape.

Perhaps he was really Harry Houdini reincarnated? In any event, Houdini (I mean "Danny") immediately called 911 and eventually told the police the brothers told him they were *"the marathon bombers and had just killed a campus officer."* How strange is that? They admitted it to a total stranger. Not surprising, though. After all, in this fable, we've been dealing with "magic" bombs, "magic" blood, and "magic" victims. Why shouldn't we conclude the tale with a "magic" confession to a stranger? Sounds like a romance novel, doesn't it?

Eventually, Tamerlan was apprehended and killed. How did he die? The official story tells us that the police caught up the brothers on April 19th, while they were still driving around in Houdini's stolen Mercedes SUV. The police managed to tackle Tamerlan, struggling to handcuff him, but then Dzhokhar got back into the SUV. Dzhokhar then allegedly tried to ram the car into the three officers, but he accidentally ran over his brother, Tamerlan, seriously injuring him, and *"contributing to his death."* After taking off in the SUV, Dzhokhar decided to abandon the vehicle, smashed his cellphones, and then hid out in a boat where he allegedly scribbled his confessions to the bombing. He was eventually captured by police, after shooting himself in the mouth. *"End of story. Don't ask questions. That's what happened. We say so!"*

Sorry, FBI/DHS/SWAT, I don't like being told what to do, so I'm going to ask some questions. How could Tamerlan have died as a result of being run over by his brother, when there is a video of him being taken into police custody naked and handcuffed? How did his body end up beaten (tortured) and eventually dead? The police claim the naked man was not Tamerlan Tsarnaev. Then what is his name? They have never released it.

The FBI claims Dzhokhar, hidden in a boat, scribbled a confession on the interior of the boat, shot at agents, and eventually tried to commit suicide by shooting himself in the mouth. Hey FBI, how was it possible for Dzhokhar, who you say was *"bleeding from multiple gunshot wounds"* inside a little boat (with no cabin or lighting) in the dark, to use a pen to inscribe an extremely long message confessing to being an anti-American radical Islamic terrorist?

Just the physical act of writing such a note with a pen on the inside of a boat, even under the best of conditions, would be very difficult. Last time I checked, a boat interior is not a good writing surface. Wait! I forgot. Despite the fact that Dzhokhar was bleeding from multiple wounds and was in total darkness, he used a "magic" pen. C'mon Feds. Seriously? We're supposed to believe this hogwash? I suppose the Feds were assisted by the Keebler Elf and Easter Bunny, too?

The photographic evidence clearly shows that Dzhokhar got out of the boat by himself and surrendered. He wasn't shot. He wasn't bloody. It's pretty unlikely that a person with his mouth and neck shot is going to get up and walk outside without assistance ... or a stretcher ... or gurney. But later on, the photos show him bloody and unconscious. Hey FBI, how did he get so bloody? And why does he still, to this day, deny involvement?

In his last Facebook post, prior to being captured (and beaten to a pulp), he wrote: *"This will be the last message before the police get me. I never done it. They set me up. Father please forgive me. I am sorry it has come to this."* Sound familiar? I can almost hear Lee Harvey Oswald saying, *"I'm just a patsy."* Can't you?

The Aftermath – Police State USA

So why didn't they just go pick them up the brothers Tsarnaev at home? After all, they knew their address. Honestly folks, I think Barney Fife could have tracked down the brothers in no time flat, and he wouldn't have even needed his lone bullet ... or Andy!

But for some reason the Feds instead preferred to roll out a paramilitary invasion and full-on lockdown of east Watertown for an entire day, complete with warrantless, unconstitutional searches. If you watched TV after the bombings, you'll remember that there was a colossal police response with over 9,000 troops (federal, state, FBI, DHS) conducting door-to-door searches to find and subdue the *"armed and extremely dangerous"* suspects. Cops unceremoniously ousted residents from their homes to set up impromptu battle stations, even aiming guns at residents who were taking photos from their own windows! Can anybody say, *"Police State USA"*? Sheesh.

Bottom line: Tamerlan is dead. Dzhokhar said they didn't do it. The Craft International agent, who happened to be wearing the exact same type of backpack (with the same insignia) as the one that exploded and who was photographed running from the scene **without** his backpack ... well ... he's not a "person of interest" because the Feds tell us that he's not a person of interest.

Oh yes, I almost forgot. About a month after the bombings, the FBI was interviewing one of Tamerlan's friends, Ibragim Todashev. During the interview, Ibragim went crazy and was waving a Samurai sword at the FBI agent, so the agent shot him. But then the story changed and he wasn't actually waving the sword. Well, actually, he didn't even have a sword. According to the FBI, who would never lie to us (except that they've already been "busted" lying about this story multiple times), Ibragim turned over a table on the FBI agent, putting the agent in "jeopardy." So the agent shot him. Seven times. In the head. I guess the agent's not in "jeopardy" any longer.

And guess what? Whatever knowledge Ibragim had about what **really** happened in Boston – whether Dzhokar and Tamerlan were actually involved or were merely "patsies" – went to the grave with him. How convenient for the Feds, eh?

What really happened? I'll admit – I don't know what happened.

But one thing I do know is that the official story stinks and they're lying to us. I'm not a betting man, but I'll bet the US "National Security State" is the real perpetrator of the Boston bombings. The complete lockdown of Boston, which removed eyewitnesses from the streets and allowed the frame-ups of the brothers Tsarnaev, is a taste of the kind of martial law and draconian repression that is in store for the American people if they do not rise up in rebellion against the criminals posing as their protectors.

What's next? The rounding up of dissidents, naturally ...

RESOURCES

Websites
http://english.pravda.ru/opinion/columnists/21-08-2013/125452-boston_fakery-0/
http://www.tomatobubble.com/boston_bomb_hoax.html
http://educate-
yourself.org/cn/bostonbombingdidyouthink20apr13.shtml
http://www.kaotic.com/media/pictures...42b556ee65.jpg
www.infowars.com/boston-authorities-in-cover-up-of-bombing-drills/
http://enfordummies.com/wordpress/where-is-jeff-bauman-the-man-
who-lost-his-legs-in-boston/
http://curezone.com/forums/am.asp?i=2074363
http://beforeitsnews.com/terrorism/2013/05/exposed-boston-bomb-
amputee-karen-rand-seen-wiping-fake-blood-on-leg-after-blast-video-
2446452.html

Movies
"Beyond Fake Death at the Boston Marathon: Northwoods Happens"
http://www.youtube.com/watch?v=t0aBZ2c0dFI
"Boston Marathon – All Fake Injuries"
http://www.youtube.com/watch?v=IWhGYZHD5xw
"Boston Bombs Bloopers and Fails"
http://www.youtube.com/watch?v=5j4XPHs0yuI
"Boston Lies!!"
http://www.youtube.com/watch?v=4tIYKHssxYU

Chapter 26

~ RUBY RIDGE ~

MONUMENTAL MYTH

On August 21, 1992, US marshals ventured onto the 20-acre property in northern Idaho known as "Ruby Ridge," which was owned by Randy Weaver. Weaver, a neo-Nazi white supremacist member of Aryan Nation, was wanted on federal weapons charges. He lived at Ruby Ridge with his wife and children and family friend, Kevin Harris. The marshals hazarded onto the property in a brave attempt to apprehend Weaver, who had missed a court date.

When the US deputy marshal attempted to serve Weaver an arrest warrant, Weaver killed him in cold blood. A firefight erupted and, within a few minutes, Sammy Weaver (Randy's 14 year-old son) and a federal agent were dead. An eleven-day standoff ensued, during which Randy's wife, Vicki, was accidentally shot and killed. In the end, despite the unfortunate deaths of Sammy and Vicki, the FBI and US Marshals apprehended a band of dangerous racists. According to the *New York Times*, the Weavers were "*an armed separatist brigade.*"

According to the press, the Weavers were "*government-hating, minority-hating, immigrant-hating, homeschooling, neo Nazis.*" Connie Chung called Weaver a "gun-runner" on national television. Ruby Ridge was yet another sad chapter in American history of "loners" and "racists" wreaking havoc with their guns, Christianity, and apocalyptic delusions.

CAN YOU HANDLE THE TRUTH?

I know Randy Weaver personally. I used to live in Kalispell, Montana, which is where he currently resides. While I lived in Montana, I was fortunate enough to speak to Randy on a couple of different occasions about what really happened at Ruby Ridge. What Randy told me was diametrically opposed to the official story. This chapter is based largely upon my conversations with Randy as well as several articles, which I list at the end of the chapter. It also contains information that I have heard from radio interviews with retired Army Lt. Colonel "Bo" Gritz and Jack

McLamb, director of the American Citizens & Lawmen Association and the most decorated officer in the history of the Phoenix police department. But before I get into what **really** happened and debunk the monumental myth, I want to give you a little background on the Weaver family.

Prelude to Ruby Ridge

In 1983, Randy and Vicki and their children had moved from Iowa to Idaho because they wanted to be self-sufficient and escape oppressive government regulation and taxation. They also wanted to homeschool their children, which was illegal in Iowa. They actually lived without electricity and a phone in their home at Ruby Ridge. Once they arrived in Idaho, Weaver visited several churches, one of which was a Christian Identity Church. Unbeknownst to Weaver, the church had ties to the Aryan Nation, which is a white supremacist group. His two visits to this church are the **only** connection Weaver had to any white supremacists groups.

Around October of 1989, Weaver was introduced to "Gus Magisono," a paid undercover ATF informant in the Aryan Nation. What Randy did not know was that "Gus" was actually an ATF informant whose real name was Kenneth Fadeley. The ATF had previously arrested Fadeley for gun-running and had offered him clemency in exchange for becoming a snitch and "ratting out" others. The official story is that "Gus" asked Randy to sell him two sawed-off shotguns that were ¼ inch shy of "legal length" for $300. After much persistence and nagging, Weaver agreed and sold him the illegal weapons.

Following the sale, Gus (the stoolpigeon) reported back to the ATF that the barrel of the guns were only 17¾ inches long, rather than the minimum 18 inches, thus they were illegal. However Randy told me that he had suspected that Gus was a rat-fink-snitch, and he made sure that both guns were of legal barrel length at the time of the sale. He said that Gus sawed them off after the sale.

Almost one year later, a couple of ATF agents approached Weaver and asked him to serve as an informant within the Aryan Nation. They told him they didn't have a warrant, but they did have incriminating conversations on tape and had proof that he had sold illegal weapons (i.e. the 17¾ inch shotguns). They threatened him with arrest and confiscation of his truck or house if he didn't cooperate. To his undying credit, Weaver invited them to "inseminate themselves." He didn't realize that nobody, I mean **NOBODY**, says "no" to the "federal gods" in the ATF. Defiance simply is not tolerated. They were going to show Weaver who was boss! Either "play ball" or "pay."

In December of 1990, Randy Weaver was indicted for manufacturing, possessing, and selling "illegal" firearms. That's right. As I just mentioned, the difference between "legal" and "illegal" was about ¼ inch per gun. Oh yes, I almost forgot, Weaver forgot to pay a $200 "tax stamp," too. **Seriously.** That's all the Feds had on Weaver. He's not really sounding like a hardened criminal any more, is he?

About a month later, in January of 1991, Randy and Vicki stopped to help a man and pregnant woman in a pickup truck pulling a camper who appeared to be having engine trouble. Little did they know that the couple was, in actuality, two undercover ATF agents. When Randy tried to help them and looked under the hood, the male ATF agent put a pistol the back of his head and informed Weaver that he was under arrest. To say *"thank you for stopping to help,"* other agents piled out of the camper and threw Vicki face down into the snow and mud. Again, we see the axiom *"no good deed goes unpunished"* in action. Randy was taken into custody and later released on an unsecured $10,000 bond, with a trial scheduled for the next month. Vicki, although she was "manhandled" by aggressive ATF thugs and treated like a common criminal, was not arrested.

Now here's where the story gets interesting. You won't hear this from the mainstream accounts. The trial was initially set for February 19, 1991, and then changed to **February** 20th in order to accommodate the ATF. But on February 7th, Karl Richins (Weaver's probation officer) sent Randy a letter instructing him to appear on **March** 20th. Did you catch that? February vs. March? The government sent Weaver a letter with an incorrect date – the wrong month!

Despite the fact that Assistant US Attorney Ron Howen **knew** that Weaver had been sent a letter with an incorrect date, he nevertheless appeared before the grand jury and got an indictment for "failure to appear" on February 20th. He asked Judge Harold Ryan to declare Randy Weaver a federal fugitive, even though they **both** knew that there had been a date "mix up." Ryan agreed with Howen and issued an arrest warrant for Weaver. The warrant was then turned over to the US marshals, whose job is to seek federal fugitives and process federal prisoners while they are in transit or at trial. That set the stage for the siege in August.

Randy told me that he never even received any court date notifications from the government. But even if he had received them, he had no plans to appear in court anyway, fearing he would be "railroaded" into prison based on false testimony, without an opportunity to defend himself. Weaver and his family hunkered down at home for the next year and a half, rarely leaving the property at Ruby Ridge. Friends brought supplies and food to the family, which by August 1992, included Sara (16), Sammy (14), Rachel (Io), and a 10-month-old baby named Elisheba.

After Weaver failed to appear in court (on the incorrect date), the federal judge issued an arrest warrant, and the Weavers were put under surveillance. A month before the standoff, Weaver had written his old Special Forces commander from Fort Bragg ("Bo" Gritz) asking for his help. Weaver wrote to Gritz that he feared the US government would destroy him and his family.

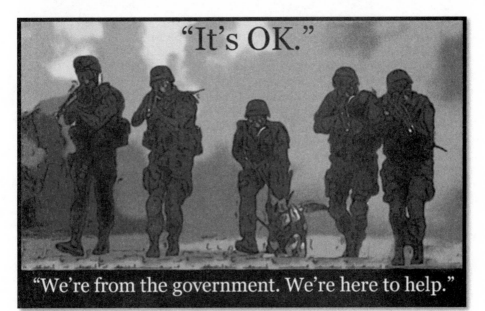

The Siege on Ruby Ridge

Let's fast forward to August 21, 1992, where the standoff at Ruby Ridge began. Please keep in mind that it all began with nothing more than Weaver's failure to appear before the court ... on an incorrect date ... for selling two shotguns ... that were ¼ inch too short ... to an ATF informant ... that entrapped him. I think that about sums it up.

The illegal siege began on August 21st when a six-man (I actually wouldn't call them "men") US marshal SWAT team, without a warrant, trespassed on the Weaver property at approximately 4 AM and began doing "recon" in preparation for a future assault on the Weavers. They were dressed in full camouflage and ski masks, carrying night vision goggles and silenced 9 mm M-16 machine guns with laser scopes. Purely "recon" is the official story; smells more like a "hit squad" to me.

Anyway, later that morning, when the family dog noticed the agents sneaking around in the woods, it began to bark wildly, so fourteen-year old Sammy and Kevin Harris grabbed their rifles. According to Randy, they initially thought the dog had come upon a wild animal and were going to kill the trapped game. Randy circled around to try to trap what they thought was an animal.

Suddenly, one of the SWAT team (dressed in "camo" fatigues) jumped out of the brush and shot the dog. Sammy, not knowing who the intruder was, returned fire. One of the marshals fired back, wounding Sammy in the shoulder. When the young boy turned around to run back to the cabin, one of the brave, courageous, valiant, heroic, federal agents (yes, that's sarcasm you smell), in keeping with the standards of valor expected of those who serve the federal Leviathan, shot him in the back, killing him instantly. Bravo! It takes a "real" man to shoot a fourteen-year old in the back as he's running away from you, posing no threat or danger. Bravo!

Two Feds in camouflage fatigues jumped in front of Randy Weaver and attempted to arrest him. Weaver (still not even aware that these were federal agents since they had never identified themselves) ran away, firing two shots into the air as a prearranged signal for Sammy and Harris to return to the cabin. In all the commotion, Randy didn't realize that Sammy was dead. Also killed was Deputy Marshal William Degan.

Later that night, Randy Weaver and Kevin Harris recovered Sammy's body and placed it in a nearby shed. As a father, I cannot even begin to imagine the stomach-turning feeling that Randy must have endured when he placed Sammy's lifeless body in the shed. During the night, FBI snipers took positions around the Weaver cabin. There is no dispute about the fact that the snipers were given illegal "shoot to kill" orders. The next day, while returning with Kevin Harris to the shed to bury his son, Randy was shot in the armpit by a sniper named Lon Horiuchi. As Randy and Kevin ran back to the cabin, without returning fire, Horiuchi shot Vicki (who was holding Elisheba) in the head, killing her instantly. Kevin Harris was also wounded by the same bullet once it shattered Vicki's skull.

Keep in mind that the FBI had not yet announced their presence and had not given the Weavers an opportunity to peacefully surrender. Minor details, though. I'm sure that the "brave" sniper Horiuchi was concerned for his own safety. Heck, those nursing mothers are dangerous! They might squirt milk in your eyes, or even worse, the baby might poop and smell up the place. I guess Vicki Weaver deserved to die. Nice job Horiuchi, you pathetic excuse for a human being. If you were even the slightest part of a man, you would make a pilgrimage to Sara's current home in Montana to express remorse for the crimes you committed against her family over twenty years ago.

Anyway, the FBI took control of the situation later that day, and imposed a news blackout and cordoned off a 3 mile radius from the cabin, forcibly evacuating all the residents. Is it just me, or does this "wreak" of Waco, which would follow the next year? Once they had "secured the perimeter," over 200 heavily armed thugs (from the FBI, ATF, and US marshal service) surrounded the Weaver cabin. I'm sorry; did I just say "thugs"? I meant "respected law enforcement agents." In any event, Weaver's cabin – or "compound" as it was labeled by the lawbreakers who besieged it and the mainstream media lackeys who peddled the official story – was surrounded by a small army of federal, state, and local law enforcement personnel.

Three days later, "Bo" Gritz and Jack McLamb arrived to negotiate a peaceful resolution to the standoff. When they arrived, they tried to calm down a group of over 100 friends and neighbors who were furious over how the Feds were handling the situation. Over the course of the next few days, the crowd grew upwards of 400 people. One week after the siege began, Gritz issued a call for outraged citizens to converge on Ruby Ridge to demand the peaceful release of the Weaver family and avert further bloodshed.

When the crowd learned of the slaughter of Vicki weaver, they became so enraged that Gritz feared they might attack the police. Officer Jack McLamb asked several skinheads at the scene to stand between the police and the crowd, which they did. When the police officers learned of Vicki Weaver's death, they were disgusted with the ATF, FBI, and US marshals.

Unbelievably, for nine days, sixteen-year old Sara had to care for her baby sister (Elishiba) as well as her ten-year-old sister (Rachel) while the shattered body of her mother decomposed underneath the table in the same room. Randy and Sara also had to endure the mocking sadism of the FBI agents who had murdered Vicki and Sammy.

One morning they were awoken by a taunting message broadcast over a loudspeaker: "*Good morning, Mrs. Weaver. We had pancakes for breakfast. What did you have? ... Why don't you send your children out for some pancakes, Mrs. Weaver?*" Seriously, is the FBI comprised of callous, cruel, cold-blooded monsters? These actions can only be described as "psychological terror."

There was finally a breakthrough in the long stand-off on August 28th when Randy agreed to speak with his old Special Forces commander, Bo Gritz, in the cabin. As previously stated, Vicki's decomposing corpse had been under the kitchen table for nine days until Gritz carried it down the mountain on August 29th. The next day, a doctor accompanied Gritz and McLamb to the Weaver cabin and told Kevin Harris, who was badly injured and bleeding, that he would die without medical attention. Harris surrendered that day.

Several events persuaded Weaver to surrender. Gritz, for whom Weaver had great respect, guaranteed his safety and that of his family. When Weaver left the cabin with Gritz, he was handcuffed and Sara and Elishiba cried as they were "escorted" down the driveway. Snipers and camouflaged agents began crawling out of the woodwork and as the Weavers noticed multiple armored carriers, helicopters flying overhead, and a massive tent city at the base of the mountain. Sarah couldn't believe her eyes. *"All this for one family,"* she muttered as tears ran down her face.

Gritz was pleased that Weaver had agreed to surrender, as the FBI had informed him that they would resolve the standoff "in their own way" if Weaver did not surrender by Monday, August 31st. Witnesses reported seeing in the vicinity a helicopter with a large external fuel tank, leading Gritz and McLamb to suspect they were prepared to burn Weaver out. Yes, indeed. In what could be seen as a "dressed rehearsal" of the holocaust at Waco's Branch Davidian refuge roughly eight months later, the Feds were getting ready to fire-bomb the Weaver cabin, thereby destroying evidence of their crimes.

I'm sure the Feds were disappointed when the Ruby Ridge standoff ended without additional bloodshed.

The Trial & Aftermath

Randy Weaver and Kevin Harris were charged with murdering Deputy US Marshal William Degan, amongst other lesser charges, and put on trial.

In his book entitled <u>Ambush at Ruby Ridge</u>, Alan W. Bock puts the trial into perspective: *"Perhaps it was inevitable that the longest federal trial in Idaho history would be followed by the longest jury deliberation in such a trial – a 20-day marathon that had news people joking about whether the jury planned to put in for retirement benefits. The eight-week trial of Randy Weaver and Kevin Harris grew out of such a bizarre set of circumstances that it's not surprising it took a while for the jurors to sort things out. It probably also took them a while to come to grips with the idea that government agencies could so blatantly engage in entrapment, lying, cover-ups, and the killing of innocent people. As one alternate juror, excused before deliberations were completed, put it: 'I felt like a little kid that finds out there is no Santa Claus.' "*

At the conclusion of the trial, the jury acquitted Harris of all charges, and found Weaver guilty only of two minor counts: 1) violating bail and 2) failure to appear in court to answer the "manufactured" weapons charge engineered by an ATF provocateur who sought to blackmail Weaver into becoming a snitch. The actual weapons charge, along with other serious charges (like murder and conspiracy), were thrown out.

In 1995, facing a lawsuit by the surviving members of the Weaver family, the government settled for $3.1 million. The *New York Times* reported, *"lawyers involved in the negotiations said the size of the settlement was a tacit acknowledgment that officials feared a substantially larger verdict if the case had gone to a jury in Idaho."* On the condition that his name not be used in any articles, one Department of Justice official told the *Washington Post* that if Weaver's suit had gone to trial in Idaho, he *"probably would have been awarded $200 million."*

Although the Weaver family received a large civil settlement (courtesy of the swindled US taxpayers), neither Horiuchi nor his supervisors were ever prosecuted for murdering Vicki Weaver in cold blood. The state of Idaho indicated their intention to prosecute Horiuchi, but apparently the prospect of doing so caused the lead attorneys to lose bladder control, so they never prosecuted him.

Incredibly, the five surviving members of the "Ruby Ridge Hit Squad" received the US marshal award for "highest valor" for murdering fourteen-year old Sammy Weaver. In the exact words of then-director Eduardo Gonzalez, they showed *"exceptional courage ... sound judgment in the face of attack, and ... high degree of professional competence."*

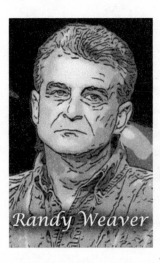

Randy Weaver

Seriously. I know, it sounds made up. But it's true. Heck, I guess if they had murdered baby Elishiba, they likely would have gotten a purple heart!

Asked in 2001 what he remembered about Ruby Ridge, Weaver said:

"There was no wind. The snowflakes were so big you could hear them when they hit the ground. The kids had three or four campgrounds around the land. They'd go out and build fires at night. And Vicki canned. She and the kids would pick huckleberries. She got top dollar 'cause she picked clean. Or she'd trade a gallon of huckleberries for our quarts of peaches. We sold firewood – me, Vick and the kids."

The incident at Ruby Ridge definitely smells like Waco, if you know what I mean. I wish I could report that these illegal, depraved police state tactics had subsided in the decades since Ruby Ridge and Waco. Unfortunately, they have been institutionalized in the "threat fusion centers" spread across the USA. These centers combine federal, state and local "law enforcement" agents in an alleged effort to combat "domestic terroristic threats" from purported "homegrown militias," where everyone from Constitutionalists to homeschoolers to Christians to Ron Paul fans to anti-fracking activists have been labeled "potential terrorists."

In the words of Timothy Lynch, director of the Cato Institute's Project on Criminal Justice, "*A new generation of young people who have never heard of Ruby Ridge are now emerging from the public school system and are heading off to college and will thereafter begin their careers in business, education, journalism, government and other fields. This generation will find it hard to fathom that the federal government could have killed a boy and an unarmed woman and then tried to deceive everyone about what had actually occurred and, in some instances, rationalize what did occur. That is why it is important to remember Ruby Ridge. Someone needs to remind the young people (and everyone else) that it really did happen – and that it will happen again if the government is not kept on a short leash.*"

RESOURCES

Websites
http://www.trutv.com/library/crime/gangsters_outlaws/cops_others/randy_we aver/1.html
http://reason.com/blog/2012/08/22/ruby-ridge-when-many-officials-realized
http://www.stormfront.org/ruby.htm
http://www.constitution.org/col/san920910.txt

Books
Ambush at Ruby Ridge (Alan W. Bock)
The Federal Siege at Ruby Ridge: In Our Own Words (Randy Weaver)
From Ruby Ridge to Freedom (Sara Weaver)

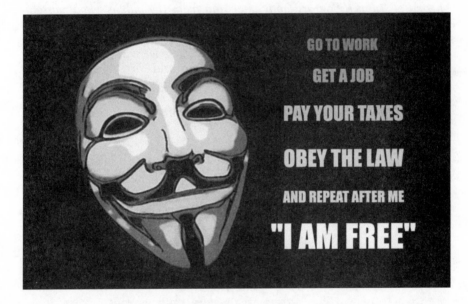

Chapter 27

~ SANDY HOOK ~

MONUMENTAL MYTH

The official story goes like this: On December 14, 2012, a 20-year-old "tech geek" (with autism/Asperger's syndrome) named Adam Lanza "snapped" and shot dead his mother, Nancy Lanza, at her home. He then loaded her car up with her guns (a semi-automatic Bushmaster AR-15 "assault rifle" and 2 pistols), then drove it across town (in Newtown, Connecticut) to his former school (the Sandy Hook Elementary School) where he shot dead 27 people, including 20 children, then turned one of his guns on himself. That's how most people "remember" the shooting, but is that actually what happened?

CAN YOU HANDLE THE TRUTH?

Let me preface this chapter with the fact that I truly feel sympathy for every parent that has lost a child. I cannot imagine the pain associated with burying a baby or small child. In light of this caveat, this chapter will be focused on exposing inconsistencies and irregularities with the official story regarding Sandy Hook as well as simply asking some questions that cannot be answered by the accepted narrative. We're on a "fact finding" mission, so difficult questions must be asked in order to find the truth.

Throughout the book, I have gone to meticulous measures to prove that the controlled mainstream media has been, and continues to be, nothing more than a "propaganda arm" for the US government. Since the event at Sandy Hook, we've been told repeatedly by the media that questioning the official story about this "shooting massacre" is as vile as racial bigotry! To take exception to what allegedly happened and actually ask questions is to make oneself an utter insensitive "conspiracy theorist" reprobate, bent on heaping insults and agony upon the grieving. So, please attempt to put aside the name-calling, since its main purpose is to squelch all discussion about the subject at hand. In all reality, the fact that researchers who were asking difficult questions were labeled "conspiracy theorists" tells me that there must be something seriously wrong with the official story.

Otherwise, they wouldn't be wasting their breath. Sandy Hook is like a "conspiracy theory on steroids!" Children were involved, so convincing people to question the facts is even more difficult than normal. Confirmed facts are in short supply, while emotion rules the day. Nevertheless, in this chapter, I will go through the overabundance of anomalies and will ask scores of unanswered questions about Sandy Hook. I will try my best **not** to tell you what to think. I will simply ask the questions and then let you decide if there are logical answers.

Anomalies with Adam and Nancy Lanza

Who was Adam Lanza? The fact is that there is nothing solid about who he actually was. Multiple public records resource sites indicate that he didn't exist since 2009 when he was student at local junior college. Adam Lanza is an enigma, at best. In todays' "information age," somewhere, somehow, everybody pops up online ... but **not** Adam! He was supposedly homeschooled but there are no records from the Connecticut Board of Education, which would have been required for him to graduate. I saw an interview with a neighbor and he said *"Nobody on the block knows him, which is odd."*

Adam supposedly smashed his hard drive, according to the official story. However, the "experts" were strangely unable to recover a single bit of data from his "smashed" hard drive. Huh? If you know anything about data recovery, you'll know that they absolutely **can** get most of the data off a badly damaged drive. There is no doubt about that. And this kid, who was supposedly a "computer genius" didn't know how to properly wipe the drive? This would have been much easier and more efficient if he wanted to get rid of his data.

Another anomaly is that Adam was allegedly found with the driver's license of his brother, Ryan. However, Ryan stated that he hadn't seen Adam since 2010. So, we're supposed to believe that Adam had Ryan's "borrowed" driver's license for over 2 years? Seriously? And since the Sandy Hook event, Ryan has never made a public statement about his brother, Adam, who allegedly weighed only about 120 pounds. Why do I mention his weight? Because the official narrative is that Adam was carrying ammunition, rifles, magazines, and full body armor that would have weighed approximately 100 pounds. Is this possible? Would he have been able to walk, much less shoot a gun and then reload, with 100 pounds of gear strapped to his 120 pound body?

My "BS" meter started beeping loudly when I learned this information...

Now here's something that it just totally bizarre and freaky about Adam Lanza's death. According to and confirmed by www.GenealogyBank.com, a database which includes the Social Security Death Index (SSDI) "death records," Adam Lanza died on December **13**, 2012 – a full day before the Sandy Hook shootings. Below is a screen capture of his SSDI record of death, which I took in January of 2013.

Adam P. Lanza: Social Security Death Index (SSDI) Death Record

Name: **Adam P. Lanza**	
State of Issue: New Hampshire	**Continue Discovering Your Family's Past**
Date of Birth: Wednesday April 22, 1992	
Date of Death: Thursday December 13, 2012	Use these links to continue exploring the Lanza family history:
Est. Age at Death: 20 years, 7 months, 21 days	
Confirmation: Proven	• **Lanza** family Recent Obituaries (1977–Today)

Interestingly, by February of 2013, the SSDI **changed** the date of death to December 14, 2012. Hmmm ... is it possible they made a mistake? Of course it is. But it's also possible that Adam died the day before the shootings and the SSDI **correctly** reported his date of death as December 13th. Just exploring the possibilities, here. Nothing more.

Where is the evidence that Adam Lanza is the Sandy Hook killer? Where are the eyewitnesses that actually saw him kill anyone? Who actually saw him brandishing weapons, carrying ammunition, or doing anything suspicious that day? Did anyone see him break into the school? These are just questions for you to ponder.

Let's look at a couple of anomalies regarding Nancy Lanza for a moment, shall we? The official story is that she was a kindergarten teacher at Sandy Hook. According to a report on Channel 9 News in Sandy Hook, which was aired live on the day of the shooting, a female reporter spoke about interviewing the Sandy Hook school nurse. When the nurse was asked about Nancy Lanza, she told the reporter: *"Nancy was beloved teacher... an absolutely loving person and a very caring experienced kindergarten teacher."*

The only problem with this testimony is that Nancy was **never** a teacher at Sandy Hook, nor even in the entire state of Connecticut. She never had a teacher's certificate. Other than the mysterious school nurse, nobody at school knew who Nancy was. *"No one has heard of her,"* said Lillian Bittman, who served on the local school board until 2011. *"Teachers don't know her."* Research shows that Nancy was actually an employee of JP Morgan Chase. Oddly, in her obituary, there was no mention of Adam.

The Car, the Weapons, and the Shooters

The official story is that Adam Lanza murdered his mother at home, stole her guns and her car and drove over to the school at Sandy Hook. The black Honda, with Connecticut license plate 872-YEO, was Nancy's car. Well ... ummm ... errrr ... it actually wasn't her car. The car is registered to Christopher A. Rodia. Who is Christopher Rodia? The raw helicopter footage of the incident showed police removing an AR-15 from trunk of Rodia's car. **All day long** the news reported that the police had found an AR-15 in the trunk and that it had **not** been used in the shooting. According to CNN, the story **all day long** was that Lanza had used a 9 mm Sig Sauer pistol and Glock 10 mm pistol and **not** an AR-15. At least that was the initial official story. But then it changed.

The evening of the event, the story mysteriously morphed into Adam using the Bushmaster AR-15 to kill all the victims and then killed himself with the same rifle. Very odd, in light of the fact that the helicopter footage clearly shows that the AR-15 was found in the trunk of Rodia's car. I guess Adam "slipped" it back into the trunk after he blew his own brains out. Was Adam related to Vince Foster? Both of them apparently had "magical" abilities to do things after they were already dead. But let's just jettison logic for a moment, and let's "flow" with the official story, OK?

Apparently the Newtown police, who must have played "hooky" on the day they learned about firearms and bullets, couldn't tell the difference between .9 mm and .10 mm rounds and .223 rounds. But once they got their story straight, the police chief was happy to inform us that Adam Lanza discharged "hundreds of rounds" of .223 ammunition. If you're not familiar with guns, the weapon that Lanza allegedly used – a .223 round with muzzle break (short barrel) – produces a deafening sound with a percussive impact on the human nervous system of 165 decibels or more. I heard an interview with a doctor of audiology who testified that the impact of 100+ rounds on the cochlear tube of the inner ear would cause an average sized man to lose balance and fall to the ground. How was (sub-average) 120 pound Adam, strapped with 100 pounds of gear, able to keep his balance after firing 100 rounds?

Initial interviews with eyewitnesses reported multiple shooters (just like Aurora, Colorado). Why have we never heard anything about the other shooters? A teacher reported that "two shadows" were observed running along the back of the school behind the gym. From the police scanner recording, we hear, with clear alarm in his voice, an officer yelling *"They are coming toward me"*... then ... *"We have a suspect proned out."* Scanner recordings also prove that the police took down at least 3 people following the shooting. Helicopter video footage shows that the police had a suspect handcuffed in the woods immediately after the incident.

The video shows the police walking a man out of the woods in handcuffs; he was wearing camo pants and a dark shirt. The evening of December 14th, CBS reported that the police had a second shooting suspect in custody and they were interrogating him. Then we never heard about him again. What about the off-duty out-of-town SWAT guy with a gun who was found hiding in the woods by first responders on the scene? We've never heard anything from him either.

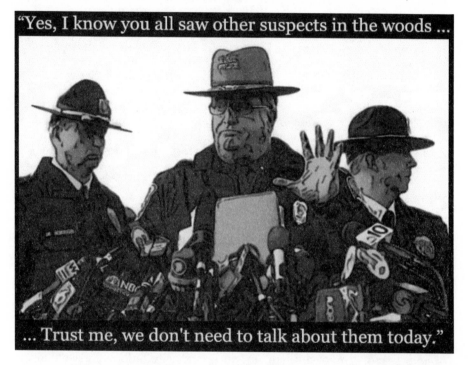

"Yes, I know you all saw other suspects in the woods ... ... Trust me, we don't need to talk about them today."

According to CBS video footage, an adult male at the school reported that he had seen a suspect "prone on the ground" in camo pants and dark jacket and saw a suspect seated in the front of a patrol car who said "*I didn't do it.*"

The Associated Press interviewed an unidentified Sandy Hook Elementary student who describes seeing a shooting suspect prone on the ground in the school's parking lot. According to the student, "*And then the police like were knocking on the door, and they're like, 'We're evacuating people! We're evacuating people!' So we ran out. There's police about at every door. They're leading us, 'Down this way. Down this way. Quick! Quick! Come on!' Then we ran down to the firehouse. There's a man pinned down to the ground with handcuffs on. And we thought that was the victim ... We really didn't get a good glance at him because there was a car blocking it. Plus we were running really quick.*"

Who were these additional suspects? Why have we never heard anything about them? Also, initial police reports were that a total of seven weapons were collected that day – three of these from the woods – where the two men had fled. Why did the official story "morph" into only 3 guns being used, and then only the AR-15?

The School Building ("Crime Scene")

Have any of you ever been to a large elementary school in the morning on a school day? I'm sure you have. What did you see? Lots of parents, cars, kids with backpacks, lunch boxes, etc. Lots of activity. But at Sandy Hook Elementary School, not a single person saw a "crazy nut job" walking up to the front door dressed in full military gear with a mask and AR-15 rifle? Not one person was in the parking lot and saw this or heard shots and called 911 or sped away to report? Really? OK, let's just assume that it was "normal" to have men in military gear, masks, and rifles at Sandy Hook, and that's why nobody reported it.

We're told that the front windows were "busted out" and that's how Adam got in the school. But when law enforcement agents arrived, they had to bust through the glass windows to get in the school. So, how did Adam get into the school? Through the front door perhaps? Not likely, since a .223 round will fragment; it will **not** penetrate a glass door like the one at the front of Sandy Hook Elementary School which was wire enforced and weighed over 200 pounds.

The initial mainstream media reports were that *"Lanza broke the glass"* and went inside the school. That's right, officially, a 120 pound developmentally disabled "computer nerd" wearing at least 100 pounds of body armor "broke through" a 200 pound wire enforced glass door. But it couldn't have been with bullets, so he must have kicked it in? Was he a closet bodybuilder? Maybe he was a clandestine superhero with magic powers? Am I missing anything? I'd like to see the video of that.

Speaking of videos, just a few months prior to the event, Sandy Hook Elementary School had installed a sophisticated camera system. And guess what? There was a camera at the front door, which was **always** locked. Protocol at Sandy Hook was that **nobody** could get inside the school unless they were recognized and "buzzed in" by the responsible school personnel. So, if Adam Lanza truly entered the school through the front door, then I'd like to see the video. Of course, no video from inside Sandy Hook has ever been released. In true "Pentagon 9/11" fashion, where are the videos? Maybe they were "accidentally" erased?

Once Lanza began his alleged "shooting spree," one would think that a mass exodus would have taken place. But did a mass evacuation of the school actually take place? Sandy Hook Elementary School was attended by 600+ students. Yet there is no photographic or video evidence of an evacuation on this scale. I've watched the live helicopter video as they describe a *"chaotic scene"* ... but there is no chaos on the video. I mean, I saw a few policemen, a police dog, and a couple dozen people or so walking around.

There was **no** panic ... **no** evacuation ... **nobody** was running. Not a single child. The helicopter reporter states, *"I have not seen any children. They are probably being kept inside because it is quite cold out here."* Huh? Hundreds of small children were being kept inside next to casualties and in harm's way of a "raving lunatic shooter," because it was too cold outside? Really?

Some folks have suggested that perhaps the videos were filmed **after** the children had already been evacuated. However, media coverage 45 minutes after the first 911 call said that none of the children had been evacuated, so that's not really a valid theory. I've looked and looked all over the internet, and nobody seems to have a real picture of events as they happened or what really happened at all. A highly circulated photo depicts students walking in a single file formation with their hands on each other's' shoulders and eyes shut. The *Newtown Bee* editor is quoted as saying she was taking photos *"left and right"* yet only this photo has emerged? Peculiarly, several of the teachers and children are wearing exactly the same outfits as they were wearing during a November drill at the school; many of the photos were posted on the school's Facebook page. Pure coincidence, I'm sure. Nothing to be concerned about...

Now, here is something that is really crazy and bizarre. On the day of the shootings, CNN's Anderson Cooper showed helicopter footage of seven police officers charging across a parking lot and toward a school. The audience is led to believe that it is "breaking news" coverage of the Sandy Hook shootings, which occurred just a few hours before. The 3-minute report posted on the CNN website was entitled "Tragedy Strikes at Elementary School." As of the writing of this book, you can still view the video online. The main problem with this video is that the school is definitely **not** Sandy Hook.

A close examination of the landscaping, diagonal lines on the asphalt, and the distinct curvature of the sidewalk reveals that no such terrain exists at Sandy Hook Elementary School. It is almost certainly video from St. Rose of Lima School, a private school less than two miles away in Newtown. According to Shepard Ambellas with www.theintelhub.com, *"Media giant CNN has now been caught airing what appears to be 'active-shooter drill footage' from another school location and passing it off as the LIVE breaking news feed of the Sandy Hook Elementary School shooting."*

I have included screen captures from the video below. Take a gander and decide for yourself. In the first picture, on the left is a "Google earth" shot of St. Rose of Lima School, and on the right is CNN footage of the shootings. The second picture shows a "Google earth" shot of Sandy Hook Elementary School. As you can see, the landscaping, asphalt, and parking lot markings don't match the CNN video footage.

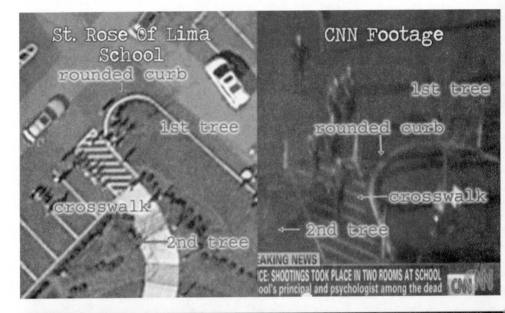

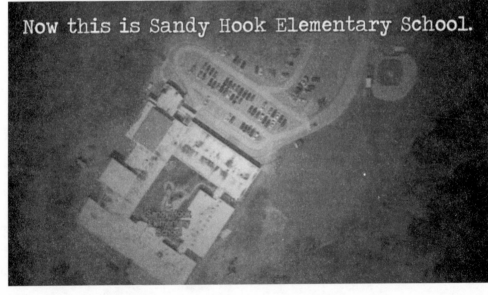

The Parkers, the "Nutty" Examiner, and the "Actor" Neighbor

One of the most outlandish features of the entire Sandy Hook event is the lack of emotion from the parents of some of the children that were allegedly killed by Adam Lanza. For instance, only a few hours after his six-year old daughter, Emilie, was murdered, Robbie Parker is seen laughing and "yucking it up" with his friends before a CNN interview. However, once the interview is about to begin, he begins to hyperventilate and appears to get "into character," almost like an actor would do before filming a "sad scene" in a movie. I have a seven-year old girl, Tabitha, and if anything of this nature had happened to her, I would have been in a hospital under heavy sedation ... almost catatonic, I'm sure. Parker's behavior is creepy, bizarre and totally out of context. Maybe he just deals with tragedy differently than the normal person. I suppose it's possible.

On December 14th, the same day as the shooting at Sandy Hook, someone created the Emilie Parker Fund page on Facebook to solicit donations for her family. If your precious six-year-old daughter had just been shot to death, would you immediately think about soliciting money from strangers for yourself? I don't think I would even be able to type a simple sentence, much less create a Facebook page.

And then there's the "nutty" medical examiner, Dr. Wayne Carver, who stated that the Bushmaster AR-15 was used to kill the small children. At point blank range, some of the children were allegedly shot 11 times; they would have been blown to pieces. Honestly, if you watch the videos of Dr. Carver, you'll quickly realize that he is an idiot. I'm not trying to be condescending to the doctor. I just can't think of another word that more accurately describes him. During one of the interviews, he laughs and jokes about the dead children. When asked what clothing the dead children were wearing, he replies, "*cute kid stuff.*" He is asked how many boys and how many girls and he says, "*I have no idea,*" while laughing like a silly schoolgirl. What's funny about dead children? I must have missed that joke. And seriously, Dr. Carver, you have "*no idea*" how many autopsies you just performed on bloody children who were wearing "*cute kid stuff*"? We're supposed to believe this ass clown?

This wouldn't be a complete chapter unless I threw in some mathematics, would it? OK, here we go. According to Dr. Carver and Connecticut State Police, Adam Lanza shot each victim between 3 and 11 times during a 5 to 7 minute span. If one is to average this out to 7 bullets per individual— excluding misses, then Lanza shot 182 times, or once every two seconds. Yet according to the official story, Lanza was the "lone nut" assassin and armed with only **one** weapon – the AR-15 that was later found in the trunk of Christopher Rodia's car.

I know, I know, it doesn't make any logical sense, but let's not worry about logic right now. Just "believe" in the enchanted butterflies and magical fairies with pixie dust. Apparently they invented the official fable about Sandy Hook.

Back to the mathematics...

So, if the misses and changing the gun's 30-shot magazine at least 6 times are added to the equation Lanza must have been averaging about one shot per second – an exceptionally skilled use of a weapon for a young man with absolutely no military training and who was on the verge of being institutionalized. Unfortunately, an accurate timeline is somewhat difficult to determine because the Dr. Carver admittedly has "*no idea*" exactly how the children were shot or how many children were shot or whether a struggle ensued.

When asked "*Did the gunman kill himself with the rifle?*" Dr. Carver replied, "*No ... I don't know yet. I'll examine him tomorrow.*" That's weird isn't it? He tells us that the shooter didn't kill himself with the rifle ... before he has even performed the autopsy. I guess a remark like this shouldn't surprise us from a medical examiner that laughs at questions about dead children and has "no idea" about how many children he had autopsied.

And then there's Gene Rosen, the wacky neighbor that said kids were in his driveway after the shooting. Strangely, Rosen not mentioned Victoria Soto (one of the teachers who was allegedly killed by Lanza), but he already knew she was 27 years old. That's weird. Do you think the kids told him that? Then he tells the sad story of the mother coming to look for her son and that night at 6:00 PM he saw that her son was on the casualty list. The only problem with this story is that the actual casualty list wasn't released for another 2 days! According to Rosen, at around 10:30 AM, he allegedly took in 6 children right after the shooting and gave them juice, stuffed animals to play with, and waited on their parents. This conflicts with the News 12 aerial footage where Rosen can be seen walking around the fire station at approximately 10:30 AM.

Oh yes, Rosen is a member of the Screen Actors Guild. In almost every interview, Rosen appears to be crying, but there's just one thing missing ... **tears**. Where are the tears? I haven't seen a single tear. Oh yes, Rosen has changed his story at least four times ... at first it was a female bus driver with the 6 kids who that told him "*there's been an incident*" and he told her "*just come in the house.*" But then it was a large man who was "*speaking harshly*" to the 6 kids before he brought them into his home. What's the truth, Gene?

It's interesting that the mainstream media condemned "conspiracy theorists" for daring to question Gene Rosen's far-fetched, implausible story.

Clearly he wasn't at two places at the same time, was he? Clearly a female bus driver didn't transform into a large man, did she? Maybe he's not only an actor ... perhaps he's also a magician? Maybe he's a time traveler, too?

"Excuse me, Sir, just one more thing. I still have one more unanswered question about Sandy Hook..."

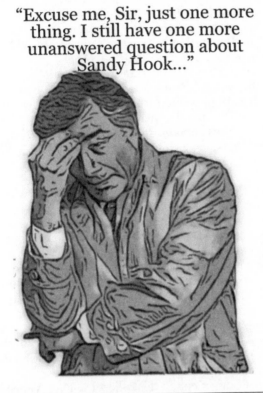

Other Problematic Questions & Uncanny Anomalies

Like my favorite detective, Lt. Columbo, I have several more intriguing questions about Sandy Hook. Here they are:

- Why didn't the teachers push the kids out of the windows and tell them to run to the fire station, which was at the end of the driveway? Why did they sit down in a circle and read stories?
- With all the shooting, why didn't any neighbors call 911? There were several neighboring homes within a couple of hundred yards.

- Did you know that there was a mass casualty drill taking place 25 minutes away from Sandy Hook at another school?
- Connecticut has an "assault weapons ban" but the initial reports that the AR-15 was "legally registered" to Nancy Lanza. How do you "legally" register an "illegal" gun?
- Dawn Hochsprung, the heroic Sandy Hook school Principal, ran out into the hall along with the school psychologist to check on a noise they heard, possibly of the glass being broken in the main entrance. They became the first casualties, we have been told. But according to the local newspaper, *The Newtown Bee*, on the day of the shooting, they spoke to Dawn Hochsprung and she had told them that "*a masked man entered the school with a rifle and started shooting multiple shots – more than she could count – more than she could count – that went 'on and on'.*" How is this possible if she was one of the first casualties?
- Why was EMS prevented from coming all the way to the school? Why were they forced to park down the street? "*You may not be able to save everybody, but you damn well try,*" 44 year old emergency medical technician James Wolff told NBC News. "*And when (we) didn't have the opportunity to put our skills into action, it's difficult.*"
- Why was the entire school put on "lock down" when there were potentially dying children inside?
- No one in the media witnessed the removal of any bodies from the school; they were somehow miraculously removed in the middle of the night in a "freezer van."
- According to the official story, the killing was tightly confined to two classrooms, near the front door and office. So why were so many children told to close their eyes while leaving the building through other exits where nothing was even close?
- The police station was 2.5 miles away. Yet from the first phone call it took 20 minutes to get there? Really? 20 minutes? The shooting lasted for only 3 minutes. So after the shooting stopped, we had 17 minutes of … what exactly?
- Why did Connecticut State Police Lt. Paul Vance threaten to arrest and prosecute people who distributed false information on the internet about the Sandy Hook event?
- Why are workers on the Sandy Hook demolition team required to sign confidentiality agreements barring them from discussing or photographing the site?
- A United Way donation page for Sandy Hook was set up on December 11th, a full three days before the event.
- An RIP Victoria Soto Facebook page was made for her on December 10th, four days before the shooting. An alert citizen managed to capture the page before it was removed. It clearly said "R.I.P. Victoria Soto" and at the very bottom, and Facebook indicated "Page created on 12/10/12." The page has been removed.

+ A tribute video was created on Vimeo over a full month before the event. It has been removed.

When the old Sandy Hook Elementary School is demolished, building materials will be pulverized on site and metal will be taken away and melted down in an effort to eliminate every trace of the building. Contractors will also be required to sign confidentiality agreements and workers will guard the building's perimeter.

WHY?

Why?

God gives us the power of reason "for a reason": **to discover truth**. The Sandy Hook event was grotesquely "circus bizarre" to say the least. Heck, the fake 2011 bin Laden killing had more evidence than Sandy Hook. After analyzing some of the anomalies and downright deceptions, the "official story" appears to be a huge stinking pile of horse manure. The facts prove that there were other shooters involved who are likely being protected by government officials. How do we know? Because the goofy coroner told us that all of the people autopsied were murdered using a .223 caliber rifle, and the videos show that the only assault rifle was found in the trunk of Christopher Rodia's car. Nevertheless, the mainstream media, who are little more than scriptwriters and teleprompter readers, still tell the tale that Lanza used an "assault rifle," despite video evidence to the contrary.

And there we have one of the reasons why Sandy Hook happened: **GUNS.** The children's bodies weren't even cold before Dianne Franken-Feinstein was talking about her total gun ban bill. The truth is that the gun grabbers want your guns! And in the aftermath of the tragedy at Sandy Hook, they put on a full court press in an attempt to disarm Mr.

and Mrs. America. Unless you just crawled out of bin Laden's cave for the first time, I'm sure you've heard the constant drumbeat for "gun control" coupled with a frenzy of fabricated fear on almost every radio and television station in the country, especially the argument that so-called "assault weapons" and large capacity magazines should be banned. When you think about it, isn't this the epitome of hypocrisy? The Obama administration sent literally tens of thousands of the "assault rifles" he now demonizes to Mexican drug cartels in Operation Fast and Furious.

Thank God, their push to disarm has failed miserably and marvelously backfired. That's right, their gutless gun grabbing crusade actually has become the single most effective gun rights **recruitment** apparatus in US history! Sales of weapons and ammunition have gone through the roof, with 2nd amendment lovers even more determined than ever to hold on to their weapons. Obviously, the gun grabbers' plans were to demonize and "shame" gun owners into somehow feeling guilty about Sandy Hook. But that never happened.

You see, the statistics are actually quite shocking, when it comes to guns and associated violent crime. On June 18, 2012, the *Washington Times* ran an article with statistics proving that violent crime decreases in areas where there gun ownership increases. Imagine that! Criminals aren't quite as bold when they know that they themselves might get shot. Nonetheless, if you happen to be aware of these statistics and dare to quote them, it's likely that you'll be lambasted as a "gun-toting right-wing nut-job."

Anthony Gucciardi did some incredible research that is directly applicable to Sandy Hook. According to 2009 FBI statistics, there are only 9,146 deaths from firearms. Of those 9,146 firearm deaths, only **348** were from rifles. Wow! This really deflates the argument that rifles are the "ultimate killing machines," doesn't it? Especially, in light of the fact that, according to Gucciardi's research, knives and cutting tools account for 1,825 deaths per year and clubs and hammers account for 611 deaths per year. Heck, even hands, fists, and feet killed 801 people in 2009.

According to a 1993 study published in the *Journal of Quantitative Criminology*, around 162,000 people per year are saved (from a **certain** life threatening situation) by using a firearm. To put that into perspective, that's 152,854 more people saved per year than are killed. And based on a 2000 study published in the same journal, US citizens defend against "**potentially** life threatening scenarios" by using a firearm an astounding 989,883 times per year!

OK, enough statistics. I told you earlier in the book that I like math and statistics! The bottom line is that the gun grabbers have proven the so-called "conspiracy theorists" to be right about claims that the US government is coming for our guns. So, when you hear the bobble-head bleached blondes in the press-titute media call something a "conspiracy theory," you may want to have a closer look.

The divergence between what is **actually** happening and what you are **told** is so vast that it pays to be guarded, cynical even, of what "your" government and "your" favorite anchor tell you.

The chances are high that it is a lie.

RESOURCES

Websites
http://moralmatters.org/2013/03/01/sandy-hook-the-real-conspiracy-theorists-by-dr-ronald-j-polland/
http://www.freedomslips.com/sandyhook.htm
http://www.storyleak.com/a-brief-and-bloody-history-of-gun-control/
http://www.stormfront.org/forum/t956386/
http://www.examiner.com/article/sandy-hook-hoax-is-falling-apart
https://archive.org/details/SandyHookOfficialStoryDebunkedevidenceICompiled

Videos
"Sandy Hook: When You're Smiling"
http://www.youtube.com/watch?v=Og_7-H86tks#t=32
"Sandy Hoax – Full Documentary"
http://www.youtube.com/watch?v=ZJLIqdFRHg0
"Sandy Hook Shooting – Fully Exposed"
http://www.youtube.com/watch?v=iJFf3ayQb8A
"Sandy Hook: CNN Used St. Rose of Lima School Drill Footage"
http://www.youtube.com/watch?v=xI0rBbLxYL0
"Sandy Hook School Shooting Hoax Exposed Sellout Medical Examiner"
http://www.youtube.com/watch?v=ShgdN8arHCc

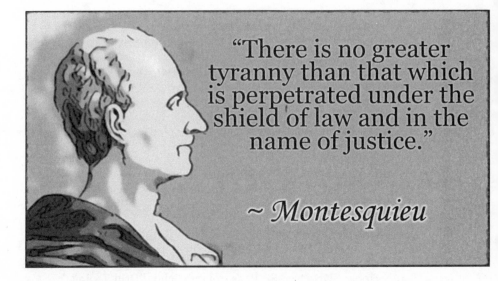

"There is no greater tyranny than that which is perpetrated under the shield of law and in the name of justice."

~ *Montesquieu*

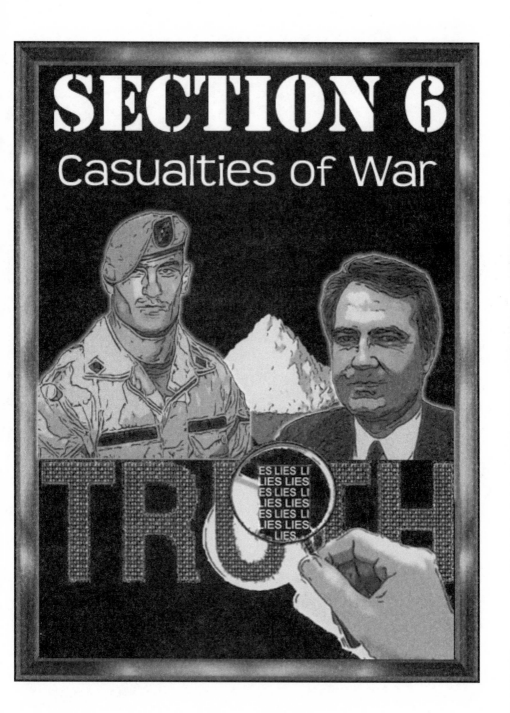

SECTION 6
Casualties of War

Chapter 28

~ PAT TILLMAN ~

MONUMENTAL MYTH

Pat Tillman. Remember him? You know, the star pro football player making a seven-figure salary with the NFL's Arizona Cardinals? Well, just a few months after the 9/11 "terrorist" attacks, Pat Tillman and his younger brother, Kevin, enlisted in the military; both qualified for the Army Rangers, one of the elite "Special Forces" units that were dispatched first to Iraq, where both brothers saw combat, and then to Afghanistan, to participate in the ongoing war with guerrillas loyal to the former Taliban regime. They both were "gung ho" to go whip some terrorist "butt."

On April 22, 2004, Pat Tillman and his team of Army Rangers were ambushed in Afghanistan. During the firefight, Tillman directed his team into firing positions and personally provided suppressive fire, while loudly encouraging his "brothers in arms" to destroy the enemy forces! Sadly, Pat Tillman was killed in the ambush. He was instantly hailed as the epitome of *"American patriotism"* and was called *"a hero"* in the media blitzkrieg that followed his death. We were reminded constantly that Tillman was a man who not only sacrificed his life for his country, but even more impressively (at least in the minds of the mainstream media) gave up millions of dollars to do so. Pat Tillman was posthumously awarded the Silver Star, the second highest military decoration for valor, with a citation declaring that he had lost his life trying to *"protect his men."* He was (and still is) portrayed as a casualty of the never-ending "war on terror," a hero who was valiantly and fearlessly gunned down in an ambush by members of Al Qaeda and the Taliban.

CAN YOU HANDLE THE TRUTH?

No matter what your opinion on the unconstitutional US wars with Afghanistan and Iraq – no matter what your theory on who was ultimately responsible for the 9/11 attacks – Pat and Kevin Tillman were clearly acting as true selfless "heroes" in the traditional sense of the word. The brothers Tillman, like most Americans, bought into the *"kill the terrorists responsible for 9/11"* babble that the mainstream media fed us every night on the news. The only difference between them and 99% of American men was that the Tillman brothers were "men enough" to actually go fight.

Michael I. Niman wrote an incredible article entitled *"Why Was Pat Tillman Really Killed?"* which was published in January/February 2006 in *The Humanist.* In this article, Mr. Niman painted a brilliant picture of the suspicious details and intricacies surrounding the murder of Pat Tillman. Since the article was an inspiration to me and was remarkably illuminating, I will be quoting (and paraphrasing) from it throughout this chapter.

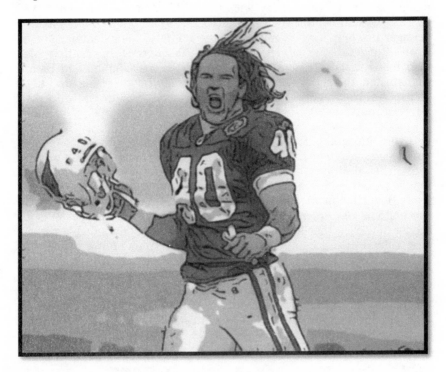

Who Was Pat Tillman?

Pat Tillman was not your ordinary, run-of-the-mill "Joe Six Pack" type soldier who joins the military for economic reasons (i.e. a steady income). You see, the American military is a volunteer army; it is comprised mostly of "economic draftees" (aka "slum soldiers"), as a description of both where they were born and where they are sent, far away from home, to be killed. This is not an indictment of American soldiers, most of whom are brave and courageous. This is an indictment of the American "war machine" that sends soldiers to their deaths so that we can steal the resources of whatever country we decide to invade.

Pat Tillman didn't join the military for a "steady income." Tillman was loyal to the USA. Heck, he was even loyal to his NFL team, the Arizona Cardinals. Some might even say he was loyal to a fault. His 224 tackles in the 2000 NFL season were a team record, and because of team loyalty he rejected a five year, $9 million offer from the St. Louis Rams for a one-year, $512,000 contract to stay with Arizona the next year. To me, that's impressive, since not many professional athletes today are loyal. Most of them are greedy and self-aggrandizing. Tillman was the exception to the rule. That's why he joined the military. He didn't need the money. He didn't need the fame. He didn't need the glory. He just wanted to fight for the country that he loved. Pat Tillman was a true American hero.

The Assassination & Cover-Up

On April 22, 2004, Pat Tillman was killed in an ambush in Afghanistan by Al Qaeda and the Taliban. At least that's how the official story goes ...

A month or so after Tillman was killed, the official story began to "morph"; the head of the Special Operations Command called a news conference to disclose that Tillman "probably" died by friendly fire. He refused to answer questions. Then, a little while later, the story changed even further; on December 5th and 6th of 2004, the *Washington Post* published a two-part series on Tillman's death based on information obtained through interviews with many of his comrades and from the internal Army investigation. The *Post* told a tale of *"mistaken decisions"* and *"botched communications"* and a *"negligent shooting"* by *"pumped-up"* Army Rangers who *"failed to identify their targets as they blasted their way out of a frightening ambush."*

Did Tillman actually die from "friendly fire"? Friendly fire refers to the accidental killing of your own guys, which happens all the time, since weapons training regarding safety and fire control are virtually non-existent in the military. On the day he was killed, Pat Tillman's platoon was traveling through a canyon in Afghanistan when a Humvee broke down. Tillman and half the platoon were ordered to continue ahead while the remainder fixed the vehicle. Tillman's unit had exited the canyon when they heard firing and explosions coming from behind, at which time Sergeant Matthew Weeks ordered him and Bryan O'Neal and an Afghan (named Thani) to go back and see what was happening. When the Humvee came within about one hundred yards of the three men, the soldiers began shooting at them, immediately killing the Afghan and wounding Tillman. Tillman and O'Neal dove behind some rocks – one of Tillman's legs was severely wounded. He threw a purple smoke grenade to show they were Americans and kept yelling at the nearby Humvee shooters. Both Tillman and O'Neal waved their arms at the shooters in the Humvee, and they stopped shooting for a moment, at which time Tillman and O'Neal thought it was safe.

In true NFL fashion, Tillman identified himself loudly, saying "*Hold your fire! I'm Pat f*****g Tillman!*" The official story is that specialist Trevor Alders "accidentally" fired his .223 rifle and hit Pat Tillman from about 100 yards away, killing him, despite the fact that both Tillman and O'Neal were in the same uniforms as the other Army Rangers and wearing the unique Kevlar helmets. Here's where the official story gets outlandish. The autopsy photos show **three** .223 holes in Tillman's forehead, in a three inch group. Could these bullet holes actually have been made from a .223 rifle at 100 yards? Nope. It would have been impossible.

Here's why: Pat Tillman would have dropped after the first head shot, making it impossible for bullets #2 and #3 to enter the head anywhere near bullet #1. The only way you can get a three inch group of three .223 bullets from 100 yards is to kill the guy with the first shot, walk over to the body, and then shoot him two more times when he's lying on the ground. But three holes in a tight little group from 100 yards? No way. No how.

"Disappearing" Evidence and the Autopsy

After Tillman was killed, evidence began to quickly and mysteriously "disappear." Less than 24 hours after he was killed, someone burned his body armor. Then, the next day, someone burned his uniform. Nothing like "*scrubbing*" the evidence, right? At some point his journal, in which wrote religiously, went missing. With that journal disappeared Tillman's voice. I wonder what scathing indictments of the "US war machine" that journal might have contained.

Meanwhile, back home in the good ole' USA, the multitude of lying liars of the Bush administration began to manufacture one of their most monumental myths, explaining how the hero Tillman was killed by enemy fire. Bush himself chimed in to announce that Tillman was "*an inspiration on and off the football field, as with all who made the ultimate sacrifice in the war on terror.*" What a bunch of nauseating, repulsive hogwash, in light of the fact that it was spewed forth out of the mouth of a cowardly, combat-avoiding, AWOL drunk who rode on his daddy's coattails to become President!

It wasn't until investigators filed a FOIA (Freedom of Information Act) request that the following information became public on July 27, 2007 and was published by the AP: "*Army medical examiners were suspicious about the close proximity of the three bullet holes in Pat Tillman's forehead and tried without success to get authorities to investigate whether the former NFL player's death amounted to a crime.*" According to the doctor who examined Tillman's body, "*The medical evidence did not match up with the scenario as described.*" The doctors (whose names were blacked out) said that the bullet holes were so close together that it appeared that Tillman was cut down by an M-16 fired from a mere 10 yards or so away. Three bullet holes ... from an M-16 ... in the forehead ... from less than ten yards. Folks, that's not "friendly fire." That's **murder**.

Upon autopsy, the medical examiners knew that the official story reeked like a dead rat and wanted the Army to investigate the possibility (probability) of fratricide, which is the crime of intentionally murdering members of your own group. The request was **denied**.

Why? ... Illegal Wars ...

Why would the US Army arrange the murder and cover-up of one of its biggest "recruiting tools"? Why would the fratricide request be denied? What were they trying to hide? Why? That's the $64,000 question, isn't it? Why would they murder Pat Tillman?

The fact of the matter is that Pat Tillman was probably the greatest recruiting asset that Bush and his team of "neocon" warmongers had. He was the "poster boy of patriotism" and was used in a ruthless, relentless PR campaign by countless military recruiters. That is, until he and Kevin were transferred from Afghanistan to Iraq in 2003. While in Iraq, they began to realize that the invasion of Iraq was immoral and illegitimate. Pat made no secret of his opinion that war in Iraq was "illegal and unjust," and according to Kevin, he was prepared to tell his story publicly at the first opportunity. So, the brothers were shipped back to Afghanistan.

Tillman had naïvely made contact with one of his favorite authors and America's leading intellectual dissident, Noam Chomsky, to discuss his plans to reveal what he knew about the lies of Bush, Cheney and Rumsfeld in the phony "war on terror." He was apparently also angry about the US Army's support of the Afghan opium trade, started up by the army after the Taliban had completely eradicated it during their four-year reign. According to Fox News, shortly after we invaded Afghanistan, the US Army authorized the Northern Alliance to resume poppy production. Yes, we were indeed guarding the poppy fields. But this should be no surprise! I've already detailed how the CIA and other alphabet agencies were at the helm of the drug trade, importing drugs, supplying the cartels, all the while the banksters launder the money. Afghanistan was no different.

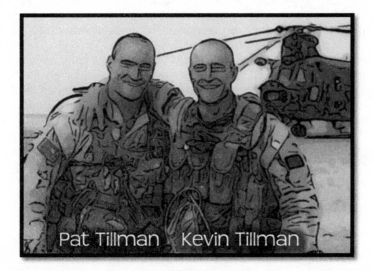

Pat Tillman   Kevin Tillman

According the *San Francisco Chronicle*, Tillman had set up a meeting with Chomsky to take place when he returned from Afghanistan. He never made it to the meeting. In the words of Michael Niman, *"This image of a Chomsky-loving, anti-Bush, anti-Iraq-war hero (at a time when most of the U.S. population supported the administration's foreign policy), flew in the face of the official Bush administration portrait of Tillman, painted by dutiful media whores like Ann Coulter ... As both wars droned on, Tillman, the picture perfect poster boy, evolved into something of a wild card. With a Chomsky meeting on the horizon there existed a very real possibility that Tillman, in the weeks leading up to the 2004 presidential election, might go public with his anti-war, anti-Bush views, dealing a critical blow to the very foundation of the Bush administ-ration's propaganda pyramid. That day never came, however."*

He continues, *"There was a lot more depth to Tillman, who was pursuing a master's degree in history, than one would normally expect of an NFL gladiator. Afghanistan had been an easier sell, but Tillman would never buy the official line on Iraq. At one point, according to a San Francisco Chronicle article published nearly a year and half after his death, he told fellow Rangers fighting in Iraq that the war was, 'so f*****g illegal.' A close friend told the paper, "That's who he was-he totally was against Bush.' ... Another friend, who served with him,* *recalled how Tillman admonished fellow Rangers to vote Bush out of office in the forthcoming presidential election."*

Pat Tillman transmuted from "neocon dream" to "neocon nightmare" and needed to be shut up before he could tell America about the lies of its leaders. America's hero was murdered, the official story was fabricated, and the facts were quickly buried. More importantly, what was buried was the complex story of Pat Tillman's opposition to the Iraq war and the Bush agenda.

Even though his intentions were courageous and admirable, the fact is, Tillman was duped (and murdered) by the Bush administration run by the "global elite" who want to establish a New World Order. Fabricated was a fairytale story of a heroic battle and tragic "mistake" which wouldn't thwart the Bush administration's global "war on terror." Tillman had waked up to the reality of the phony war, so the only option was to murder Tillman. It didn't have to happen that particular day. It just had to happen sometime when there were guns going off to make it a "mistake." It was as good a day as any to kill Pat Tillman, because he had to be killed.

There is no doubt that the Army Rangers shot Pat Tillman deliberately and with malice on April 22, 2004. They shot and wounded him first and then waited while he popped purple smoke to let them know he was "friendly." Then they started shooting again and didn't stop until he was dead. Pat Tillman was an idealist and a patriot. According to Henry Makow, Ph.D., he sacrificed his life for a country that has been subverted by an international financial cartel which holds trillions of its "debt" – a cartel intent on folding the US into a veiled world government tyranny to ensure that this "concocted" debt is paid. The cartel controls the media, politicians, professors, corporations, and generals. Wars are a profitable way of distracting the public from the real enemy within and increasing the debt to the bankster cartel.

The Tillman Family Speaks

Six weeks after Pat Tillman was assassinated, with the mythic version of his heroic death firmly embedded in the American conscious, and with the Tillman story safely buried in the ashbin of "old news," the Army finally told Tillman's family that the official cause of death was "fratricide." In other words, they admitted that the Rangers had murdered Tillman. Of course, the family already suspected this, due primarily to the enormous cover-up and incredible, inconsistent lies that they were told by the Army.

According to Jon Krakauer's book, <u>Where Men Win Glory: The Odyssey of Pat Tillman</u>, the extensive cover-up that followed Pat Tillman's death included the military ordering Tillman's comrades to lie to his family at the funeral. In June 2005, Tillman's father passionately condemned an army investigator, writing, "*I assume, therefore, that you are part of this shameless bullshit. I embarrassed myself by treating you with respect (on) March 31, 2005. I thought your rank deserved it and anticipated something different from the new and improved investigation. I won't act so hypocritically if we meet again.*" He later added, "*In sum: F**k you ... and yours.*"

Back in 2008, Mary Tillman, Pat's mother, wrote a book entitled <u>Boots on the Ground by Dusk</u> in which she suggested that her son was deliberately murdered by his fellow Rangers, reserving most of her anger for General Stanley McChrystal, who led the lying cover-up of the murder.

I want to end this chapter with a long quote by Kevin Tillman, which was part of an article he wrote on October 20, 2006, entitled "*After Pat's Birthday.*" I honestly don't know how this could be any more poignant.

"*Somehow we were sent to invade a nation because it was a direct threat to the American people, or to the world, or harbored terrorists, or was involved in the September 11 attacks, or received weapons-grade uranium from Niger, or had mobile weapons labs, or WMD, or had a need to be liberated, or we needed to establish a democracy, or stop an insurgency, or stop a civil war we created that can't be called a civil war even though it is. Something like that. Somehow our elected leaders were subverting international law and humanity by setting up secret prisons around the world, secretly kidnapping people, secretly holding them indefinitely, secretly not charging them with anything, secretly torturing them.*

Somehow that overt policy of torture became the fault of a few "bad apples" in the military. Somehow back at home, support for the soldiers meant having a five-year-old kindergartener scribble a picture with crayons and send it overseas, or slapping stickers on cars, or lobbying Congress for an extra pad in a helmet. It's interesting that a soldier on his third or fourth tour should care about a drawing from a five-year-old; or a faded sticker on a car as his friends die around him; or an extra pad in a helmet, as if it will protect him when an IED throws his vehicle 50 feet into the air as his body comes apart and his skin melts to the seat.

Somehow the more soldiers that die, the more legitimate the illegal invasion becomes.

Somehow American leadership, whose only credit is lying to its people and illegally invading a nation, has been allowed to steal the courage, virtue and honor of its soldiers on the ground.

Somehow those afraid to fight an illegal invasion decades ago are allowed to send soldiers to die for an illegal invasion they started.

Somehow faking character, virtue and strength is tolerated.

Somehow profiting from tragedy and horror is tolerated.

Somehow the death of tens, if not hundreds, of thousands of people is tolerated.

Somehow subversion of the Bill of Rights and The Constitution is tolerated.

Somehow suspension of Habeas Corpus is supposed to keep this country safe.

Somehow torture is tolerated.

Somehow lying is tolerated.

Somehow reason is being discarded for faith, dogma, and nonsense.

Somehow American leadership managed to create a more dangerous world.

Somehow a narrative is more important than reality.

Somehow America has become a country that projects everything that it is not and condemns everything that it is.

Somehow the most reasonable, trusted and respected country in the world has become one of the most irrational, belligerent, feared, and distrusted countries in the world.

Somehow being politically informed, diligent, and skeptical has been replaced by apathy through active ignorance.

Somehow the same incompetent, narcissistic, virtue less, vacuous, malicious criminals are still in charge of this country.

Somehow this is tolerated.

Somehow nobody is accountable for this.

In a democracy, the policy of the leaders is the policy of the people. So don't be shocked when our grandkids bury much of this generation as traitors to the nation, to the world and to humanity. Most likely, they will come to know that somehow was nurtured by fear, insecurity and indifference, leaving the country vulnerable to unchecked, unchallenged parasites.

Luckily this country is still a democracy. People still have a voice. People still can take action. It can start after Pat's birthday."

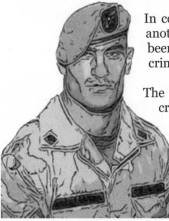

In conclusion, the sad saga of Pat Tillman is yet another instance where the American public has been fed a monumental myth to cover up a criminal act of the US government.

The lies and the propaganda are endemic, the crimes are never-ending, the bodies are countless, and the ruined lives are innumerable.

Pat Tillman was a true American hero.

May he rest in peace.

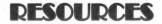

RESOURCES

Websites
http://www.thehumanist.org/humanist/articles/Niman.JanFeb06.html
http://theconspiracyzone.podcastpeople.com/posts/39815
http://www.truthdig.com/report/item/200601019_after_pats_birthday
http://henrymakow.com/pat_tillman_-_hero_or_dupe.html
http://www.veteranstoday.com/2011/12/18/the-assassination-of-cpl-pat-tillman-usa/

Movie
"A Pat Tillman Tribute – A Tale of Deceit, Lies, and Murder"
http://www.youtube.com/watch?v=p2TzA4zum-c

Books
Where Men Win Glory: The Odyssey of Pat Tillman (Jon Krakauer)
Boots on the Ground by Dusk (Mary Tillman)

Chapter 29

~ GARY WEBB ~

MONUMENTAL MYTH

In 1996, journalist Gary Webb wrote a series of articles, entitled *"Dark Alliance,"* that forced a long-overdue investigation of a very dark chapter of recent US foreign policy – the Reagan-Bush administration's protection of cocaine traffickers who operated under the cover of the Nicaraguan Contra war in the 1980s.

For his brave reporting at the *San Jose Mercury News,* Webb paid a high price. He was attacked by journalistic colleagues at the *New York Times,* the *Washington Post,* and the *Los Angeles Times,* amongst other well-known publications. Under this media pressure, Webb was demoted; he quit his job, got divorced, and was severely depressed.

On December 10, 2004, Webb committed suicide by shooting himself in the head ... **twice.**

CAN YOU HANDLE THE TRUTH?

Gary Webb was found with two bullet holes to the head. It was suicide ... *"an open and shut case..."* That's what the coroner said. You know what I want to know? I want to know who told the coroner to say it was "suicide." Obviously, somebody told him. And somebody told them. And so on. And so on. I want to follow the chain upwards until arriving at the group who ordered the hit. I'll betcha it's an "alphabet agency" with a three-letter acronym. There comes a time when you just have to stand back and take a look at the big picture. This is one of those times.

Two Bullets to the Head = Suicide?

The official story is that Webb shot himself in the head, realized that he was still alive, and then shot himself again? So, I guess the first shot (which entered his head just behind his right ear and blew out his lower left jaw and entire left side of his face) must have missed his brain? Webb then must have had the "presence of mind" – after half his face had been blown away – to shoot himself a second time through the brain, killing himself instantly. That's truly amazing! Webb certainly was determined wasn't he?

Michael Ruppert, former L.A. cop, thinks so. Quoted in the *Sacramento Bee* regarding the two bullets to the head, Ruppert said: *"In death Gary proved to be as determined and single-minded as he had been in life ... Here are the facts: Gary Webb fired two shots from a .38 caliber revolver into his own head. (A suicide) ... open and shut."* **Wow.** I guess that explains it. Webb was so tremendously "determined" and "single-minded" that he shot himself twice. Case closed. Don't question.

Forgive me if I don't buy it. It almost reminds me of the good ole' *"dog ate my homework"* line. It's total nonsense. Pure poppycock! Hey, how about a more logical conclusion: Somebody shot Gary Webb twice in the head. It was a "hit." How's that? Pretty simple, eh? That way you don't have to "make stuff up" to cover up what was obviously a **murder**.

Rewind to 1996 ...

Gary Webb was the quintessential investigative reporter – a persistent inquisitor with instinctively "crazy-good" skills. *"Dark Alliance"* – Gary Webb's 1996 series in the *San Jose Mercury News* – alleged that Nicaraguan drug traffickers had sold literally tons of crack cocaine in Los Angeles and funneled millions of dollars in profits to the CIA-supported Nicaraguan "Contras" during the 1980s.

Remember "Ollie" North? Well, he was one of the military leaders in the Reagan administration's "proxy war" in Nicaragua, better known as the Contra War, which culminated in humiliation for Reagan and the CIA when it was revealed they had been trading arms to Iran in exchange for the release of American hostages in Lebanon. The money Iran paid for American missiles was passed through covert back channels to the Nicaraguan Contras fighting against the socialist Sandinista government. Better known as the Iran-Contra scandal, all of this was, of course, against US policy.

The term "Contras" was a generic label given to the various rebel groups opposing Nicaragua's Sandinista government. It was short for *"la contrarrevolución,"* or in English, *"the counter-revolution."*

Iran-Contra wasn't the first big scandal, however, involving the CIA-sponsored war in the shadowy jungles of Central America. A year before news of Iran-Contra made headlines, two AP reporters (Robert Parry and

Brian Barger) broke a story saying the Nicaraguan Contras were exporting drugs to the USA to help pay for the war effort. Of course, the mainstream media virtually ignored the story. Then along came Gary Webb ... who wanted to break this story wide open. And he did. Some might say he broke it "way too wide open" for his own good.

Here is a quote from Webb's original *"Dark Alliance"* article: *"For the better part of a decade, a San Francisco Bay Area drug ring sold tons of cocaine to the Crips and Bloods street gangs of Los Angeles and funneled millions in drug profits to a Latin American guerrilla army run by the US Central Intelligence Agency ... This drug network opened the first pipeline between Colombia's cocaine cartels and the black neighbor-hoods of Los Angeles, a city now known as the crack capital of the world."*

Does that sound like an accusation that would enrage the CIA? Especially if it were true? Now you're starting to get the picture aren't you?

Rewind to 1995 ...

According to Susan Paterno, in her article entitled *"The Sad Saga of Gary Webb,"* published in the *American Journalism Review* in June/July 2005, in 1995, *"Gary Webb received a call from Coral Baca, a twenty-something woman he once described as all 'cleavage and jewelry.' Baca, a strange, shadowy character in the novel of Webb's life with alleged ties to a Colombian drug cartel, wanted Webb to investigate how 'a guy who used to work with the CIA selling drugs' had framed her drug-dealing boyfriend. Webb was uninterested in the boyfriend but intrigued by the CIA. He used Baca as a tour guide through the world of West Coast drug trafficking, racking his brain to remember the details of what had happened in Nicaragua a decade earlier while he was covering state government in Ohio. He called his editor at the Mercury News, Dawn Garcia, and read her the grand jury testimony of Oscar Danilo Blandón, a Contra supporter somehow connected to cocaine dealing in South Central Los Angeles. Garcia told him to find out more. Webb did what he did best: He dug and dug and dug, scribbling notes from indictments, detention-hearing transcripts, docket sheets, US Attorney motions."*

She continues, *"He returned to Sacramento and spent a week sitting in the California State Library in front of a microfiche copier, a roll of dimes on the table next to him, 'growing more astounded each day,' he said, sifting through Congressional records, US Customs and FBI reports, internal Justice Department memos, many showing 'direct links between the drug dealers and the Contras ... It almost knocked me off my chair.' Back in his office, Webb called Jack Blum. 'Why can I*

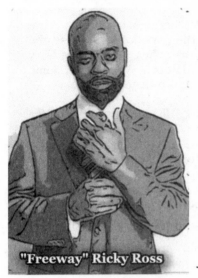

"Freeway" Ricky Ross

barely remember this? I read the papers every day,' Webb asked. 'It wasn't in the papers, for the most part,' Blum said. 'The big papers stayed as far away from this as they could ... It was like they didn't want to know.' Intrigued, Webb kept digging. Pretty soon he connected Nicaraguan cocaine supplier Blandón to a Los Angeles drug dealer named Ricky Donnell Ross, aka 'Freeway' Ricky Ross. From there, he quickly found a Los Angeles Times article about Ross, written by Jesse Katz, with the headline: 'Deposed King of Crack.' The Times called Ross a 'master marketer,' the 'key to the drug's spread in L.A ... the outlaw capitalist most responsible for flooding Los Angeles streets with mass-marketed cocaine.' Ka-ching. Pay dirt."

Webb quickly put the pieces of the puzzle together, connected the dots, and drafted a memo to his superiors in which he stated, *"While there has long been solid – if largely ignored – evidence of a CIA-Contra-cocaine connection, no one has ever asked the question: Where did the cocaine go once it got here? Now we know."*

He anxiously swallowed the red pill and officially entered the matrix. He traveled to Nicaragua and into the shadowy underworld of the Contra rebels and the CIA, chasing Blandón from California to Florida and back, following the cocaine supply route through the filthy streets of South Central Los Angeles, all the way to "Freeway" Ricky Ross.

Eventually, Webb sent a four-part series to his editors, which they loved. The series of articles is what ultimately became "Dark Alliance" in which Webb revealed the shocking results of his year-long investigation into the roots of the crack cocaine epidemic in America, specifically in Los Angeles, proving that for the better part of a decade, a Bay Area drug ring sold tons of cocaine to Los Angeles street gangs and funneled millions in drug profits to the CIA-backed Nicaraguan Contras.

Gary Webb officially took his readers down the rabbit hole as far as humanly possible, and not surprisingly, the response was intense. Quickly, Webb became a celebrity, entertaining six-figure book and movie deals and going on radio and TV shows while the mainstream media agonized.

Another Pulitzer for Webb?

In the wake of Webb's "Dark Alliance" series, which ignited a firestorm of controversy, there were protests at the CIA headquarters, and the NAACP and Congressional Black Caucus demanded an explanation. Of course, as we've seen throughout history, no good deed goes unpunished, and Gary Webb was certainly no exception. So, what was his "reward" for this amazing journalistic accomplishment? Did he win another Pulitzer Prize?

He should have, no doubt. But when black leaders began demanding a full investigation of Webb's allegations, the mainstream media obeyed their "masters," began to circle the wagons, and formulated their counterattack against Webb's indictments. They interviewed former CIA agents to refute the drug charges, calling Webb a "nut job" and a "liar." Yes, taking cues from their controllers, the mainstream media attacked Webb and accused him of falsifying his research and misleading his readers. Of course, these were false accusations, but since when does the truth matter to the liars in charge?

Webb became the target of outright media ridicule and mockery, which had a predictable effect on the executives of the *San Jose Mercury News*: they retreated. Webb was left twisting in the wind. On May 11, 1997, the executive editor (Jerry Ceppos) published a front-page column saying the series *"fell short of my standards."* He criticized the stories because they *"strongly implied CIA knowledge"* of Contra connections to US drug dealers who were manufacturing crack-cocaine. *"We did not have proof that top CIA officials knew of the relationship."* No doubt Ceppos was carrying out orders, directly or indirectly, issued by sinister figures higher up the food chain.

The final insult: Gary Webb was eventually reassigned to a small office in Cupertino, far from his family, where he was relegated to the "dust bin," writing about obituaries and weddings. He eventually resigned in disgrace, watched his career collapse, and got divorced. However, in true Webb fashion, within a year of resigning from the *San Jose Mercury News*, Webb transformed his "Dark Alliance" series into a book: Dark Alliance: The CIA, The Contras, and the Crack Cocaine Explosion.

Internal Investigations & Hitz

But the story of the CIA-funded Contras trafficking cocaine wasn't new. Despite his personal hardships, Gary Webb had set in motion internal government investigations by the CIA and the Department of Justice, probes that confirmed that scores of Contra units and Contra-connected individuals, including high-level CIA agents, were implicated in the drug trade.

The CIA's defensive line against Webb's allegations began to break when they published "Volume One" of Inspector General Frederick P. Hitz's findings on January 29, 1998. Despite a largely exculpatory press release and conveniently eclipsed by the Monica Lewinski scandal, Hitz's findings admitted that not only were many of Webb's allegations true but that he actually **understated** the seriousness of the drug crimes and the CIA's knowledge and involvement in importing drugs to the gangs of Los Angeles.

In his research, Hitz found CIA files evidence that proved the spy agency knew from the first days of the Contra war that its new clients were involved in the cocaine trade. Hitz concluded that there had indeed been a clandestine agreement between the CIA and the Department of Justice from 1982 to 1995 that authorized both agencies to ignore, with impunity, drug trafficking by CIA "*agents, assets and non-staff employees.*"

"*A murmur coursed through the room as Hitz's admission sunk in,*" wrote Gary Webb. "*No wonder the US government could blithely insist there was 'no evidence' of Contra/CIA drug trafficking. For thirteen years – from the time Blandón ... began selling cocaine in L.A. for the Contras – the CIA and Justice Depatment had a gentleman's agreement to look the other way.*"

Back to the Literal "Smoking Gun"

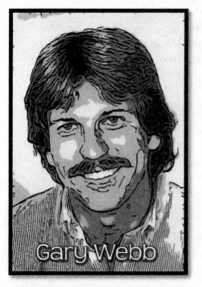

Gary Webb

If Gary Webb committed suicide with **two** shots to the head via a .38 caliber pistol, then I've got a bridge I'd like to sell you in the desert of New Mexico. Seriously, that's the official story ... the monumental myth. Webb was so depressed that he ended it all. And he was "*persistent in death*" just like he was "*persistent in life.*" That's right. He shot himself behind his right ear and blew out his lower left jaw and entire left side of his face. But that wasn't a "fatal" shot, so he gathered his nerves for a second time, then pulled the trigger again! Luckily, the second time was a success.

Are we seriously supposed to believe this bunch of hot air? Hey, maybe Webb hired

"Lucky the Rabbit" to kill him. Yeah, that's the ticket!

Speaking of hares, that's not the only "rabbit tale" we're supposed to believe. I haven't even mentioned the "note" for the movers. You see, Gary Webb was in the process of moving when he was "suicided." Yeah, he picked an odd time to commit suicide – right in the middle of a big move. And we're told that he was so concerned about the movers (who would inevitably find his bloody corpse) that he sympathetically left them a note on the outside door warning them not to enter. The note said: "*Please do not enter ... call 911 and ask for an ambulance.*" How kind of Gary to be so concerned with the movers' potential post-traumatic stress!

Question: Why "*ask for an ambulance*" if he planned to kill himself? And while we're on the topic, how strange it is that he didn't call the movers to cancel the move? I mean, why the dramatic note? Let me think. Hey, maybe the moving company actually sent someone that was involved with the "suicide"? Like an alphabet agency agent? That would be a great way for the moving company to avoid investigation, wouldn't it? Rather than finding a bloody body, which would certainly give rise to questioning and scrutiny, they found a "note" and called someone else to find Webb's body. No questions asked. The perfect crime. Think about it.

This reminds me of the 1970s television show "Welcome Back Kotter." Remember when Epstein would want to get out of school? He would bring a (forged) note to school and it would always be signed "*Epstein's mother*" (rather than her actual name). **Of course**, Epstein wrote the note. And, of course, somebody else wrote the "warning" note to the movers. Definitely not Gary Webb, that's for sure. I mean, c'mon, he's about to commit suicide and he still has the presence of mind to warn the movers and make sure they "*do not enter*" and "*ask for an ambulance*" so they don't have any PTSD from viewing his gory corpse? Huh?

Did someone else write the note? I think you know the answer ... Gary Webb's alleged "suicide" by two shots to the head is similar to Karen Silkwood's car "accident" which resulted in her death. It's about as believable as Vince Foster's "suicide" – we'll talk about Vince in the next chapter.

The "Chilling Effect"

Why did they murder Gary Webb? **Easy answer**: To put a chill in the spines of those who might want to "dissent" from the party line and expose the corruption that is so rampant in the US government. To say, "*...look, we can do what we want, when we want, wherever we want, with whomever we want, and there is nothing anyone can do about it. If you don't believe us, then just take a look at poor 'wacko' Gary Webb* *who dared to challenge us. Imagine what he must have gone through to fire that second shot into his own face ... (sardonic laughter) ..."*

The CIA has forever been involved in the drug trade. That's no secret. Just search for Operations Pegasus, Amadeus, and Watchtower; they speak volumes about the illicit nature of the CIA's covert operations in South and Central America. We don't know all the "who's" and the "why's," but the incontrovertible truth is that the CIA commits murder. They perform assassinations. These are known facts. No doubt some of those murders and assassinations have been covered up as "suicides." Like Gary Webb.

Is there any doubt that Gary Webb was one of those unfortunate folks who have been "suicided" by the government? You see, Gary Webb was right. The CIA **is** a criminal organization tied to assassinations, drug trafficking, money laundering, investment fraud, and other illegal machinations. You've heard the old saying, *"You can't fix a problem until you admit that there **is** one."* How true. Regarding the CIA's unlawful activities, we will never solve the "CIA problem" until we first admit that it exists.

> *RIP, Gary Webb. What you did was courageous, brave, honest, and true. You "blew the whistle" on the nefarious activities of the CIA. But the "system" doesn't like whistleblowers.*

Want proof? Oliver North (a traitor) is considered a "true American patriot" and was "rewarded" with his own spot on Fox News.

Gary Webb is dead. Go figure.

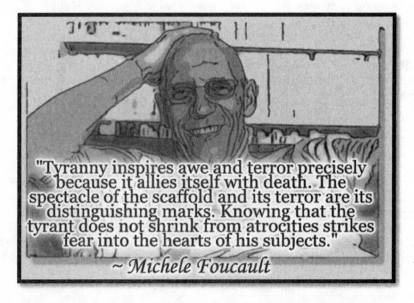

"Tyranny inspires awe and terror precisely because it allies itself with death. The spectacle of the scaffold and its terror are its distinguishing marks. Knowing that the tyrant does not shrink from atrocities strikes fear into the hearts of his subjects."

~ *Michele Foucault*

RESOURCES

Websites
http://www.narconews.com/darkalliance/
http://www.ajr.org/article.asp?id=3874
http://www.consortiumnews.com/2004/121304.html

Movie
"Dark Alliance: The CIA, the Contras, and the Crack Cocaine Explosion"
– Gary Webb interview
http://www.youtube.com/watch?v=JKE2XL24FG4

Book
Dark Alliance: The CIA, The Contras, and the Crack Cocaine Explosion
(Gary Webb)

"Bad men need nothing more to compass their ends than that good men should look on and do nothing."

John Stuart Mill

Chapter 30

~ VINCE FOSTER ~

MONUMENTAL MYTH

On a muggy night in July 1993, Vince Foster was found dead in a park near Washington DC from an apparent gunshot wound to the mouth. His father's .38 caliber revolver was at his side. It was the same method of suicide used by a Marine officer in the film "A Few Good Men" which Foster was known recently to have watched. In the movie, the officer had killed himself because he was distraught about testifying against his commanding officer. In real life, Vince Foster was distraught at the prospect of being grilled about the shady affairs of Hillary Clinton. It was a clear case of suicide.

CAN YOU HANDLE THE TRUTH?

Before we get started dissecting the "monumental myth" regarding Vince Foster's death, I want to give credit where credit is due. Pat Shannan wrote a brilliant article entitled *"Vince Foster Was Murdered – 'Suicide' Was Fixed,"* from which I greatly benefited, and I'll be quoting from it throughout. Richard L. Franklin also wrote a meticulous article entitled *"101 Peculiarities Surrounding the Death of Vince Foster,"* and I will also be quoting from it. Both articles are referenced at the end of the chapter.

Vince Foster was a Deputy White House Counsel during the first few months of President Bill Clinton's administration and also a law partner and friend of Hillary Rodham Clinton. Before the Clintons moved to Washington DC, while in Little Rock, Vince and Hillary were partners in the Rose Law Firm while Bill was governor of Arkansas. Naturally, when the Clintons moved to the White House, Vince Foster came, too. But Foster's position at the White House did not sit well with him. Just days before his death, following a public speech stressing the value of personal integrity, he had confided in friends and family that he was thinking of resigning his position; he had even written an outline for his letter of resignation. Foster had scheduled a private meeting with Bill Clinton for the very next day after his death (July 21, 1993) at which it appeared Foster intended to resign.

According to Foster's secretary, approximately six hours before his death, Foster mailed a letter to his mother. Foster was a "southern gentleman" and was extremely well-mannered. And he loved his mother. Despite this, his letter to his mother, sent only hours before he allegedly killed himself, does not contain a single hint whatsoever that this would be his last communication with his mother. The fact is that Foster's behavior during the last days preceding his death indicates he had no intention of killing himself. He had made plans with his good friend, James Lyons, to get together in Washington DC on July 21st, which was the day after he died. Foster called Lyons two days before his death to confirm their Wednesday appointment. Not exactly the behavior you would expect from a man about to kill himself, is it?

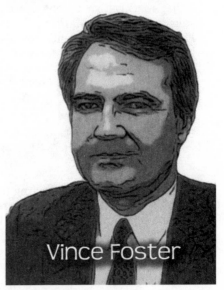

Vince Foster

And then there was Sharon Bowman, Foster's sister, who traveled 1,000 miles to Washington DC to visit her brother, only to arrive the day of his death. Vince had talked to Sharon and promised her an exciting personal tour of and lunch at the White House. It seems apparent he was really looking forward to seeing his sister. Yet he supposedly killed himself on the day of her arrival? **Seriously**? What an unbelievably cruel "joke" to play on your sister!

Did I mention that Vince Foster was the attorney that represented the Clintons in the buyout of their Whitewater shares. And that was where this whole mess started ... with Whitewater. Remember Whitewater?

What Was Whitewater?

"Whitewater" is the popular name for a failed 1970s Arkansas real estate venture by the Whitewater Development Corporation, in which Governor (later President) Bill Clinton and his wife, Hillary, were partners. Whitewater was backed by the Madison Guaranty Savings and Loan, which went bankrupt in 1989. The controlling partners in both the land deal **and** the bank were friends of the Clintons, James and Susan McDougal.

Vincent Foster represented the Clintons in the buyout of their Whitewater shares. Foster was also the keeper of the files of the Clinton's

Arkansas dealings, including Whitewater, and had indicated in a written memo that *"Whitewater is a can of worms that you should NOT open!"*

Not surprisingly, accusations of impropriety against the Clintons and others soon surfaced, regarding improper campaign contributions, political and financial favors, and tax benefits. Claiming that relevant files had "disappeared" (they were "miraculously" found at the White House in 1996), the Clintons denied any wrongdoing.

In 1996, the McDougals and Jim Guy Tucker (Bill's successor as governor of Arkansas) were found guilty of fraud in the Whitewater case. The Monica *"I didn't have sex with that woman"* Lewinsky scandal soon followed, and queries about the Clinton's alleged unlawful activity with Whitewater soon vanished.

Oh yes, Susan McDougal was pardoned by President Clinton in January of 2001, just a few days before he left office. In other words: *"You took the fall and didn't implicate me or Hillary in Whitewater – now I'm going to pardon you even though we're all guilty and everybody knows we're guilty. Thanks."*

Back to the "Official Story"

On July 20, 1993, at approximately 1 PM, Deputy White House Counsel, Vince Foster, left his office for the last time. Reminiscent of Arnold Schwarzenegger's cyborg character in "The Terminator," his last words to his secretary, Deborah Gorham, were *"I'll be right back."* Unlike the cyborg, Foster never returned. That was the last time he was seen alive.

According to the official narrative, Foster took his White House pager and left for lunch. After giving a Secret Service agent a welcoming smile and a friendly "hello," he drove his car out of the White House parking lot for the last time. Perhaps Foster was carrying the revolver (that would figure so prominently in his immediate future) and he merely had to smuggle it into the White House past several metal detectors and Secret Service agents. Or perhaps he left it in the car and it only had to survive the "once-over" by an ammunition sniffing dog.

Did I mention that the new FBI director, Louis Freeh, was being sworn in that day?

Yep, all the cars in the parking lot were checked multiple times by the team of dogs. Or perhaps he just drove home to get the revolver. Then, Foster drove to some unidentified location and rolled around on a carpet for a while. Why do I say this? Well, carpet fibers were later found all over his clothing, so he must have had a fetish for rolling around on carpets. Yeah, that's the ticket. It certainly couldn't be due to the fact that Foster was killed and then stuffed into the carpeted trunk of his own car. More on that in a moment. Anyway, after the carpet adventure, Foster was overcome with the desire to visit Fort Marcy Park, an obscure park on the other side of town, to end his life. According to his family, he had never visited the park before.

We're told that Foster arrived at the park, surveyed the scene, and then either sprouted wings and flew to the intended location of his demise, or maybe he merely levitated, or perhaps he "tip toed" like a ballet dancer. Whatever he did, and however he did it, Foster magically managed to walk 700 feet across grass and dirt without getting any dirt or grass on his shoes. Navigating the never-before-visited Fort Marcy Park grounds like a seasoned professional, he arrives at the perfect location to end his life: the edge of a hill with weeds up to his face.

In his remarkable article, *"Vince Foster: The Case for Suicide,"* Zach Nguyen dissects the absurdity of the "official story" in evocative, sardonic, and satirical details: *"... ignoring the mosquitos that were out in full force on the hot July day, (Foster) attempts to shoot himself in the side of the neck. Finding that this does not seem to do the trick, he jams his thumb into the trigger guard, wraps his fingers around the barrel, stuffs it so far down his throat that he very nearly swallows the gun, and somehow manages to pull the trigger. The sharp (bang) of the .38 caliber revolver fell on deaf ears – no one in the surrounding area heard anything. Foster's teeth and mouth remained miraculously undamaged, while an astoundingly small amount of gunpowder residue was found in his mouth. The bullet disappeared. Foster's heart stopped instantly – almost no blood was found on the ground or on his body."*

Nguyen continues, *"... at this point, Vince Foster comes back to life, remembering that he has forgotten his car. He walks to wherever he parked it, but is forced to hotwire it, because his car keys have mysteriously disappeared (they were not found until Foster's body was safely in the morgue). He then drives back to Ft. Marcy, parks his car, and resumes his position on the grassy slope, being careful to lay his body out perfectly straight and flat. He then throws the gun away. Confidential Witness 1 discovers the body, notes the lack of a gun, and leaves to phone the authorities. Foster gets up, retrieves the gun, and resumes his position. The authorities arrive, taking pictures of the body that are all immediately lost or 'over-exposed' in the FBI labs."*

You know, .38 caliber revolvers certainly are popular. Gary Webb and Vince Foster both used a .38 revolver to commit "suicide." Wow! What a coincidence! That about covers it. The "official story" ... the "monumental myth" ... "the fabricated fable from the lying liars in charge." Of course Vince Foster was murdered. Or, as I've previously called it, "suicided."

The Autopsy – "Suicide"?

Yes, the death was ruled a suicide. Don't ask questions. Why? Because we say so! Virtually the entire case for supposed suicide rests firmly on the autopsy done by Dr. James C. Beyer, a pathologist for Fairfax County, Virginia. At first glance, the autopsy report seems typical. The conclusion is that Vincent Foster died of a *"single gunshot wound entering the roof of the mouth and exiting the back of the skull."* Case closed. However, upon closer inspection, several small "problems" become apparent.

First of all, Dr. Beyer didn't actually examine the body at Fort Mercy Park. His co-worker, Dr. Donald Haut, was the one who truly examined Foster's body at the park, assisted by John Rolla. On page two of Dr. Haut's signed report, the wound track is described as a *"gunshot wound mouth to neck."* This corroborates the eyewitness testimony of EMS Technician Richard Arthur, who described the gunshot wound in some detail, placing it under the right ear. This is also consistent with the report of Ambrose Evens-Pritchard, who described a photograph of that wound.

This begs the question: Was there **really** an exit wound out the back of Foster's head? Nobody who saw the body (prior to Beyer) reported a gunshot wound out the back of the head. Nobody. As a matter of fact, EMS Sergeant Gonzales stated he did **not** see a gunshot wound out the back of the head. John Rolla did not report a gunshot wound out the back of the head. Another EMS Technician, Cory Ashford, testified that he was certain there was **not** an exit wound at the back of the head while Vince Foster was at Fort Marcy Park! You see, Ashford helped lift Foster's body into a body bag. While doing so, he cradled Foster's head against his stomach. Ashford's white shirt remained immaculate following this contact. And he didn't have to wash his hands.

There was no exit wound ... at least not until Foster's body arrived at Dr. Beyer's morgue. Then, the neck wound that was seen by Haut and Arthur "magically" vanishes and the wound out of the back of the head "magically" appears. Do you get it? That means that the autopsy conclusion was false. Thus Dr. Beyer was lying. Thus nothing he says can be trusted.

Of course, Beyer's history wasn't the most reassuring; he was the Virginia version of the infamous Dr. Fahmy Malek, whom I talked about briefly in the "War on Drugs" chapter. Remember Malek? He was the Arkansas medical examiner who ignored clear evidence of homicide in the deaths of Don Henry and Kevin Ives and in one case ruled that a man who had been beheaded was dead of natural causes and man that shot himself five times committed suicide. Basically, Dr. Beyer's "modus operandi" was to assist in covering up murders by ruling them to be "suicide." Malek and Beyer were both a "piece of work," as my Dad used to day.

Hillary Clinton says she had no idea Vincent Foster, whom she describes as her "best friend," was seriously depressed before he was found dead of a gunshot wound in Fort Marcy Park. *"I will go to my grave wishing I had spent more time with him and had somehow seen the signs of his despair,"* she writes. *"But he was a very private person, and nobody – not his wife, Lisa, or his closest colleagues, or his sister Sheila, with whom he had always been close – had any idea of the depth of his depression."*

Hey Hillary! Maybe that's because he was **not** depressed.

Maybe that's because he did **not** commit suicide.

The Enigmatic Stranger Who Stumbled On the Crime Scene

In an April 30, 2008 article entitled *"Vince Foster Was Murdered – 'Suicide' Was Fixed,"* Pat Shannon did a tremendous job of "connecting the dots" regarding what really happened that afternoon, specifically regarding what Patrick Knowlton saw, so I'll be paraphrasing quite a bit in this section.

Vince Foster left his White House office saying, *"I'll be back"* ... but he never returned. A few hours later, Patrick Knowlton, a building contractor having completed a hot day's work, finished a cold beer with friends and headed home. Little did Patrick Knowlton know that he would stumble into history that day, when at 4:30 PM, he wheeled his car into the parking area of Fort Marcy Park.

As he pulled into the park, his car was parked between a late model blue-grey sedan (which was occupied by an "eerie" man who was closely watching the front entrance) and an unoccupied mid-1980s brown Honda sedan with Arkansas license plates. As Knowlton emerged from his car, the strange man in the blue-grey sedan, who *"looked like he was out of a James Bond movie,"* gave him a menacing look, which unnerved him.

"Why did Knowlton get out of the car?" Good question.

He had to pee. So, he headed into the woods. The strange man watched him intently as he walked about 75 feet down the footpath's left fork to the first large tree. This was in the opposite direction from where Foster's body would soon be recovered. While *"relieving himself,"* Knowlton heard the man close his car door, but he couldn't see the parking lot and hoped the man was not pursuing him.

According to Pat Shannon, *"As he walked back to the parking lot, he scanned the area with a new sense of awareness, but did not see the man. He purposefully in order to maintain space until he learned the man's whereabouts walked directly to the driver's side of the Honda and then around the back of it, observing and remembering several items in the back seat. He then was comforted to see that the stranger was back behind the wheel of his own car but still staring fixedly at him.*

Shannon continues, *"Of the five things Patrick witnessed at the park and in the car, the 'rust-brown' Honda itself is the most relevant and became the root of Knowlton's future troubles. It was not Vince Foster's car! When Foster's body was discovered approximately 70 minutes after Patrick left the park, the autopsy and other forensic evidence showed Foster had been dead for much longer than that."*

When he heard later about the death of Vince Foster, Knowlton called the FBI to offer his testimony. However, Knowlton claims that the FBI, specifically Special Agent Lawrence Monroe, fraudulently altered his statements to indicate that he saw Foster's car (a late model silver Honda) in the parking lot.

You see, according to the official story, Foster had already driven to Fort Marcy Park to kill himself, so his silver Honda should have been in the parking lot at that time. Knowlton and his attorney, John Clarke, found testimony from two additional witnesses corroborating that the Honda in the parking lot was an old brown Honda, not a late model silver Honda. One thing was for sure – Knowlton was not going to be coerced into lying by the FBI.

So, since he wouldn't lie, the FBI launched a campaign to harass and intimidate Knowlton. Teams of agents harassed him 24 hours a day and threatened him. He was followed constantly. His phone rang in the middle of the night, and agents knocked on his door at 4 AM. Eventually, he filed a civil suit. The Knowlton civil suit is very important. The facts of harassment are telling.

Why did several unknown persons commit multiple crimes in order to hinder the investigation into the death of Vince Foster? And why are these people allowed to remain "unknown"? It kind of shoots holes in the official story, doesn't it? As I've said before, if you have nothing to hide, then why are you hiding something?

"Eighty times the Office of Independent Counsel made specific points and eighty times they lied."

~ *John Clarke — attorney for Patrick Knowlton*

The Looting of Foster's Office

While the US Park Police (a unit not equipped for a proper homicide investigation) studied the body, Foster's office was looted. White House aides freely went in and out, ransacking and removing potentially key evidence. Wasn't his office technically part of a crime scene? Wasn't this a gross violation of police procedures? Why was this criminal interference with a police investigation tolerated?

According to Sr. Robert Gates, in his book, The Conspiracy That Will Not Die, *"Secret Service agent Henry O'Neill watched as Hillary Clinton's chief of staff, Margaret Williams, carried boxes of papers out of Foster's office before the Park Police showed up to seal it. Amazing when you consider that the official identification of Vincent Foster's body by Craig Livingstone did not take place until 10PM! Speaking of Craig Livingstone, another Secret Serviceman saw him remove items from Vincent Foster's office in violation of the official seal. Witnesses also saw Bernard Nussbaum in Foster's office as well. Three witnesses noted that Patsy Thomason, director of the White House's Office of Administration, was desperate to find the combination to Vincent Foster's safe. Ms. Thomason finally opened the safe, apparently with the help of a special 'MIG' technical team signed into the White House in the late hours. Two envelopes reported to be in the safe by Foster's secretary Deborah Gorham, addressed to Janet Reno and to William Kennedy III, were never seen again. When asked the next day regarding rumors of the safe opening, Mack McLarty told reporters Foster's office did not even have a safe, a claim immediately shot down by former occupants of that office."*

He continues, *"The next day, when the Park Police arrived for the official search of Vincent Foster's office, they were shocked to learn that Nussbaum, Thomason and Williams had entered the office. Conflicts channeled through Janet Reno's Department of Justice resulted in the Park Police merely sitting outside Foster's office while Bernard Nussbaum continued his own search of Foster's office. During this search, he opened and upended Vincent Foster's briefcase, showing it to be empty. Three days later, it would be claimed that this same briefcase was where the torn up suicide note was discovered. The boxes of documents removed from Foster's office by Hillary Clinton's chief of staff, Margaret Williams, were taken to the private residence area of the White House! Eventually, only 54 pages emerged. One set of billing records, under subpoena for two years, and thought to have originated in Foster's office, turned up unexpectedly in the private quarters of the White House, with Hillary's fingerprints on them!"*

So, who ordered the office looting?

The "Investigation"

Remember Kenneth Starr?

He worked for the Office of Independent Counsel (OIC) and spearheaded the make-believe charade (err ... umm ... I mean "investigation") that followed. Well, in October 1994, Starr appointed assistant US attorney, Miquel Rodriguez, to take charge of the grand jury investigation into Foster's death. But Rodriguez was not a "yes man." He actually investigated the incident. And he determined that the official story was nothing but a fairytale, a fable, a monumental myth. In his own words, *"I was told what the result was going to be from the get-go,"* Rodriguez said. *"This is all so much nonsense; I knew the result before the investigation began, that's why I left. I don't do investigations to justify a result."*

He continued, *"Everyone makes a very big mistake when they believe a lot of people are necessary to orchestrate some results,"* he said. *"All people need to know is what their job is, not why – be a good soldier, carry out the orders. There are a lot of people, starting at the very night the body was investigated, all the way down the line ... told to do certain things"* who *"don't necessarily know the big picture."*

The official story is that there were multiple investigations. But Rodriguez said this is very misleading. *"In fact, all of the investigations were done by the same people, the FBI."* Rodriguez told Starr he wanted to summon FBI agents before the grand jury to compel sworn testimony concerning their handling of evidence. He also wanted to bring in private experts to evaluate the evidence. Since he wanted to get to the truth, Starr agreed.

Err ... ummm ... wait. **Rewind!** I stand corrected.

What really happened was that Starr refused both requests and told him to wrap up the investigation as quickly as possible. When Rodriguez snubbed this request and continued searching for the truth, Starr forced him to hand in his resignation. That's right. Less than six months after Rodriguez was hired by Starr to lead the investigation, he was forced to resign.

Then there was the issue of Starr's Honda sedan – you know ... the silver sedan that was **not** seen at the park by eyewitnesses. Well, that's not all that is odd about the car. The driver's seat was pushed forward to a position appropriate for a person about 5' 8" tall. Did I mention that Foster was nearly 6' 5" tall? It would have been extraordinarily difficult for Foster to have driven his car with the seat in this position. Despite this, and despite the fact that nobody ever saw the Honda at the park, the official story is that Foster drove his car to Fort Marcy Park. The possibility that somebody else drove Foster's car has been steadfastly rejected.

At least four witnesses saw a briefcase lying on the front seat of the car after the police had arrived. George Gonzalez, a medical technician, described it as *"a black briefcase-attaché case."* Mysteriously, the briefcase vanished and was never seen again. But don't be concerned about that, because evidence regularly disappears from crime scenes and we shouldn't be alarmed. Plus, it probably wasn't important anyway.

Family, Friends, & Experts Don't Buy the Myth

Back in Little Rock, Foster's friends weren't buying it. Doug Buford, friend and attorney, stated, *"... something was badly askew."* Foster's brother-in-law, a former congressman, also did not accept that depression was what had been behind the "suicide," stating *"That's a bunch of crap."* And Webster Hubbell, former Clinton deputy attorney general, phoned a mutual friend to say, *"Don't believe a word you hear. It was not suicide. It couldn't have been."*

Outside experts who were not connected to the official investigation also had their doubts. Vincent J. Scalise (former NYC detective), Fred Santucci (former forensic photographer for NYC), and Richard Saferstein (former head of the New Jersey State Crime Lab) investigated the "suicide" of Vince Foster and arrived at several conclusions:

- The position of Foster's arms and legs were radically inconsistent with suicide.
- Neither of Foster's hands was on the handgrip when it was fired. This is also inconsistent with suicide.
- The investigators noted that in their 50 years of combined experience they had *"never seen a weapon or gun positioned in a suicide's hand in such an orderly fashion."*
- Foster's body was in contact with one or more carpets prior to his death. The team was amazed that the carpet in the trunk of Foster's car had not been studied to see whether he had been carried to the park in the trunk of his own car.
- The lack of blood and brain tissue at the site suggests Foster was carried to the scene.

Honestly, the lack of blood is the single, strongest evidence that Vince Foster did not put the .38 caliber revolver into his own mouth and pull the trigger. If he had actually shot himself, the blowback from the gunshot would have coated the gun, hand, and white sleeve of Foster's shirt with a spray of blood and organic matter. But the (few) photos show **no** blood ... anywhere. That's right. The FBI lab report reveals that even with the most sensitive chemical test available, **no** blood was found on the gun that Foster allegedly inserted into his mouth and fired. Not a single drop!

For those of you who are unfamiliar with handguns, a .38 caliber weapon firing a high-velocity slug normally makes a large exit hole and produces a huge pool of blood. And following a fatal shot to the brain, the heart keeps pumping until it runs out of blood, possibly lasting up to two minutes, thusly expelling a massive quantity of blood. It appears that the US government wants us to believe that the laws of physics were "suspended" at the Vince Foster "suicide" scene, resulting in no blood and no organic matter. I don't buy it, and neither should you. The lack of blood raises two questions: (1) Did Foster die somewhere else? (2) Was he shot in the head after he was already dead? Just questions, that's all. Think about 'em.

But the lack of blood wasn't the only issue with the crime scene. The handgun also provided some challenges to the official story. You see, Foster's fingerprints were **not** on the gun. I guess he wiped it clean **after** he killed himself. Yeah, that's what happened. He cleaned it ... post mortem. Actually, the FBI tried to "explain" this by claiming that the lack of fingerprints was due to a lack of sweat on Foster's hands. Let's see, the temperature on July 21, 1993 in Washington DC was 95°F, with a heat index of 103°F. No sweat on his hands? Sure, FBI, that makes sense.

Regarding the photos – we have very little photographic evidence of the crime scene. The 35mm photographs taken by the Park Police were supposedly "underexposed" in the laboratory. In addition to the 35mm photos, many more of the Polaroids of the crime scene simply vanished. But that's normal in a suicide investigation. Photographs sometimes just "grow legs" and walk off. It happens.

Seriously? We're supposed to believe this crap? Maybe they were stolen by fairies with magic "pixie dust"? Or, better yet, maybe poodle-sized leprechauns took the photos? Perhaps they're buried with Jimmy Hoffa.

The "Suicide" Note & "Spin Machine"

Ah yes. The "suicide" note. No single item connected to Foster's death has aroused as much controversy as the so-called "suicide" note. The note, allegedly written by Foster, was discovered in his briefcase several days after he died. The problem was that Bernard Nussbaum, in controlling the Park Police search of Foster's office, had shown them that same briefcase empty just two days before. Perhaps it was a "magic" suicide note? You know ... a note that is written with "invisible ink" and suddenly "appears" several days after it's written. Sort of like a "time lapse" invisible ink "magic" note? That's the official story.

Here's something else strange about the "suicide" note. It was torn into over two dozen tiny pieces. All but one of the pieces was found in one of Foster's briefcases. Guess what? The missing piece was from the lower right-hand corner, the precise spot where Foster's signature would have appeared. How convenient. And no fingerprints were found on the note despite the fact Foster allegedly had torn it to shreds. Only Bernie Nussbaum's palm print was found. I guess Foster must have worn gloves to tear up the note. And why would he tear it up in the first place? What's the purpose of a suicide note if it's shredded into dozens of pieces? And what was Bernie Nussbaum doing handling critical evidence?

When you couple these anomalies with the fact that the White House did not even report the existence of the "suicide" note for almost 2 days after it was allegedly discovered, this seems quite bizarre, does it not? Adding another odd aspect to the note was the great pains taken to conceal it from the public. Even though the text itself had been published, the FBI made it clear that the public was not allowed to view actual photos of the note ... even in response to a Freedom of Information Act Request! Hey, FBI, if you've got nothing to hide, why are you hiding something?

Eventually, someone on the inside "leaked" the note and the *Wall Street Journal* published it. Once the note was available to the public, James Dale Davidson, editor of *Strategic Investment*, a premier world financial newsletter, commissioned three of the world's top document examiners and forensic handwriting experts to inspect the note. All three experts determined that the note is a forgery; it was **not** written by Foster. As a matter of fact, one of the experts, Reginald Alton of Oxford University, is arguably the most eminent handwriting expert in the world. He judged the forgery to be *"the clumsy work of an amateur."*

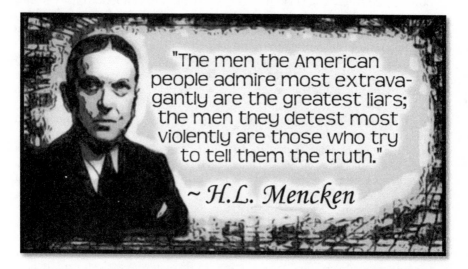

"The men the American people admire most extravagantly are the greatest liars; the men they detest most violently are those who try to tell them the truth."

~ *H.L. Mencken*

After Foster was killed, the "spin machine" went into action. Much like what happened immediately after the 9/11 events, before Foster's body was even cold, the mainstream media began to help craft the official story that Foster had indeed been depressed, despite the fact that he had concealed it from everyone around him, including his wife. Leading the propaganda machine was CBS and "60 Minutes" with several hit pieces directed at anyone who questioned the government's official narrative.

Then A&E stepped up to the "propaganda plate" and took a swing with "Inside Investigations" hosted by Bill Kurtis. In this ludicrous and misleading report they attempted to deceive – sorry, did I say "deceive"? – I meant to say they attempted to "illuminate" the audience on why there were no fingerprints on the gun by explaining that the deep grooves of a modern automatic pistol simply do not provide the surfaces needed to capture fingerprints. I guess they must have "forgotten" that Foster's body was **not** found with a modern automatic pistol with deep grooves and heavy texturing, but with a smooth metal .38 caliber revolver.

Yeah, they just "overlooked" this fact. A mere mistake, I'm sure.

A Few More Anomalies

As I mentioned, the new FBI director, Louis Freeh, was being sworn in at the White House on the day that Vince Foster was murdered. Since it's the White House, there are video cameras everywhere. This is a key point. The White House is the most secure private residence in the world, equipped with a sophisticated entry control system and video surveillance system. You know what's odd? No logbook entry shows he checked out of the White House on July 20, 1993. And there isn't a single video of Foster leaving the White House either, at least not on his own two feet that is. But these videos were never inspected during the "investigations" after the murder.

So, if he didn't leave the White House on his own cognizance, then somebody must have carried him. So who brought Foster's body from the White House to Fort Marcy Park? Did I mention that Fort Marcy Park was adjacent to the CIA Headquarters? I'm sure that is just a coincidence. Strangely, the first witness to find Foster's body insisted that there was no gun near the body. Even stranger, the memory in Foster's pager had been erased. And then the Park Police turned it over to the White House within hours of finding it. It is blatantly illegal to give away key evidence, especially to associates of the victim. Coworkers of murder victims are inevitably suspects in homicide investigations. Any officer turning over physical evidence to potential suspects would normally face serious charges. Instead, praise and promotions were heaped on the Park Police by a grateful White House. Cheryl Braun, for example, was promoted to sergeant. Hmmm ...

And then there were the eyewitnesses that kept changing their stories:

- Park Police Investigator John Rolla changed his story.
- Then Park Police Officer Kevin Fornshill changed his story.
- Then Firefighter Todd Hall changed his story.
- Then John Rolla again changed his story again.
- Then he changed it again.
- Then Paramedic Richard Arthur changed his story.
- Then Firefighter Jennifer Wacha changed her story.
- Then Dr. Donald Haut changed his story.
- Then Investigator Renee Abt changed her story.
- Then Park Police Technician Peter Simonello changed his story.

↓ Then Park Police Investigator Christine Hodakievic changed her story.

But I'm sure that's nothing to worry about, because material witnesses at a potential homicide scene frequently change their story. That's all part of "routine" investigative procedures.

Oh yes, I almost forgot. Foster could not have driven to the park. Last time I checked, in order to drive a car, the keys are necessary. And Foster's car keys were not in his pocket at the scene when Park Police officer John Rolla searched his pockets for personal effects. Officers Cheryl Braun and Christine Hodakievic watched while Rolla carefully searched Foster's front and back pockets. Rolla found nothing. Foster's wallet and credit cards were found in his Honda, but his car keys were missing. Amazingly, the car keys were eventually found in Foster's pockets at the morgue, following a visit from two White House aides (Craig Livingstone and William Kennedy). What do you know? The Vince Foster story has not only "magic" notes, but also "magic" keys. Amazing!

Lastly, nobody heard a shot! Five homes are located an average of 490 feet from the crime scene, yet nobody in the neighborhood heard a shot. The residence of the Saudi Arabia ambassador is 700 feet from the crime scene. Guards at the residence heard no shot.

Conclusion

This is the crux of the monumental myth (aka "suicide theory") put forth by the US government: that Vince Foster, under stress, on a hot July day in 1993, put the barrel of a .38 caliber revolver into his mouth and pulled the trigger, blowing his brains out, yet did not leave blood or fingerprints on that gun, nor were there any blood or brains at the scene of the "suicide." Did I miss anything?

Folks, the official story is a fairytale invented by government "magicians" who deftly bamboozle the American populace with sleight-of-hand card tricks in order to fool us into believing that Vince Foster committed suicide. Just like Gary Webb, the "official story" has been revealed to be a "monumental myth."

Webb was murdered. Who did it? I have no idea, and probably never will, due to the colossal government chicanery. But we're being lied to ... again.

Foster was also preparing a "Waco report" when he died. This has been confirmed by veteran British journalist, Ambrose Evans-Pritchard, in his book, The Secret Life of Bill Clinton. I wonder what was in that Waco report? Incriminating evidence against the Clintons? A detailed account of criminal activity in the Whitewater scandal? I guess we'll never know.

Don't like that you've read in this chapter? No worries. Turn back on the television. Watch CNN or MSNBC. Remain asleep.

RESOURCES

Websites
http://www.rense.com/general81/vince.htm
http://whatreallyhappened.com/RANCHO/POLITICS/FOSTER COVE
RUP/foster.php
http://prorev.com/foster.htm
http://www.wnd.com/2003/07/19870/
http://www.coffeeshoptimes.com/foster.html
http://www.wnd.com/2003/07/19870

Video
"The Strange Death of Vince Foster"
http://www.youtube.com/watch?v=rCiiB1 OGUE

Book
The Conspiracy That Will Not Die (Sr. Robert Gates)
The Secret Life of Bill Clinton (Ambrose Evans-Pritchard)

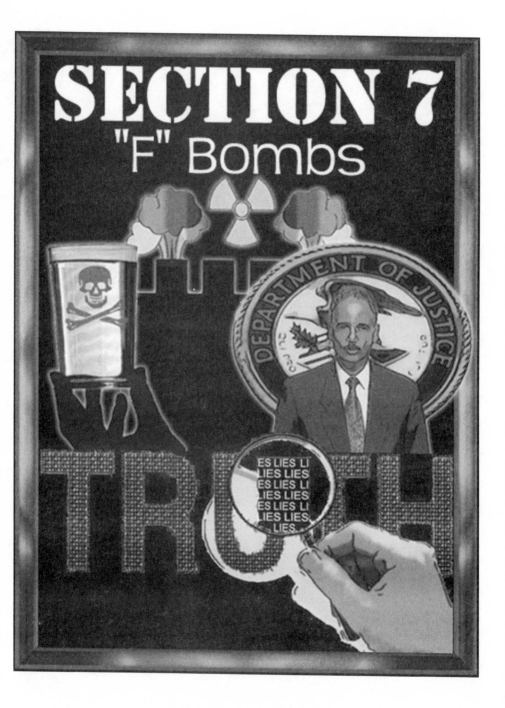

SECTION 7
"F" Bombs

Chapter 31

~ FLUORIDE ~

MONUMENTAL MYTH

Fluoride prevents tooth decay and is essential for healthy teeth and gums.

CAN YOU HANDLE THE TRUTH?

There's nothing like a glass of cool, clear water to quench your thirst. But the next time you turn on the tap, you might want to question whether that water is in fact, too toxic to drink. If your water is fluoridated, the answer is likely "yes."

For decades, we have been told a lie, a lie that has led to the deaths of hundreds of thousands of Americans and the weakening of the immune systems of tens of millions more. This lie is called fluoridation. It's a **hoax** ... a **con** ... a **scam**.

Drinking any amount of fluoride is dangerous to your health and has **never** been proven to prevent tooth decay. It's actually the biggest scientific fraud ever to be promoted by national and international governments. That's right. A process we were led to believe was a safe and effective method of protecting teeth from decay is in fact a fraud. In the words of Dr. Robert Carton, former scientist for the EPA, *"Fluoridation is the greatest case of scientific fraud of this century, if not of all time."*

Fluoride ... what exactly is it? Fluoride is any combination of elements containing the fluoride ion. In its elemental form, fluorine is a pale yellow, highly toxic and corrosive gas. In nature, fluorine is found combined with minerals as "fluorides." Fluorine compounds ("fluorides") are listed by the US Agency for Toxic Substances and Disease Registry as among the top 20 of 275 substances that pose the most significant threat to human health. They are cumulative toxins.

The most pervasive type of fluoride being added to municipal water is hydrofluorosilicic acid.

- **What if** you found out that hydrofluorosilicic acid is a neurotoxic industrial waste by-product of the aluminum, steel, cement, and phosphate fertilizer industries?
- **What if** you found out that it damages the immune, digestive, and respiratory systems as well as the kidneys, liver, brain, and thyroid?
- **What if** you discovered that there is no scientific evidence that fluoride is a beneficial additive to water, and in fact that there is overwhelming scientific evidence that proves, without a doubt, that fluoride is harmful?
- **What if** you found out that all federal health agencies have known these facts for years, but have kept it a secret?

Yes, unfortunately, all of the "what ifs" above are true. Fluoride is poison. Some of the most harmful attributes of fluoride are that it inhibits enzyme activity, paralyzes white blood cells, and causes collagen to break down. Enzymes, the immune system's leukocytes, and collagen are all fundamental in fighting cancer. And all three are adversely affected by fluoride.

Dr. John Yiamouyiannis, a biochemist and president of the Safe Water Foundation, was one of two researchers who first determined the fluoride-cancer link. Yiamouyiannis warns: *"Fluoride is a poison! . . . It has been used as a pesticide for mice, rats and other small pests. A 10-pound infant could be killed by 1/100 of an ounce, and a 100-pound adult could be killed by 1/10 of an ounce of fluoride. The Akron Regional Poison Center indicates that a 7-ounce tube of toothpaste contains 199 mg. of fluoride, more than enough to kill a 25-pound child."*

In 1977, epidemiological studies by Dr. Dean Burk, former head of the National Cancer Institute's cell chemistry section, and Dr. Yiamouyiannis showed that fluoridation is linked to about 10,000 cancer deaths yearly. According to Dr. Burk, in his book, <u>Fluoride, The Aging Factor</u>, *"Fluoride causes more human cancer, and causes it faster, than any other chemical."*

A 2005 Harvard School of Dental Health study found that fluoride in tap water directly contributes to osteosarcoma (bone cancer) in young boys; *"boys exposed to fluoride between the ages of five and 10 will suffer an increased rate of osteosarcoma – bone cancer – between the ages of 10 and 19,"* according to a *London Observer* article about the study. Interestingly, Harvard Professor Chester Douglass initially downplayed the connection, stating that there was *"no relationship."*

However, Douglass was investigated for scientific misconduct when it was discovered that he was, in fact, the editor-in-chief of *The Colgate Oral Health Report*, a quarterly newsletter funded by Colgate-Palmolive Company, which, by the way, just happens to make fluoridated toothpaste. Purely coincidence, I'm sure. No conflict of interest, there, right? Eventually, Douglass published a letter stating, "*We are also finding some positive associations between fluoride and osteosarcoma.*" Wow, that's diametrically opposed from "*no relationship,*" isn't it? I guess he was forced to tell the truth once the bloodhounds were on his scent.

In the mid-1980s, the largest study ever conducted on fluoridation and tooth decay was performed by the World Health Organization, using data from 39,000 school children in 84 areas around the country. The results showed no statistically significant difference in rates of tooth decay between fluoridated and non-fluoridated cities. Surprised? I'm not. But that's not all. A 1989 study by the National Institute for Dental Research concluded that 12% of children living in areas artificially fluoridated (between one and four parts per million) developed dental fluorosis, a permanent discoloration and brittling of the teeth.

As if causing cancer and ruining/discoloring your teeth weren't enough, there has been credible documentation showing other debilitating effects of fluoride. Dr. Phyllis Mullenix proved that fluoride had an adverse effect on the brain. As a result she was told that her work was "*no longer relevant to dentistry*" and fired. Studies have repeatedly linked fluoride to brain damage and reduced IQ. Peer-reviewed studies showing adverse effects on the thyroid gland were ignored as were studies linking fluoride to damage of the pineal gland. The pineal gland is located between the two hemispheres of the brain and is responsible for the synthesis and secretion of melatonin. Melatonin affects jet lag, sleep patterns, and aging and by the time old age hits, the buildup of fluoride in the pineal gland is in very high concentrations.

In early 2010, two separate stories out of India reveal that children are being blinded and crippled partly as a result of fluoride being artificially added to their drinking water. In the Indian village of Gaudiyan, well over half of the population has bone deformities, making them physically handicapped. Children are born normally, but after they start drinking the fluoridated water, they begin to develop crippling defects in their hands and feet.

It is well-known that fluoride prevents iodine absorption and causes thyroid disorders. Did you know that endemic "dental fluorosis" areas have been shown to be the same as those affected with iodine deficiency? Iodine deficiency causes brain disorders, miscarriages and goiter, among many other diseases. Other health risks associated with low to moderate doses of fluorides are bone fractures, joint pain, skeletal abnormalities, and increased lead absorption.

What is adding insult to injury is the fact that ingesting fluoride has little to no effect in preventing tooth decay. Dubious studies by the American

Dental Association ("ADA") have suggested fluoride **may** have a hardening effect on the enamel when it is applied topically, but even if that's the case (which is unclear), they have failed to confirm its benefit when consumed systemically. Ingesting fluoride to prevent tooth decay makes about as much sense as ingesting sunscreen to prevent a sun burn.

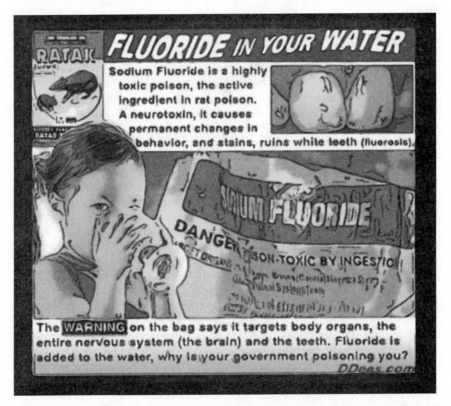

The fact that fluoride accumulates in the body is the reason that US law requires the Surgeon General to set a "maximum contaminant level" (MCL) for fluoride content in public water supplies as determined by the EPA. It boggles my mind that thousands of brainwashed dentists proudly proclaim fluoride to be the "wonder nutrient" that prevents cavities and promotes healthy teeth and gums. Let me ask you a question. How can a poisonous waste product and a cumulative toxin be described as a "nutrient?" I want to be crystal clear: fluoride is **not** an essential nutrient for your health – dental or otherwise. Not a single process exists in your body that requires fluoride. None. Zero.

Let's attempt to get to the bottom of this monumental myth, shall we? But first, you had better put on your "history cap" and grab a cup of water (non-fluoridated, of course) to prevent your mouth from becoming overly "parched" as we travel back in time almost a century. In case you weren't aware of it, when one travels back in time, a recurrent side effect is dry mouth coupled with hair that grows backwards, so keep the water handy and don't try to comb your hair while reading this chapter.

In the 1920s, aluminum manufacturing, due largely to the thriving canning industry, was booming. But it was also a big producer of toxic fluoride waste. The biggest dilemma was the cost to safely dispose of this hazardous waste, since it was extremely expensive. A company in Pittsburgh, ALCOA, had some revolutionary ideas on how to cut the costs of disposal. At that time, the US Public Health Service (PHS) was under the jurisdiction of Treasury Secretary Andrew W. Mellon, who just happened to be the founder and major stockholder of ALCOA.

In 1931, a PHS dentist named H. Trendley Dean (aka the "father of fluoridation") was dispatched to over 300 small towns in Texas where water wells contained high concentrations of fluoride, which was most likely calcium fluoride (CaF_2). His mission was to determine how much fluoride people could tolerate without sustaining obvious damage to their teeth. What he found was startling: teeth in these high-fluoride towns were often discolored and mottled. However, he also theorized that there "*appeared to be*" a lower incidence of cavities in communities having about one part per million (1 PPM) fluoride in the water.

Dean used a strategy called "selective use of data" to try to prove his theory. He chose to use the data from only 21 communities to "*back into his number.*" That's what we call it in the accounting world when you know the desired answer and use only numbers which will support your desired answer, and then you reach your predetermined conclusion. Dean totally disregarded the other 270+ localities that showed no correlation between fluoride and cavities.

Later, in 1955, Dean admitted (under oath) that fluoride does **not** work as a remedy for tooth decay (*Fluoride*, Vol. 14, No. 3, July 1981). Then in 1957, he had to admit at AMA hearings that even water which contained a mere .1 (1/10th) PPM could cause dental fluorosis. Moreover, there has never been a single double-blind study to indicate that fluoridation is effective in reducing cavities. Not one!

But ALCOA didn't let the facts get in their way! ALCOA-funded scientist Gerald J. Cox learned of Dean's findings, and devised a way for ALCOA to actually profit from fluoride. He proposed that this "*apparently worthless by-product*" might reduce cavities in children (despite no evidence). He haughtily declared that fluoride was good for your teeth, and in 1939, he proposed that the USA should fluoridate its water supplies. That's right, not by a doctor, not by a dentist, but by a scientist who was working for the largest producer of fluoride in the entire USA.

The aluminum industry had already been marketing their toxic fluoride waste as an insecticide and rat poison, but they wanted a much larger market. But they had a minor roadblock. In the 1944 *Journal of the American Dental Association*, the ADA warned that *"the potentialities for harm (from fluoridation) far outweigh those for the good."* In 1945, two Michigan cities were selected for an official "fifteen-year" comparison study to determine if fluoride could safely reduce cavities in children, and fluoride was pumped into the drinking water of Grand Rapids. In 1946, despite the fact that the official fifteen-year experiment in Michigan had barely begun, six more American cities were allowed to fluoridate their water. The two-city Michigan experiment was abandoned before it was half over, with the results "inconclusive." This is the only scientifically objective test of fluoridation's safety and benefits that was ever performed.

In 1947, Oscar R. Ewing, a long-time ALCOA lawyer, was appointed head of the Federal Security Agency, a position that placed him in charge of the PHS. Under Ewing, a national water fluoridation campaign began. The public relations strategist for the water fluoridation campaign was none other than Sigmund Freud's nephew Edwin L. Bernays, known as the "Father of Spin." Bernays pioneered the application of Freud's theories to advertising and government "half-truths."

In his book Propaganda, Bernays argued that scientific manipulation of public opinion is the key. He stated, *"A relatively small number of persons pull the wires which control the public mind."* The government's fluoridation campaign was one of his most enduring successes.

Bernays' techniques were simple. Pretend there is some favorable research by using phrases like *"Numerous studies have shown..."* or *"Research has proven..."* or *"Scientific investigators have found..."* but then never really cite anything (since they had **ZERO** scientific studies to cite). Say it long enough and loud enough, and eventually people will believe it. If anyone doubts or questions the lies, attack their character and/or their intellect.

Bernays never strayed from his fundamental axiom to *"control the masses without their knowing it."* He believed that the best brainwashing takes place when the people are unaware that they are being manipulated. So, under Bernays' spell, the popular image of this insecticide and rat poison was transformed into a beneficial provider of gleaming smiles, absolutely safe, and good for children. This was a brilliant marketing move by ALCOA! Rather than having to pay extremely high costs to safely dispose of this toxic waste, ALCOA (and other aluminum manufacturers) could now sell it to municipalities for a huge profit! Any opponents were quickly and permanently engraved on the public mind as crackpots, quacks, and lunatics.

Fluoridation allows a community to do to everyone what a doctor can do to no one: **force** a patient to take a particular medication. Civil liberties, human rights, and informed consent are all violated when public water is used as a vehicle to deliver any sort of toxic chemical into our bodies; whether it is claimed to be a benefit or not.

On April 12, 2010, *Time Magazine* listed fluoride as one of the *"Top Ten Common Household Toxins"* and described fluoride as both *"neurotoxic and potentially tumorigenic if swallowed."* Truth be told, in almost every country in the world (including the USA), it's against the law to "mass medicate" an entire population with a substance that everyone admits is toxic. However, in the USA, we do it anyway...

Remember the chapter on the Rockefellers and their Nazi connection? Well, fluoride also has the same connection to the Nazis. Charles Elliot Perkins, research scientist sent by the US government to take charge of the I.G. Farben drug/chemical plants in Germany, confirmed this fact when he discovered that *"the real purpose behind water fluoridation is to reduce the resistance of the masses to domination, control and loss of liberty."* In his report to the Lee Foundation for Nutritional Research in October of 1954, he said, *"Repeated doses of infinitesimal amounts of fluoride will in time reduce an individual's power to resist domination, by slowly poisoning and narcotizing a certain area of the brain, thus making him submissive to the will of those who wish to govern him."*

One of the things I find so interesting about this debate on fluoride is that dentists and doctors will leap to defend this practice at every opportunity. Why? Is it because there's good scientific evidence that fluoridation is somehow beneficial to the public? **NO**. It's because they've been told to support it by the Medical Mafia (specifically the AMA and ADA). All of this is so bizarre that a reasonable person can only conclude these doctors and dentists are operating on auto-pilot. They are parroting whatever "talking points" that they are given.

And to top it off, they are typically extremely arrogant about the whole thing. They act as if they are qualified to talk about this one single nutritional deficiency and its effects on the entire human body because they are dentists. In fact, dentists have no qualifications to talk about the effects of fluoride on the human nervous system, the blood supply, chronic disease, behavioral disorders, or other physiological effects.

Dentists are really only qualified to talk about what's happening with your teeth – not drugs or chemicals that you ingest and that have a systemic effect. Neither are medical doctors qualified to talk about nutrition. As I've already mentioned, at best they have a few hours of education on nutrition and are largely illiterate about the relationship between nutritional deficiencies and chronic disease. The bottom line is that you have a whole group of so-called *"experts"* that know nothing about the subject, yet grandstand and claim to be the authorities on it.

In an illuminating article published on NaturalNews.com in September of 2013, Mike Adams revealed some shocking information about fluoride. You see, there was a story published in *The Independent* which was entitled, *"Revealed: Government let British company export nerve gas chemicals to Syria."* In the article, it was reported that *"The Government was accused of 'breathtaking laxity' in its arms controls last night after it emerged that officials authorised the export to Syria of two chemicals capable of being used to make a nerve agent such as sarin a year ago."*

What, exactly, are those two dangerous chemicals that need to be controlled via "arms control" regulations to prevent the manufacture of sarin gas? Well ... ummm ... they would be ... drum roll please ... **sodium fluoride** and potassium fluoride!

So, yes, it appears that we do indeed live in the "medical matrix," because the same toxic chemical (sodium fluoride) that is force fed to the US population in what the CDC and FDA refer to as a "public health victory" is openly and frequently referred to as a "chemical weapon" when sold to Syria. Mike Adams states: *"According to US Secretary of State John Kerry, any government "regime" that uses chemical* *weapons against its own people should be bombed / invaded / overthrown by a coalition of other United Nations members. By his own definition, then, the United States of America should now be invaded by the UN because the government uses a deadly chemical weapon – sodium fluoride – on its own people. By implication, then, John Kerry is now calling for the UN to bomb the USA. As the international media now confirms, **sodium fluoride is a chemical weapon,** and this chemical weapon is used against the American people every single day in the water supply, a favorite attack vector for terrorists."* Well said, Health Ranger!

In summary, what started out as an experimental program almost a century ago, without any health studies done whatsoever, turned out to be a "cash cow" for industries that previously had to dispose of this toxic waste to the tune of millions of dollars a year.

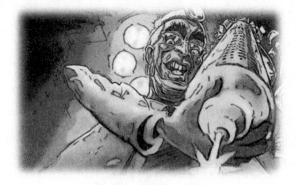

RESOURCES

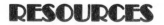

Websites
http://fluoridealert.org/
www.naturalnews.com/041883_Syria_chemical_weapons_sodium_fluoride.html
http://fluoride.mercola.com

Video
"The Hidden Agenda: The Fluoride Deception" – Dr. Stan Monteith
http://www.youtube.com/watch?v=dbj4zdYZnJc

Book
Fluoride, The Aging Factor (Dr. John Yiamouyiannis)
The Case Against Fluoride (Dr. Paul Connet)
The Fluoride Deception (Christopher Bryson)

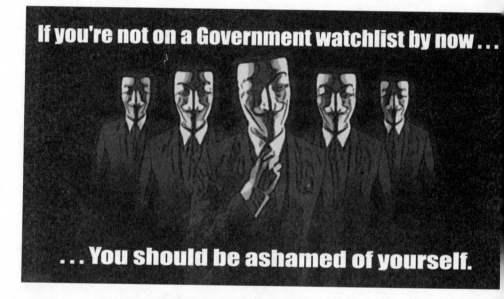

Chapter 32

~ FUKUSHIMA ~

MONUMENTAL MYTH

On March 11, 2011, there was a 9.0 earthquake which caused a massive tsunami that crippled the cooling systems at the Tokyo Electric Power Company (TEPCO) nuclear plant in Fukushima Daiichi, Japan. It also led to hydrogen explosions and reactor meltdowns that forced evacuations of those living within a 20 km radius of the plant. It was the largest nuclear disaster since the Chernobyl disaster of 1986. The explosions were bad, but the danger is over. Japan will eventually return to normal. Nuclear radiation is basically harmless. It won't affect the rest of the world.

CAN YOU HANDLE THE TRUTH?

It's been over 2½ years since the initial meltdown, and the *Wall Street Journal* is estimating that it may take at least 40 more years to clean it up! The entire northern hemisphere is being contaminated from this out-of-control flow of "death and destruction." Fukushima is a nightmare of epic proportions. Samples of radioactivity in air, water, precipitation, and milk, taken less than a month after the initial meltdowns, indicated levels hundreds of times above normal.

Is Fukushima the greatest environmental disaster of all time? It certainly appears so, in light of the fact that Japanese officials recently admitted that, each and every day, over 600,000 pounds (almost 72,000 gallons) of radioactive water from Fukushima enters the Pacific Ocean. This massive quantity of water contains radioactive nuclides (isotopes of elements with a higher than normal amount of nucleons that are prone to radioactive decay) such as tritium, plutonium, uranium, iodine-131, cesium-135 and 137, and strontium-89 and 90. These radioactive nuclides will outlive everyone reading this book ... by a long shot!

Michael Snyder has written several marvelous articles about Fukushima, including "*11 Facts About the Ongoing Fukushima Nuclear Holocaust That Are Almost Too Horrifying To Believe*" and "*28 Signs That The West Coast Is Being Absolutely Fried With Nuclear Radiation From*

Fukushima." Since I benefited tremendously from his research, I have quoted and paraphrased Mr. Snyder's work throughout.

What Really Happened?

After the earthquake on March 11, 2011, the 11 operating nuclear power reactors at Fukushima Daiichi all "tripped" as designed, and the nuclear fission process was stopped.

"What is fission?" Good question. I'm glad you asked.

Fission is a process by which an unstable atom breaks into smaller atoms, releasing energy as it does. What makes an atom **un**stable is the number of neutrons in its nucleus. In nature, elements show up with a different count of neutrons – these are called "isotopes" of the element. For example, a nucleus made of one proton is hydrogen, but when it has a proton and a neutron, then it's called "deuterium" (an isotope of hydrogen). When it has two neutrons and a proton, it's called "tritium" (another isotope of hydrogen).

But even after the fission process was stopped, the fuel in the reactors continued to produce considerable amounts of heat, thus the main goal after the reactors tripped was to keep water circulating over the fuel rods to keep them cool and prevent damage. The reactor at Fukushima was surrounded by a concrete outer building designed to keep fissile material (capable of sustaining a chain reaction of nuclear fission) isolated from the outside world. The earthquake resulted in loss of power, thus the pumps didn't work, and the water couldn't be pumped. But the back-up generators kicked in and all was well. At least until the tsunami hit and knocked out all the back-up generators.

At Fukushima Daiichi, all of the reactors (except Reactors #1, #2, #3, and #4) were brought into "cold shutdown" with water circulating as required. But these were the oldest reactors, and the loss of power to the pumps led to water in the pressure vessel boiling and the fuel heating up immensely, bursting the zirconium alloy cans that contain the fuel pellets. On March 12, 2011, the concrete outer buildings of Reactor #1 exploded. Then on March 14, 2011, the same thing happened at Reactor #3. A few days later, a crack was detected in Reactor #2.

And today, over 2½ years later, Reactor #4 is teetering on the edge of collapse. Seismicity standards rate the building at a zero, which means that even a minor earthquake could send it into a heap of rubble. And sitting at the top of the building (in a pool that is cracked, leaking, and hazardous even without an earthquake) are 1,535 fuel rods, some of them full of "fresh fuel" that was ready to go into the reactor when the earthquake and tsunami hit.

Dr. Arnie Gundersen (a nuclear engineer who used to build spent fuel pools) explains that there is no protection surrounding the radioactive fuel in the pools. He warns that if the fuel pools at Reactor #4 collapse due to an earthquake or other event, people should get out of Japan, and residents of the West Coast of America and Canada should shut all of their windows and "stay inside for a while." According to Reuters, the combined amount of cesium-137 contained in the 1,535 nuclear fuel rods still at Reactor #4 is **14,000** times greater than what was released when the USA dropped atomic bombs on Nagasaki and Hiroshima at the end of World War II.

While speaking at the public hearing of the Budgetary Committee of the House of Councilors on March 22, 2012, Japan's former Ambassador to Switzerland, Mr. Mitsuhei Murata, stated that if the crippled building of Reactor #4 (with 1,535 fuel rods in the spent fuel pool 100 feet above the ground) collapses, not only will it cause a shutdown of all six reactors but will also affect the common spent fuel pool containing 6,375 fuel rods which are located only 150 feet from Reactor #4.

In both cases, the radioactive fuel rods are not protected by a containment vessel. Believe it or not, they are open to the air! Should they collapse, the result would be a global catastrophe like we have never seen before. In the words of Mr. Murata, "Such a catastrophe would affect us all for centuries." This assertion is confirmed by most trustworthy experts like Dr. Arnie Gundersen and Dr. Fumiaki Koide.

As a matter of fact, anti-nuclear physician, Dr. Helen Caldicott, says that if the fuel pool in Reactor #4 collapses, she will evacuate her family from Boston and move them to the Southern Hemisphere. And she lives on the East Coast! What about those living on the West Coast? Wow! That's a telling statement, isn't it?

Founder and host of Nuked Radio, Christina Consolo, in a 2013 interview with RT, stated: "We have three 100-ton melted fuel blobs underground, but where exactly they are located, no one knows. Whatever 'barriers' TEPCO has put in place so far have failed. Efforts to decontaminate radioactive water have failed. Robots have failed. Camera equipment and temperature gauges ... failed. Decontamination of surrounding cities has failed. If and when the corium reaches the Tokyo aquifer, serious and expedient discussions will have to take place about evacuating 40 million people. We have endless releases into the Pacific Ocean that will be ongoing for not only our lifetimes, but our children's lifetimes."

The Cover-Up

From day one, doctors in Japan helped perpetuate the Fukushima cover-up. Sick patients are **not** being told their illnesses are from exposure to radioactive contamination. Scientific reports showing radiation health damage to humans are forbidden to be published. Heck, the Fukushima Radiation Health Risk Advisor (aka "Propaganda Minister"), Dr. Shunichi Yamashita, has been promoting bizarre beliefs like *"laughter will remove your radiation phobia."*

Yes, you read that correctly. The Japanese "expert" told the Japanese people that radiation would not affect "happy" people who laughed a lot! **How absurd!** Is he related to Tokyo Rose? Hey, maybe they should also follow after tiny leprechauns riding unicorns that can lead them to a huge pot of gold at the end of a magic rainbow! Or maybe they should sprinkle magic pixie dust over their beds at night to protect from radiation. Yeah, that's the ticket!

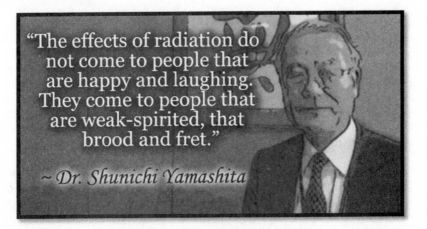

"The effects of radiation do not come to people that are happy and laughing. They come to people that are weak-spirited, that brood and fret."

~ Dr. Shunichi Yamashita

According to Dr. Arnie Gundersen, *"We're seeing scientist after scientist ... writing to us saying that they've got good science and they're being ostracized in Japan and being forbidden from publishing scientific reports that show radiation health damage to Japanese people. So basically the government is sitting on the scientific community and preventing good science from being done. Same as the doctors, the doctors have contacted us as well. They say they've been told not to tell their patients that their illness is radiation induced. So these guys have an oath as a doctor to be honest with their patients, and yet they're basically ignoring their own oath and helping perpetuate a cover-up in the Japanese government."*

Reminiscent of the US government's reaction to 9/11, specifically with the first responders, the Japanese authorities committed numerous atrocities in an effort to "save face," sending hundreds of heroic people to go into the reactor buildings to "stabilize" the plant. Sadly, these people were basically sent to their death, as many of them have since died. This would have been acceptable if their mission were a voluntary one to "save the world," but their mission was to "save face" for the Japanese government and the owners of the plant.

Check this out! Rather than evacuating the area around Fukushima, Japan chose to raise its acceptable radiation-exposure rate by **20 times**!

And the USA is no different than Japan. Just like 9/11 and Waco and Oklahoma City and JFK and the financial crisis and the Gulf oil spill, the US government focused all their energy on covering up the truth. Only two weeks after the Fukushima incident, the EPA responded by increasing acceptable radiation levels and pretending that radiation is good for us. Just like DDT, I can just hear the EPA trolls singing *"Radiation is good for Me-e-e!"* ... kind of like Ann Coulter did a few years ago.

But it's not just the bobble-head bleached blonde idiots like Ann Coulter saying this. Government scientists from the Pacific Northwest National Laboratories and pro-nuclear hacks like Lawrence Solomon are saying this. That's right. Incredibly, since Fukushima, government scientists and mainstream media shills have been engaged in a propaganda campaign focused on "reexamining" old studies that show that radioactive substances (like plutonium and uranium) cause cancer to argue that they actually help prevent cancer.

Hey, maybe they could begin spreading the theory that the Easter Bunny lays golden eggs and gives them to Santa Claus and the elves to give to "good" children at Christmas time. That makes about as much sense as telling us that plutonium and uranium prevent cancer. Are we living in the matrix? Let's go back to the EPA changing allowable radiation limits.

A 2013 update to the 1992 EPA manual is being planned, and if the "hare-brained" wing of the EPA has its way, here is what it means (please brace yourself for these preposterous increases):

- A nearly 1000-fold increase for exposure to strontium-90
- A 3000 to 100,000-fold hike for exposure to iodine-131
- An almost 25,000 rise for exposure to radioactive nickel-63

It's sickening to me that, in order to deceive the good people of the USA, the government constantly changes the rules and definitions in order to "win." Sort of like it's some sick game to them.

Oh yes, I almost forgot. Right after the 2011 explosions at Fukushima, the EPA pulled 8 of its 18 radiation monitors in Washington, California, and Oregon. I wonder why. Were they giving readings that were too high? *"The government is our friend ... they would never cover anything up!"* **Really?** Please remember that our beloved government has covered up numerous nuclear meltdowns (like Canoga Park, Santa Susana, and Three Mile Island) for half a century to protect the nuclear power industry. So, it sure appears that there is a concerted effort (by the USA and Japan) to suppress the truth about nuclear meltdowns, especially Fukushima.

For instance, until recently, TEPCO maintained that *"no tainted water is leaking from the facility."* Really, I guess it must be "magic water," eh? You know ... magic water that miraculously doesn't leak from a facility that is full of cracked and deteriorating containment buildings. Over the past 2½ years, thousands of tons of water have been poured over the plant.

That's right, I said *"over the plant."* This was done according to some fantasy that the "magic water" would somehow find its way through cracks in the walls of the building and refill the pools. Realistic? Ummm ... about as realistic as expecting a monkey with a piano to play Beethoven's 5th Symphony. In reality, even if some water gets to the pools, the pools are cracked. The water becomes radioactive and goes into the water table, the ocean, and the atmosphere.

It's important to remember that with nuclear reactors, the "spent" fuel rods remain highly radioactive. As a matter of fact, everything in the reactor becomes radioactive. That includes the heavy water, the closed system recirculating water, and the shielding. And stopping the chain reaction is not as simple as turning off a light or a car engine. It is a lengthy, complex process that is not instantaneous. All the while, radioactive materials are being released into the air and water.

Dead Sea Creatures & Human Health Effects

These radioactive materials are continually building up in the food chain. How? Researchers from the *Japan Agency for Marine Earth Science and Technology* reported in early 2012 that they had detected radioactive cesium in plankton collected from all 10 points in the Pacific they checked. Plankton, and the radiation they contain, moves right up the food chain through fish, whales, and seals when larger fish eat smaller fish.

Something is causing Pacific herring along the west coast of Canada to bleed from their gills, fins, tails, bellies, and eyeballs. And something is causing starfish off the west coast of Canada and Washington state to literally melt. Could Fukushima be responsible? I know ... that's a rhetorical question. An MSNBC article in April of 2012 reported that seals and polar bears were found to have "external maladies" that consisted of fur loss and open sores – obvious signs of radiation burns from the Fukushima meltdown. Fukushima radiation appears to be causing an epidemic of dead and starving Sea Lions in California. And just last year, according to the French newspaper *Le Monde*, a fisherman caught a fish that contained **2,500 times** the legal limit for radiation in seafood!

But there's more. Tissue samples were taken from 15 Bluefin tuna caught in August of 2011 (five months after the meltdowns), and **all 15** contained measurable amounts of cesium-134 and cesium-137. And unlike some other compounds, radioactive cesium does not quickly sink to the sea bottom but remains dispersed in the water column, from the surface to the ocean floor. Fish can swim right through it, ingesting it through their gills. And then it is continually ingested right up the food chain. Also remember that large fish like tuna are migratory, crossing the ocean multiple times per year. In other words, all Pacific migratory fish are likely contaminated. **Question**: Why have contaminated Alaskan Halibut been found even though halibut don't migrate? I'll tell you why. The radioactive plumes don't just fall on land. Think about it.

According to Michael Synder, *"Back in 2012, the Vancouver Sun reported that cesium-137 was being found in a very high percentage of the fish that Japan was selling to Canada: 73% of mackerel, 91% of halibut, 92% of sardines, 93% of tuna and eel, 94% of cod and anchovies, and 100% of carp, seaweed, shark and monkfish."* Daniel Hirsch, a nuclear policy lecturer at the University of California-Santa Cruz, told *Global Security Newswire*, *"We could have large numbers of cancer from ingestion of fish."*

A recent study at the German *Marine Research Institute* indicated that the entire Pacific Ocean will be contaminated with radiation by the year 2018. Here's one of the big problems: You can't see or smell nuclear radiation and its health effects (like cancer) don't occur immediately. But it's a fact that radiation causes cancer. That's not even up for debate. We all know this. So, I wonder how many people will develop cancer from this disaster. How many people will eventually die from exposure to the radiation from Fukushima? Some experts are not afraid to use the word "billions."

Truth be told, peer-reviewed scientific studies have already provided evidence of increased mortality in North America and thyroid problems in infants on the West Coast of the USA. And, as I've already mentioned, the radiation leaking from the Fukushima plants contains radioactive Iodine-131, which can cause thyroid cancer. If you aren't already taking it, you should consider taking an iodine supplement, which will saturate the thyroid with non-radioactive iodine. This, in turn, makes it difficult or impossible for radioactive iodine to be absorbed by the thyroid. If the gland has enough iodine in it, the thyroid doesn't absorb any radioactive iodine and it is flushed out of the system in urine. Children are considered the most vulnerable to this form of radiation exposure, which is usually absorbed by eating contaminated food or drinking contaminated milk or water. After the 1986 Chernobyl nuclear accident, thyroid cancer rates in children in the Ukraine increased substantially.

"So, how do you measure radiation?" I'm glad you asked. However, I'm just going to touch on the specific measurements for radioactivity (like "becquerels" and "curies"), but I want to focus on the fact that radioactive nuclides (like cesium-137) are lethal at the atomic or molecular level, they disintegrate atoms, and they produce enormous amounts of energy. One **becquerel** is equal to one atomic disintegration per second. One **curie** is defined as that amount of any radioactive material that will decay at a rate of 37 billion disintegrations per second. So one curie equals 37 billion becquerels. According to a professor at Tokyo University, 3 gigabecquerels of cesium-137 are flowing into the port at Fukushima Daiichi every single day! How much is a gigabecquerel? 10 **billion** becquerels!

According to Steven Starr, senior scientist and Director of Physicians for Social Responsibility, radioactive nuclides *"...emit radiation, invisible forms of matter and energy that we might compare to fire, because radiation burns and destroys human tissue. But unlike the fire of fossil fuels, the nuclear fire that issues forth from radioactive elements cannot be extinguished. It is not a fire that can be scattered or suffocated because it burns at the atomic level – it comes from the disintegration of single atoms. Thus, radioactivity is a term which indicates how many radioactive atoms are disintegrating in a time period. We measure the intensity of radioactivity by the rate of the disintegrations and the energy they produce."*

I remember talking to someone right after the 2011 radiation releases and explosions at Fukushima, and he said, *"We don't need to worry about radiation. There's radiation on all the food we eat. It's everywhere."* While it's factual that naturally occurring radioactive nuclides (like as potassium-40) are found in bananas and other fruits and vegetables, equating potassium-40 to man-made radioactive nuclides (like cesium-137) is a false comparison since naturally occurring radioactive elements are very weakly radioactive, whereas man-made radionuclides are much more potent. For instance, potassium-40 has a specific activity of 71 ten millionths of a curie per gram, while cesium-137 has a specific activity of 88 curies per gram. Let me pull out my calculator. OK, got it. That means that cesium-137 emits roughly 12.4 **million** times more radiation per unit than does potassium-40. This is like comparing a single match to an atomic bomb. Which one of these would you rather have in your bananas?

Steven Starr explains that *"as little as one third of a gram of cesium-137, made into microparticles and distributed as a smoke or gas over an area of one square kilometer, will make that square kilometer uninhabitable. Less than two grams of cesium-137, a piece smaller than an American dime, if made into microparticles and evenly distributed as a radioactive gas over an area of one square mile, will turn that square mile into an uninhabitable radioactive exclusion zone. Central Park in New York City can be made uninhabitable by 2 grams of microparticles of cesium-137. Hard to believe, isn't it?"*

According to Dr. Jose Benavente, *"Radiation exposure damages DNA, motor nerve cells, and other internal structures of our cells, which can lead to cancer and other diseases. Cells of the immune system and red blood cells are produced in the bone marrow. These are bone marrow stem cells. Cell division and proliferation goes on rapidly in the bone marrow and because there is a tremendous amount of cell division going on in the bone marrow – more than almost any other place in the body – the bone marrow is particularly sensitive to radiation. When the DNA of the cells is damaged by the radiation the cells lose their ability to replenish themselves. This is why people receiving radiation treatment tend to lose their hair, and this is why your immune system is rapidly depleted by exposure to radiation."*

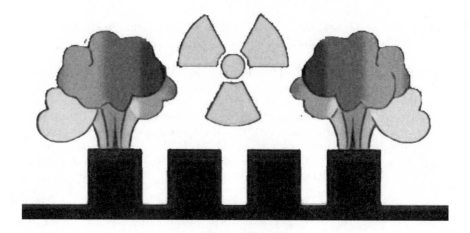

Is Fukushima an ELE (Extinction Level Event)?

Is the Fukushima disaster the equivalent of an "open air Auschwitz"? Is it a potential extinction level event ("ELE")? Well, the fact of the matter is that globally, sperm counts are down, immune system diseases are escalating, mutations are occurring in all life forms. Yes, I believe the evidence supports the assertion that Fukushima Daiichi has the potential to be an ELE.

You see, the Fukushima reactors used "dirty fuel," a combination of plutonium and uranium (aka "MOX" fuel), which means Japan is going to be a "dead zone" for centuries. With MOX fuel, **one** fuel rod has the potential to kill 2.89 **BILLION** people. And there are over 1,500 fuel rods in Reactor #4 alone! Do the math. That means that if Reactor #4 melts down and collapses, and the fuel rods are compromised, it would have the potential to kill over 4.3 **TRILLION** people! Last time I checked, there were only about 7 billion people on the entire earth. The bottom line is that if Reactor #4 collapses, we would face a massive ELE from the release of radiation. Yale Professor Charles Perrow is warning that if the cleanup of Fukushima is not handled with 100% precision that humanity could be threatened *"for thousands of years."*

That is, if we aren't in one already. Nuke experts like Dr. Arnie Gundersen and Helen Caldicott are prepared to evacuate their families to the southern hemisphere if that happens. It is **that** serious. So now you know, if you didn't before. We are in big trouble. Let me reiterate. This isn't just about Japan. The cold, hard reality of the matter is that this is truly a disaster that is planetary in scope. Keep in mind that Tokyo beat Madrid and Istanbul to host the 2020 Olympics. I'm not a betting man, but if I were, I'd bet that by 2020, Tokyo is uninhabitable. The Olympics will **not** be held in Tokyo.

Former UN advisor, Akio Matsumura, was told that if the fuel pool at Reactor #4 collapses or the water spills out, so much radiation will spew out for 50 years that no one will be able to approach Fukushima. Even more dramatically, Matsumura writes: *"It is no exaggeration to say that the fate of Japan and the whole world depends on Number 4 reactor."* Ambassador Murata also informed the world that the total numbers of the spent fuel rods at the Fukushima Daiichi site is in excess of 11,000. This number is confirmed by US Department of Energy data.

The jet stream, and a highly dynamic portion of our atmosphere called the troposphere, have been swirling around massive amounts of radioactive particles and settling them out, mostly in rain, over the entire northern hemisphere, especially the west coast of North America, from Alaska down to Baja and even further. Please do your own research, keeping in mind that the nuclear "propaganda machine" is well armed and funded, and the global internet is being systematically "sanitized" of truthful information about the Fukushima global disaster and subsequent cover-up.

Let me ask you a few questions.

- Are you breathing the air?
- Are your children breathing?
- What about the radioactive nuclides in your drinking water?
- And in the rainwater?
- And in the fish you are eating?
- And in your vegetables?
- And the milk supply?

Keep in mind that it's been happening every second of every day ... for the past 2½ years. Are you beginning to understand the enormity of the problem?

In the words of my good buddy, Liam Scheff: *"I'd move to France...if they didn't have more nuclear power there than anywhere in the world. I wonder if I can learn to speak Penguin? I understand Antarctica is nice, this time of year."* I'm with you Liam. If Reactor #4 collapses, we may be heading back to Panama or New Zealand!

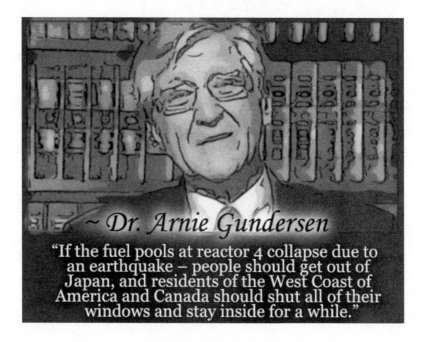

~ *Dr. Arnie Gundersen*

"If the fuel pools at reactor 4 collapse due to an earthquake – people should get out of Japan, and residents of the West Coast of America and Canada should shut all of their windows and stay inside for a while."

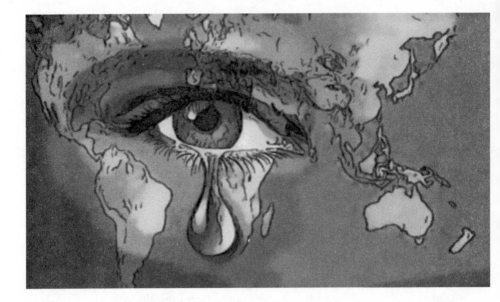

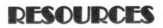

RESOURCES

Websites

http://endthelie.com/2012/04/21/fukushima-is-falling-apart-are-you-ready
http://askaboutfukushimanow.com/
http://www.washingtonsblog.com/2012/04/the-largest-short-term-threat-to-humanity-the-fuel-pools-of-fukushima.html
http://thetruthwins.com/archives/11-facts-about-the-ongoing-fukushima-nuclear-holocaust-that-are-almost-too-horrifying-to-believe
http://thetruthwins.com/archives/28-signs-that-the-west-coast-is-being-absolutely-fried-with-nuclear-radiation-from-fukushima
http://www.ratical.org/radiation/Fukushima/StevenStarr.html

Video

"New Fukushima Dangers the Government isn't Telling You" – Anthony Gucciardi
http://www.youtube.com/watch?v=cEFfpkBjdGw

Chapter 33

~ FAST & FURIOUS ~

MONUMENTAL MYTH

Operation "Fast and Furious" was launched in 2009 by top Department of Justice (DoJ) officials, in collaboration with the FBI, the DEA, and the Bureau of Alcohol, Tobacco, and Firearms (ATF) as part of a strategy to identify and eliminate arms trafficking networks. Instead of prosecuting the individual "straw purchasers" who buy guns for the cartels, ATF agents would track the guns to the top bosses of Mexico's powerful drug cartels.

CAN YOU HANDLE THE TRUTH?

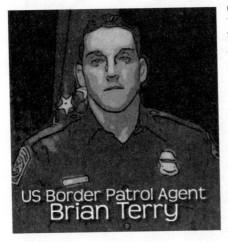

US Border Patrol Agent
Brian Terry

Operation Fast and Furious was a US government program authored by the Obama administration to arm violent Mexican drug cartels with weapons from the USA.

Between 2009 and 2011, ATF agents allowed more than 2,000 firearms to "walk" across the border. As many as 1,700 of those weapons have since been lost, and more than 100 corpses have been found at bloody crime scenes on both sides of the border, including the 2010 murder of a US Border Patrol agent (Brian Terry) in Arizona.

The program's purpose, according to a report from the US House Oversight and Government Reform Committee, "... *was to wait and watch, in hope that law enforcement could identify other members of a trafficking network and build a large, complex conspiracy case.*" Unfortunately, the report indicated that the ATF had **no** way of physically tracking the weapons, and once purchased, the guns were lost in the network of Mexico's drug cartels, where they could **not** be identified. Sending the guns to a place where they were *"impossible to track"* and *"could not be identified"* certainly sounds like a strange way to *"identify members of a trafficking network,"* doesn't it? Hmmm ... perhaps there were other motives? More on that thought in a moment.

So, in essence, under the direction of the Obama administration, the DoJ and the ATF "ran" thousands and thousands of guns across the border and watched them go directly into the hands of some of the most evil people on earth – the Mexican drug cartels – despite the fact that their intentions were **not** to actually track the guns nor to identify dangerous members of the cartels. Did I miss anything? Meanwhile, at the exact same time, the US government was allowing good, honest, decent, just, law-abiding American gun dealers to be defamed and maligned. How's that for nauseating? Sick yet? Disgusted? I am.

So who was actually responsible for authorizing and overseeing this operation? The details are slowly surfacing, but many emails and documents point to the US Attorney General, Eric Holder. I'm not surprised, because Holder's intentions have been known for years. Check out the graphic below, which is based upon a quote from Holder in 1995.

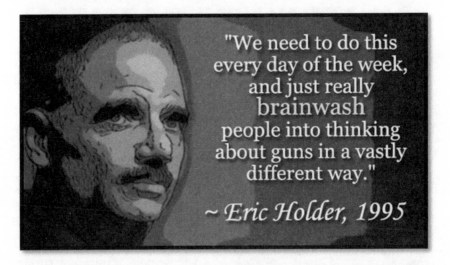

"We need to do this every day of the week, and just really **brainwash** people into thinking about guns in a vastly different way."

~ *Eric Holder, 1995*

In 2011, when Attorney General Eric Holder testified under oath before a Congressional committee that, *"I probably heard about Fast and Furious for the first time over the last few weeks."* However, Fox News broke the story on released government documents which proved that Holder was actually aware of Fast and Furious in 2010. **Oops.** Another pesky "oversight" by Holder, I'm sure. Holder was actually held in "criminal contempt" of Congress for refusing to hand over approximately 80,000 documents requested by the House Oversight Committee.

Of course, Holder was only doing what his boss, Barry Soetoro, I mean Barak Obama, told him to do. What exactly were his orders? Well, that's still a mystery. You see, Obama has never explained the details of what occurred to anybody, not the media, not investigators, not Congress. On the same day that Holder was charged with contempt, Obama asserted "executive privilege" and refused to answer any questions.

I guess if you're Obama, you have to *"know when to fold 'em and when to Holder 'em."*

When asked about the operation, Obama stated that he knew nothing about Fast and Furious. That's odd. Because in the 2009 stimulus package, Obama set aside $10 million for "gun tracing" and "gun enforcement programs" and freely discussed this in his joint press conference with Mexican President Felipe Calderon in February of that same year. During a news conference in March of 2009, Holder's underling, Deputy Attorney General David Ogden said Obama ordered and Holder expanded "Project Gunrunner" in Mexico as part of the DoJ's "Southwest Border Initiative." The project began in 2005 under Bush. Fast and Furious became operational under Project Gunrunner in 2009.

So, Obama is lying ... again. *"Would you like some fries with that whopper, Mr. President?"* But don't be concerned – he only lies when he opens his lips. In reality, multiple White House officials, including Obama, had been briefed about the scheme and knew that the supposed "targets" of the alleged "investigation" were drug lords already on the FBI's payroll.

In 2011, the Obama administration **was** forced to release more than 1,300 pages of documents related to Fast and Furious. The subpoenaed records exposed desperate email communications between senior officials about how vigorously to defend the operation, as well as concerns about the legitimacy of some of the proposed defenses. The documents showed that DoJ officials were apprehensive that if the administration were to cooperate with the congressional investigation, Congress would press for even more information. Not surprisingly, the mainstream media has continued to ignore the most important elements of the scandal, pretending that it was basically a "bungled" operation in which low-grade employees inadvertently "lost" the weapons.

Why would the media play along with this charade? Because if they admitted to the nefarious nature of this operation, then they would also have to admit to its palpable purpose: **grabbing our guns**. You see, there are many people in power that want to disarm America. That's just a fact. It's not speculation. It's real. They don't want you to have guns, regardless of what the US Constitution says. The only problem with their traitorous "gun grabbing" plans is that the overwhelming sentiment of Americans is to maintain the 2nd Amendment.

The vast majority, and I'm talking vast majority, of Americans do **not** want any more gun control legislation. Period. But, apparently, that doesn't matter either. They're going to try to disarm America, whether we like it or not!

You think I'm nuts? You think I'm making this up? Nah! I'm not. Official documents showed that the violence from Fast and Furious — US law enforcement agents killed and hundreds of Mexicans massacred — **was** indeed used as a pretext to push more gun control in the USA. The emails exposing the Obama administration's foul scheme to use the bloodshed to assault the 2nd Amendment backed up the assertions I just made. Tyrants always want to take away guns from the citizenry ... always ... without exception ... it's part of history. Unfortunately, our schools don't teach real history any longer. And as George Santayana famously observed, *"Those who forget the past are condemned to repeat it."*

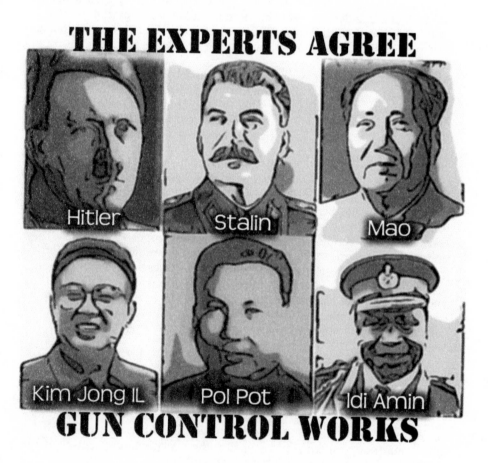

C'mon. If you're really "awake," it's obvious, isn't it? The true purpose of Fast and Furious was to create "anti-2nd Amendment" sentiment in the USA resulting from news stories where everybody was "traumatized" and "stunned" and "shocked" about all the weapons purchased by Mexican drug cartel members in America.

Comments like the following would ensue:

- *"It's too easy for Mexican gangs to purchase guns in the USA!"*
- *"Our gun laws are too lax!"*
- *"We need protection from heinous crimes!"*

You see, the United Nations (UN) has been working for a long time on tactics to disarm and control Americans. The purpose of the UN Arms Trade Treaty (UN-ATT) is to regulate the transfer of weapons. That obviously requires that all guns be registered and tracked by governments. Of course, they don't really want to track the guns, per se. They want to track the gun **owners**. You and me!

April 19, 1775
An English attempt to confiscate guns from Americans triggered a successful revolution

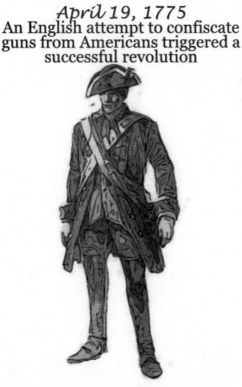

Hey Congress ... that's a hint.

Clearly, the purpose of Fast and Furious was to scare Americans about firearms crossing the Mexican border (the "problem") and get the public to cry out for protection (the "reaction"). And the UN-ATT was the legislation they had already prepared to offer as a "solution." Does this technique sound familiar?

Remember the Hegelian Dialectic which I mentioned earlier in the book? *"Thesis, antithesis, synthesis"* (aka *"problem, reaction, solution"*) – where a problem is manufactured usually with a ready-in-the-wings antithesis (reaction) so that the resulting synthesis (solution) can take society further toward a knee-jerk direction that it doesn't really want to go. Bingo! That's the intended consequence of Fast and Furious.

Secretary of State, John Kerry, signed the UN-ATT in September of 2013. Constitutionally, it doesn't really matter that the Secretary of State signed the treaty. And even if Obama eventually signs the treaty, it still has to be ratified by the Senate. But it's important to note that the US Constitution doesn't require 2/3 of the Senate to approve. It only requires 2/3 of the Senators **present** to approve.

Will "Dirty" Harry Reid schedule a vote during a recess to get it ratified? I certainly hope not, but I wouldn't put it past him. And don't forget traitor Senator, Diane Feinstein, who made her intentions crystal clear in a 1995 "60 Minutes" interview on CBS: *"If I could have gotten 51 votes in the Senate of the United States for an outright ban, picking up every one of them . . . Mr. and Mrs. America, turn 'em all in, I would have done it. I could not do that. The votes weren't here."*

More gun laws are not the answer. Period.

Why is it so difficult to comprehend that every time a new law is passed, good folks lose more liberty? When the people lose liberty, the government becomes bigger, more authoritative and invasive. Is there a lucid, rational person out there who **really** believes that "grabbing our guns" will keep weapons out of the hands of criminals? Seriously?

Does anyone **really** believe that if the US government made owning a gun illegal or put tighter restrictions on gun ownership that murderers, gangs, and those who basically have a disregard for human life will throw them away or willingly turn them in?

C'mon. If you do, then you're delusional, irrational, and naïve, all wrapped up in one package. Or maybe you should stop smoking crack. Better yet, try laying off the "Loony Toons" and "California Sunshine" and "Window Pane" (street names for LSD).

Speaking of drugs, alcohol (yes, it's a drug) prohibition did not work in the 1920s, yet the arrogance (and pure malevolence) of certain lawmakers seems to cause them to believe they are wiser than those of the past, and they can make gun prohibition work in the 21st century.

For those in our country who wish to disarm the American people and have us eventually turn in our guns, I leave you with the legendary words of King Leonidas I in response to the Persian King Xerxes' demand that the Spartans surrender their weapons at the Battle of Thermopylae:

"Molon Labe!" ("ΜΟΛΩΝ ΛΑΒΕ!") ... Which translated means ...
"Come and get them!"

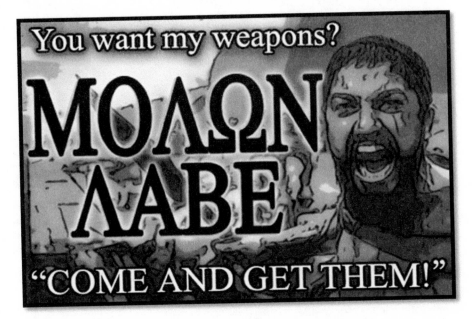

RESOURCES

Websites
http://www.thenewamerican.com/usnews/crime/item/15533-obama-s-fast-and-furious-gun-running-scandal-grows
http://www.infowars.com/the-untold-story-behind-the-fast-and-furious-scandal/
http://www.politico.com/story/2013/09/fast-and-furious-doj-documents-97604.html

Videos
"Fast and Furious: Obama's Watergate"
http://www.youtube.com/watch?v=kD-2KxJbsx8
"Could Fast and Furious Scandal Bring Down Obama?"
http://www.youtube.com/watch?v=BLT2lEZr2Do

CONCLUSION

What? The book is finished? Wow. I can't believe it. Hopefully you've been entertained, educated, and challenged by the contents herein. It was fun for me to write, and I hope it was enjoyable to read. Well, maybe "enjoyable" isn't the correct word. Maybe "enlightening" is a better choice. Yeah, that's the correct word. I hope you have been enlightened and awakened to the monumental myths that we have been told by the Medical Mafia and mainstream media.

We live in the "matrix" where lies abound and myths take precedence over truth. Because we live in a world where endless spin, propaganda, and manipulation are ubiquitous, it's quite easy for the "powers that be" to deceive people, especially in light of the fact that the mainstream media monkeys seem to live by the axiom: *"See no evil, hear no evil, report no evil"* when it comes to actually broadcasting their rampant dishonesties and deceptions.

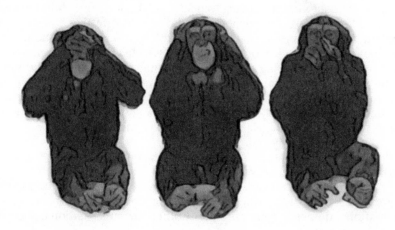

In the words of Mark Twain, *"... it's easier to fool people than to convince them that they've been fooled."*

I agree with Mr. Clemens completely. That's why I wrote the book.

The controlled mainstream media are like worn-out old dogs, loyally fetching "official myths" on command and dropping them like bloody bones at the feet of an gullible and naïve public. Eventually, however, the myths unravel, cracks appear, and the truth begins to squeeze out. The "light switch" in their brain is flipped to the "on" position and those who were previously deceived begin to open their eyes and admit that they have been fooled. They begin to hate the lies and thirst for truth. That's when the official "unplugging" from the matrix begins.

When the government's popularity diminishes sufficiently, despite the support of the controlled mainstream media, even old dogs can come up with new tricks, reviving the lost art of investigative reporting. I'm one of those "old dogs" attempting to come up with new tricks.

"*What new trick?*" you might ask. I'm telling the (unpopular) truth in a period of virtually omnipresent lies and widespread deceit, which is no easy task. It's not a "new trick" for me, as I've always been someone who is bound by conscience and truthfulness. But it's definitely a "new trick" for most people who are considered to be "mainstream" journalists.

George Orwell couldn't have been more accurate when he said, "*In a time of universal deceit, telling the truth is a revolutionary act.*" It reminds me of an old proverb: "*It's hard to accept the truth when the lies were exactly what you wanted to hear.*"

I told my wife that this book was going to be the one that got me killed, so if you hear about me committing "suicide" by shooting myself in the head **twice** (like Gary Webb purportedly did) or committing "suicide" by **beating** and **torturing** myself like Officer Terry Yeakey (Oklahoma City Policeman) allegedly did, or committing "suicide" by shooting myself in the head and then wiping off the fingerprints after I'm dead (like Vince Foster allegedly did) ... don't believe it. If I die in suspicious circumstances, then you can rest assured that "they" got to me. Honestly, I'm not worried about it in the least. God is sovereignly controlling all things and I'm his kid, so He's watching out for me. ☺

God gives us the power of reason "for a reason," to discover truth. By definition, monumental myths are **not** true. They're contrary to reality. They turn truth on its head. They point fingers the wrong way. They're pretexts for militarism, wars, mass killing and destruction, sickness, occupations, domestic repression, and other extremist national security state measures.

Hopefully, this book has helped you understand and appreciate why I said in the introduction that most monumental myths are not really as much of a "*riddle wrapped in a mystery inside an enigma*" as they are a "*furtive foothill of foul-smelling feces wrapped in a fairytale inside a fable of fabrications and falsehoods.*"

I hope that this book has inspired you to think for yourself, so that when the next false flag occurs (yes, there will be more false flags), you will not "blindly believe" everything that the bimbo bobble-head bleached blonde on television tells you.

Don't believe their "explanations" of the pictures and videos. It's all staged!

Why? Because it works. The "sheeple" gulp in the propaganda. They swallow it "hook, line, and sinker."

Since the invention of television, untold billions of people have been relying on a "television anchor" to "explain the pictures." And even if the official explanations make no plausible sense, most folks believe them because "they" told us so, and we all know that "they" would never lie. As a result, scores of people, like lemmings, follow one another right off the proverbial cliff. It's time to end the insanity.

And this doesn't just apply to television. It also applies to the "anchors" in the "health" care (which some folks refer to as "sickness perpetuation") industry. *"Well, Mr. Smith,"* the M.D. says, as he pins an X-ray to the wall. *"See this thing? Right here? This lump? We'll need to start chemo immediately, we'll follow up with several rounds of radiation, and then, just in case, we might want to remove a large chunk of your brain. Then, as a preventative measure, we may need to remove an eye."*

If you find yourself in this position, say **NO!!!!**

God gave us all brains. I hope and pray that this book has inspired you to use yours.

Be inquisitive. Be brave. Always question authority. Be suspicious of the official story. Read between the lines. Look for the motive. Keep an open mind. Seek for the truth. Share with others.

I leave you with a quote from one of our Founding Fathers, Thomas Jefferson: *"All tyranny needs to gain a foothold is for people of good conscience to remain silent."*

Maranatha and God bless.

"And ye shall know the truth, and the truth shall make you free."

John 8:32

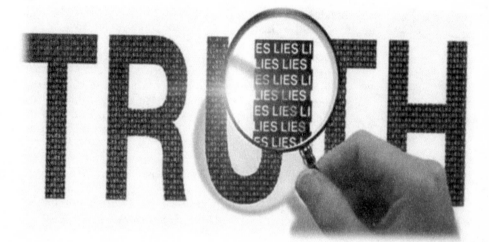

"Ye are of your father the devil, and the lusts of your father ye will do. He was a murderer from the beginning, and abode not in the truth, because there is no truth in him. When he speaketh a lie, he speaketh of his own: for he is a liar, and the father of it."

John 8:44